DIETARY MANAGEMENT OF

FOOD ALLERGIES & INTOLERANCES

A COMPREHENSIVE GUIDE

Second Edition

DIETARY MANAGEMENT OF

FOOD ALLERGIES & INTOLERANCES

A COMPREHENSIVE GUIDE

Second Edition

Janice Vickerstaff Joneja, Ph.D.

J.A. HALL PUBLICATIONS LTD.
Vancouver, British Columbia, Canada
www.HallPublications.com   e-mail: info@hallpublications.com

This publication is designed to provide authoritative and accurate information in regard to the subject matter contained herein. Expert professional advice from a competent medical practitioner should be sought when following the advice contained in this book. The publisher is not engaged in rendering professional medical services.

Revised: Table 18-1: Level of Nickel in Common Foods

Canadian Cataloguing in Publication Data

Joneja, Janice M. Vickerstaff
    Dietary management of food allergies and intolerances: a comprehensive guide

2nd ed.
Includes bibliographical references and index.
ISBN 0-9682098-2-3

    1. Food Allergy--Diet therapy. 2. Food allergy
I. Title

RC588.D53J66 1998   616.97'50654   C97-907709-4

J.A. Hall Publications Ltd.
9500 Erickson Drive Suite 502
Burnaby, British Columbia
Canada,   V3J 7B5

Printed in the U.S.A.

DEDICATION

To Raj, Sunil, and Nalini

Contents

Preface   i

     Note to the Reader   ii

     Note on Terminology   iii

     Design of the Book   iv

Part I Introduction

1   What is Food Allergy?   1

     Immunological Mechanisms of Allergy   1

     Allergy as an Inflammatory Process   3

     Examples of Allergic Symptoms and Conditions   4

     Factors Contributing to the Expression of Allergy to Foods   5

     What is Food Intolerance?   7

2   Adverse Reactions To Food Additives   11

3   Anaphylactic Reactions to Foods   15

4   Allergenic Cross-reactivity   19

5   The Allergenic Potential of Foods   23

     Table 5-1: Food Additives from Potentially Allergenic Foods   24

Part II Diagnosis and Detection of Food Allergens and Reactive Chemicals in Foods

6   Food Allergy Tests   29

7   Elimination and Challenge Test   35
    Method: Exposure Diary   39
    Sample Food Diary   40
    Method: Challenge Phase   41
    Method: Sequence of Testing Foods   43
    Method: Challenge Test Check List   56
    Challenge Test Checklist   57

8   Rotation Diets   67
    Method: Use of The Rotation Diet Table   69
    Sample Four Day Rotation Diet   71

Part III Specific Food Restrictions

9   Important Nutrients in Common Allergens   73
    Table 9-1: Important Nutrients in Common Allergens   74
    Table 9-2 Summary: Important Nutrients in Common Allergens   75
    Table 9-3: Alternative Sources of Nutrients   76

10   Milk Allergy and Lactose Intolerance   79
    Milk Allergy   80
    Table 10-1: Levels of Individual Proteins in Cow's Milk   80
    Lactose Intolerance   83
    Table 10-2: Lactose Content of Foods   86
    Method: Milk-free Diet   89
    Milk-free Diet   90
    Method: Lactose Restricted Diet   92
    Phase I - Restriction of Lactose   92
    Table 10-3: Levels of Lactose in Normal Serving Sizes of Common Foods and Beverages   94
    Feeding the Lactose Intolerant Infant   95
    Phase II - Determining Lactose Tolerance Levels   96
    Method: Calcium   98
    Table 10-4: Daily Calcium Requirements   100
    Table 10-5: Dietary Reference Intake Values for Calcium and Vitamin D[2]   101
    Table 10-6: Non-Dairy Sources of Calcium   102

11 Egg Allergy   105
    Method: Egg-free Diet   107
    Egg-free Diet   109

12 Grain Allergy   111
    Grain Restricted Diets in the Management of Allergy   113
    Method: Restricted Grain Diet   116
    Restricted Grain Diet   119
    Method: Wheat-free Diet   122
    Wheat-free Diet   124

13 Peanut Allergy   127
    Method: Peanut-free Diet   129
    Peanut-free Diet   130

14 Soy Protein Allergy   133
    Method: Soy-free Diet   135
    Soy-free Diet   136

15 Avoidance of Multiple Food Allergens   139
    Method: Diet Free From the Ten Most Common Allergens*   139
    Diet Free of Milk, Egg, Wheat, Corn, Soy, Peanut, Nuts,
      Chocolate, Fish, and Shellfish   140

16 Yeast and Mold Allergy   143
    Method: Yeast and Mold Restricted Diet   146
    Yeast and Mold Restricted Diet   146

17 Biogenic Amines   149
    Tyramine Sensitivity   150
    Method: Tyramine Restricted Diet   153
    Tyramine Restricted Diet   154
    Histamine Sensitivity   158
    Method: Histamine Restricted Diet   160
    Histamine Restricted Diet   160

18 Nickel Allergy   165
    Method: Nickel Restricted Diet   174
    Nickel Restricted Diet   174

19   Tartrazine and Other Food Coloring Agents   177
       Table 19-1: Artificial Food Coloring Agents in General Use (USA)   177
       Table 19-2: Examples of the Use of Colors in Foods   179
       Method: Diet Restricted in Tartrazine and Other Food
        Coloring Agents   181
       Tartrazine and Other Food Color Restricted Diet   182

20   Sensitivity To Salicylates   187
       Table 20-1: Level of Salicylates in Some Common Foods and Beverages   190
       Method: Salicylate Restricted Diet   200
       Salicylate Restricted Diet   200

21   Benzoate Sensitivity   205
       Benzoic Acid and Sodium Benzoate   205
       Benzoyl Peroxide   206
       Adverse Reactions to Benzoates   206
       Table 21-1: Level of Benzoates in Common Foods   208
       Method: Benzoate Restricted Diet   213
       Benzoate Restricted Diet   215

22   Butylated Hydroxyanisole and   219
       Butylated Hydroxytoluene   219
       Method: Butylated Hydroxyanisole (BHA) and Butylated
        Hydroxytoluene (BHT) Restricted Diet   221
       BHA and BHT Restricted Diet   222

23   Sulfite Sensitivity   225
       Method: Sulfite Restricted Diet   228
       Sulfite Restricted Diet   229

24   Monosodium Glutamate (MSG) Sensitivity   233
       Method: Monosodium Glutamate (MSG) Restricted Diet   239
       Monosodium Glutamate (MSG) Restricted Diet   239

25   Nitrate and Nitrite Sensitivity   241
       Method: Nitrate and Nitrite Restricted Diet   243
       Table 25-1: Level of Nitrates and Nitrites in Some Meats and Vegetables   243

Part IV Pediatric Allergy

26   Pediatric Allergy   245
       Method: Preventive Measures to Reduce Food Allergy in Infants   254

Egg, Milk, Dairy, and Peanut Restricted Diet for Pregnant and
   Breast-feeding Women   258
Method: Feeding the Allergic Infant Solid Foods After Six Months of Age   260
Table 26-1: Sequence of Adding Solid Foods for the Allergic Infant   263
Composition of Infant Formulae   264
Table 26-2: Composition of Infant Formulae   264

Part V Therapeutic Diets for Specific Conditions

27   Disaccharide Intolerance   269
   Method: Disaccharide Restricted Diet   273
   Disaccharide Restricted Diet   276
   Phase I: Restriction of All Types of Disaccharides   276
   Disaccharide Restricted Diet   276

28   Crohn's Disease   281
   Method: Diet For Crohn's Disease   286
   Phase I Diet For Crohn's Disease   288

29   Irritable Bowel Syndrome   291
Table 29-1: A Comparison of Dietary Starch Fed and Recovered After
   Digestion in the Small Intestine of Humans   294
Method: Diet For Irritable Bowel Syndrome (IBS)   297
Diet For Irritable Bowel Syndrome   299

30   Urticaria and Angioedema   305
   Method: Histamine Restricted Diet for Control of Urticaria / Angioedema   309

31   Diet and Migraine   311
   Method: Test Diet for Migraine   319
   Test Diet for Migraine   319

32   Attention Deficit Disorder with Hyperactivity (ADDH)   325
   Method: Hyperactivity Test Diet   328
   Test Diet For Hyperactivity   331

33   Diet and Asthma   335

34   Diet and Eczema   337

35   Diet and Nocturnal Enuresis (Bed Wetting)   339

Part VI Appendices

I   Few Foods Elimination Test Diet   341

      Suggested Menus   344

      Recipe List   346

      Elimination Test Diet Recipes   348

      Nutritional Content of Recipes   374

II   Irritable Bowel Syndrome (IBS) Diet General Guidelines   377

      Recipes   382

III   Cookbooks with Recipes Suitable for Allergen-restricted Diets   409

      Sources of Allergy Recipes for Children   416

Preface

The dietary management of food allergies and intolerance can be a tremendous challenge for the clinician and dietitian. It is, however, far more challenging, confusing, and frustrating for the allergic or intolerant person whom we are trying to help. Adverse reactions to foods can impose enormous pressures on sufferers and their families. People who are in danger of a life threatening anaphylactic reaction, and their families, live in continual fear of exposure to the allergen, and must maintain constant vigilance in seeking out and avoiding foods that contain the "enemy allergen." This view of food as a lethal threat often leads to an obsessive preoccupation that results in extreme anxiety states, a phobia to food, and nutritional depletion.

Even when the allergy is not life threatening, nutritional, economic, and social stresses can compromise the quality of life of food-sensitive persons and their families. In situations where the reaction is not clinically visible (e.g., when no hives, nasal congestion, or asthma attacks occur), observers tend to discredit the sufferer's complaints, causing frustration and psychological stress to the food-sensitive person. A definitive diagnosis becomes necessary for the sufferer to establish credibility. In these situations, people often turn to practitioners of alternative medicine and rely on tests that are not scientifically sound, in an attempt to validate their reactions.

The management of food allergy is possibly more demanding than any other area in dietary practice, principally because there are no definitive laboratory tests to determine food sensitivities. Because many different immunological and physiological reactions contribute to the symptoms of adverse reactions to foods, no single test could possibly detect them all. We have little to guide us initially in planning an appropriate diet. Clients often come to the dietitian having followed a nutritionally unsafe diet, believing that if they avoid "the wrong foods" for long enough, their symptoms will go away and they will feel better. Sometimes this does happen. However, if a very restricted diet is followed for an extended period of time, the resulting semi-starved state leads to suppression of the immune system. At this point, the symptoms of allergy, which are caused by a hyper-responsive immune system, do disappear. But the person's suppressed immune system is now less able to fight infections and other health threats.

Detecting and eliminating specific antagonistic foods, and designing a nutritionally sound diet to ensure the optimum health of the food-sensitive person, is the ultimate aim in food sensitivity management. This process is often tedious and time consuming, and requires tremendous knowledge, skill, commitment, and dedication, from both the food-sensitive individual and the dietitian. However, when a person who has been feeling chronically sick suddenly feels well for the first time in many years, as so often happens, the rewards for both practitioner and client more than justify the time and effort of the endeavor. Managing food sensitivities can be the most gratifying of all fields of dietary practice because the results (and rewards) are immediate. The practitioner does not have to wait months or years to see results, as is the case in many areas of dietary practice.

This book is designed to provide the information and tools that are required to detect food-sensitivities and design nutritionally adequate diets to ensure the best possible health for food-sensitive persons. There is no short cut to understanding the complexities of adverse reactions to foods. Many factors besides foods influence the expression of symptoms, and each affected person must be treated individually, taking into account medical history, lifestyle, and adverse reactions to both food and non-food factors (such as airborne and environmental allergens). Although people with food allergies frequently request a "hypoallergenic diet," no such thing exists. What may be "hypoallergenic" for one person could be life-threatening for another.

This book does not contain "diets" for specific conditions. Instead it provides the most complete information currently available to enable clinicians and dietitians to design appropriate diets for their clients, who are undeniably and unavoidably unique in their reactions and needs. The ultimate goal is to assist the health care practitioner to equip these people with the tools they need to obtain optimal nutrition and quality of life in spite of their food sensitivities.

Note to the Reader

This book is designed for the health care practitioner involved in counseling patients or clients in the management of adverse reactions to foods. It takes a great deal of time, energy, and dedication on the part of both the health care practitioner and the person suffering the adverse reaction, to detect the foods, food components, and food additives that are responsible for, or contribute to, a food sensitivity.

Ultimately, people are responsible for taking care of their own health, and people who have food sensitivities are often the best detectives for finding the sources of their problems. Food-sensitive people may try to use this book to determine their food sensitivities on their own. We caution against using the book without the involvement of a qualified health care professional.

The information provided here is as up-to-date, accurate, and practical as possible in a field that moves very quickly and is full of controversy. However, no book can substitute for advice and treatment from a physician and qualified health care provider. No treatment protocol in this book should be undertaken without the approval of a physician. Any strategy suggested should be discussed with and managed by a physician and, for maximum benefit, implementation should be supervised by a registered dietitian/nutritionist.

The author and publisher disclaim responsibility for any adverse consequences resulting from the use of any of the drugs, diet plans, or procedures mentioned in this book.

Trade names of food products are used only as examples. The names given are not meant as a complete list of all available formulations, nor as recommendations for any particular product.

Note on Terminology

There is a great deal of confusion in the literature on food allergy and intolerance because the familiar term "food allergy" is used interchangeably and synonymously with "food intolerance" and "food sensitivity" in non-medical and non-scientific articles and books. In other words, "food allergy" popularly refers to any reactions that appear to result from eating food.

In scientific literature, food allergy is a very specific term which refers *only* to a reaction of the immune system that results in clearly defined symptoms. Conventional allergists will take the definition even further, and distinguish between different responses of the immune system to food by limiting the use of the term "allergy" (or "atopy" which means the same thing) to those immune reactions which are mediated by IgE antibodies, designated a Type I hypersensitivity reaction (see page 1). Other clinical conditions caused by a reaction of the immune system to foods or other allergens (Type II, III, and IV hypersensitivity reactions [see page 2] are designated "immune-mediated reactions").

Reactions in which there is no causative role for the immune system, but which are a result of a physiological response of the body to a food or food additive, are referred to as "non-immune-mediated reactions" in medical and scientific literature.

There is an important reason why there should be a clear distinction between these terms. The diagnosis and management of a Type I hypersensitivity reaction (allergy) and a non-immune-mediated reaction (intolerance) can sometimes be quite different, and it is important for the clinician to be able to distinguish between them.

In this Book

Food allergy means a hypersensitivity reaction of the immune system, and may be a Type I, Type II, Type III, or a Type IV reaction. At present, there is no test which will readily distinguish these reactions when food is the trigger. There is little point in using separate terms in practice.

Food intolerance refers to any non-immune-mediated reaction. The term is usually used when the trigger is a man-made chemical, such as a food additive, or a naturally occurring component of food, which the body is unable to process adequately. The resulting symptoms can be loosely equated with a reaction to a drug.

Food sensitivity refers to an adverse reaction to a food, which encompasses both allergy, immune-mediated, and non-immune-mediated responses.

Adverse reaction to a food or food additive is synonymous with the term "food sensitivity".

Design of the Book

This book is designed as a practical tool for practitioners in the field of food allergy and intolerance and for individuals experiencing adverse reactions to foods. The scientific data has been kept to the minimum that will provide a comprehensive overview of the current knowledge in each area. For those who wish to pursue a specific topic in greater depth, key references have been provided, rather than extensive lists of research papers in the field. The references will direct the interested reader to further relevant information.

The book is divided into six parts, made up of individual chapters dealing with specific topics of food allergy and intolerance.

Part I is an introduction to the mechanisms responsible for food allergies and intolerance, the nature and allergenic potential of food antigens, and the cross-reactivity of antigens in foods.

Part II deals with the detection of the foods, food components and additives that are responsible for food sensitivities. Detailed instructions are provided for elimination and challenge tests to determine the reactive foods.

Part III discusses a variety of conditions resulting from food allergies and intolerance to naturally occurring chemicals and food additives and provides guidelines for their dietary management.

Part IV discusses food allergy and intolerance in childhood, since the prevention and management strategies for adverse reactions to foods in infants sometimes differ significantly from those in adults.

Part V discusses a variety of specific conditions and includes guidelines for therapeutic diets for management of the conditions. In most cases, adequately controlled trials have not yet been carried out. These diet strategies may be considered somewhat controversial.

Part VI consists of appendices: the Few Foods Elimination Diet, recipes for the Elimination Diet, a nutritional analysis of the recipes, a diet plan and recipes for Irritable Bowel Syndrome, and a list of cookbooks and other aids which will help in the implementation of the dietary strategies suggested in the book.

Part I

Introduction

1

What is Food Allergy?

Food allergy is a response of the immune system to a component of food, almost invariably a protein or a molecule linked to a protein, that the immune system recognizes as foreign to the body. A more accurate term for food allergy is food hypersensitivity.

Food allergy is common in infancy, with a prevalence of 1 to 3%,[1] but only represents a small proportion of food reactions in the adult. Sometimes food allergy is lifelong.

Immunological Mechanisms of Allergy

Hypersensitivity reactions involve a series of specific events and result in clinical symptoms.[2] Four distinct hypersensitivity reactions are recognized, and each type involves different components of the immune system. As far as is known, food allergy can be mediated by Type I, Type III, or Type IV hypersensitivity, or possibly by a combination of these types. Readers who want more detailed information on these mechanisms can find it in *Understanding Allergy, Sensitivity and Immunity: A Comprehensive Guide*, by the author.[2]

Type I Hypersensitivity

Type I hypersensitivity involves IgE antibodies, mast cells, and other granulocytes. The symptoms resulting from this type of reaction are traditionally referred to as atopy, and the allergic individual as atopic. For this type of hypersensitivity, the person must be sensitized by a first exposure to the allergen.

Thereafter, events occur sequentially, as follows:

First exposure - "Sensitization"
- B-cell lymphocytes produce allergen specific IgE antibodies.
- IgE molecules couple with receptors on the surface of mast cells (in tissues) and basophils (in blood).
- No symptoms are observed on first exposure to the allergen.

Subsequent exposure to the same allergen
- Allergens complex with cell bound IgE molecules. Each allergen bridges two IgE molecules; thus, to be allergenic, a food molecule must be large enough to form this bridge. Allergens are normally 10 to 40 kilodaltons in molecular size.
- A series of reactions involving cyclic AMP and GMP takes place at the cell surface.
- Calcium enters the cell.
- Mast cells release intracellular granules that contain:

    Preformed inflammatory mediators (e.g., histamine), which can cause symptoms immediately (typically within a few minutes but possibly up to two hours after exposure).

    Chemotactic chemicals that attract more granulocytes (eosinophils and neutrophils) to the site, which in turn release similar inflammatory mediators that augment the immediate reaction.

    Enzymes that act at cellular membranes to produce secondary inflammatory mediators, especially arachidonic acid metabolites such as prostaglandins and leukotrienes, which cause additional symptoms, especially smooth muscle contraction (e.g., the bronchospasm typical of asthma).

- Antigen-specific B-cells produce more allergen specific IgE.

Type III Hypersensitivity

This type of reaction involves IgM and IgG antibodies and chemicals formed in the complement cascade. Steps in the reaction are:

- T-cell lymphocytes recognize the antigen as foreign after it is "processed" by macrophages.
- IgM and later, IgG are produced in response to the antigen.
- Antigen-antibody complexes are formed.
- The complement cascade is triggered.
- Anaphylatoxins formed in the complement cascade cause the release of inflammatory mediators.

In some food allergies, a Type III hypersensitivity reaction may be the initial response (e.g., as in milk allergy) or may be a secondary response following an initial Type I hypersensitivity reaction.

Symptoms typically occur at the site where the antigen enters the body (e.g., asthma occurs in the lungs in response to inhaled allergens; gastrointestinal symptoms are in response to foods). The Type III hypersensitivity reaction is sometimes called an anaphylactoid reaction.

Type IV Hypersensitivity

Type IV hypersensitivity involves T-cell lymphocytes and cytokines. This reaction is called a contact allergy because the reaction continues as long as the allergen is in contact with body cells. T-cell lymphocytes respond to the allergen, causing the release of cytokines, which act on body tissues.

With this type of hypersensitivity, allergenic foods cause an immediate reaction when they come into contact with the lips, tongue, mouth, and gastrointestinal tract. Nickel allergy, an example of a Type IV hypersensitivity, is usually identified by reactions resulting from skin contact with the metal in jewelry, watch bands, and other metal objects. However, increased levels of nickel due to ingestion of foods containing nickel may be responsible for a form of dermatitis that resembles eczema (see *Nickel Allergy*, page 165).

Allergy as an Inflammatory Process

Regardless of the type of hypersensitivity reaction involved, the symptoms of allergy result from the release of inflammatory mediators. These chemicals act on body tissues to cause the clinical condition. Each inflammatory mediator released in the hypersensitivity reaction has its own effect.[3]

Histamine, for example, increases the permeability of capillaries (small blood vessels), causing fluid to move from the vessels into tissues and produce swelling. Rhinitis (inflammation of nasal tissue causing "stuffiness") is due to fluid buildup in tissues in nasal passages. Excessive fluid in the skin causes urticaria (hives) and angioedema (tissue swelling). Histamine also causes itching and vasodilation (widening of capillaries), resulting in flushing or reddening of the skin. Prostaglandins cause vasodilation and vasoconstriction. Leukotrienes cause contraction of smooth muscle and are largely responsible for the bronchospasm of asthma. Bradykinin, in conjunction with prostaglandins, causes pain. The combined effect of these chemicals constitutes the allergic response.

Sometimes these inflammatory mediators are released, or their levels are enhanced, by mechanisms that are independent of the immune system. This situation is usually considered to be intolerance rather than allergy.

Examples of Allergic Symptoms and Conditions[2]

Respiratory Tract

Allergic or perennial rhinitis (nasal congestion, hay fever)
Rhinorrhea (runny nose)
Allergic conjunctivitis (itchy, watery, reddened eyes)
Serous otitis media (earache with effusion)
Asthma (wheezing, difficulty breathing)
Laryngeal edema (throat tightening due to swelling of tissues)

Skin

Atopic dermatitis (eczema)
Urticaria (hives)
Angioedema (swelling of tissues, especially the mouth and face)
Pruritus (itching of skin, eyes, ears, and mouth)
Contact dermatitis (rash due to contact with an allergen)

Digestive Tract

Diarrhea	Abdominal bloating and distension
Constipation	Abdominal pain
Nausea	Indigestion
Vomiting	Belching

Nervous System

Migraine	Lack of concentration
Other headache	Tension-fatigue syndrome
Spots before the eyes	Irritability
Listlessness	Chilliness
Hyperactivity	Dizziness

Other

Urinary frequency	Low grade fever
Bed wetting	Excessive sweating
Hoarseness	Pallor
Muscle aches	Dark circles around the eyes

Anaphylaxis

Anaphylaxis (or anaphylactic reaction) is an intense, immediate allergic response that involves several organ systems. Symptoms can include urticaria, angioedema, pruritus (itching), rhinitis, bronchospasm (difficulty in breathing), hypotension (reduced blood pressure), tachycardia (increased heart rate), nausea, and diarrhea. Severe cases can lead to cardiovascular collapse due to anaphylactic shock and death.

Incidence of Allergy

Allergy can be considered an inappropriate reaction of the immune system. Simplistically, the immune system is responding to substances that are usually harmless to the body, from which no adverse effects would result if the immune system were unresponsive. This unnecessary response of the immune system can result from several factors, which often act in combination. One of the most important factors is an inherited tendency.

For all allergies, whether caused by allergens that are ingested (foods), inhaled (pollens, dust, animal dander, or mold spores), injected (wasp or bee venom), or contacted (dust or animal dander), the estimated likelihood of a person having allergies, or the potential to develop them, has been estimated to be:[4]

  5-15% if neither parent has allergies
20-40% if one parent has allergies
40-60% if both parents have allergies
60-80% if both parents have the same allergy
25-35% if one sibling has allergies.

Factors Contributing to the Expression of Allergy to Foods

Although the potential to develop allergy is inherited, the development of overt symptoms often depends on a number of additional factors that expedite the abnormal immune response. The most common factors include the following physiological conditions:

Increased Permeability of the Intestinal Mucosa

An increase in the permeability of the cells lining the digestive tract allows food allergens to contact cells of the immune system. In contrast, fully developed, intact intestinal mucosal cells exclude the larger (and therefore potentially allergenic) molecules.

Increased permeability can be due to a number of causes, including:

Immaturity

The digestive lining is hyperpermeable in the early months of life,[5] and gradually matures over the first three to four years. As a result, children under five years of age are particularly vulnerable to food allergies. Most sensitization to food allergens occurs within this period, especially during the first year. If the foods most commonly allergenic can be avoided during this vulnerable period, food allergy may be avoided or greatly reduced.

Inflammation in the digestive tract

Inflammation of the gastrointestinal tract (enteritis) can result from infection or some other pathology. Inflammation compromises the integrity of the lining of the digestive tract and may allow food allergens to enter the circulation and gain access to cells of the immune system.[6]

Combined Allergic Reactions

Concurrent allergic reactions, such as a respiratory tract response to an airborne inhaled allergen, can increase the allergic reaction to a food. The combination of inflammatory mediators from the respiratory and intestinal reactions may result in symptoms, even though the level of inflammatory mediators from the food alone is insufficient to cause clinical expression of the reaction.

This concept of a combined inflammatory insult may also explain the observation that certain foods eaten in combination result in an allergic reaction, whereas either eaten alone does not cause a reaction.

Enhanced Uptake of Food Allergens

Alcohol can increase the rate of uptake of an allergen from the digestive tract, reducing by as much as half the time normally needed for the absorption of certain food components. Consuming an alcoholic drink at the same time as an allergenic food may cause a dramatic rise in the level of a food allergen at a reaction site, thus provoking allergic symptoms even though no symptoms result from eating the food alone.[7]

Exercise

Vigorous exercise after eating an allergenic food sometimes results in an allergic reaction even though eating the food without exercising produces no response.[8] The physiological mechanism responsible is unknown, but may relate to accelerated food uptake or increased body temperature during exercise.

Changes in Hormone Levels

Changes in levels of hormones such as estrogen, progesterone, and possibly testosterone, appear to affect the responsiveness of the immune system to allergens.[9] It has been suggested that this effect is expressed at the level of the T-suppressor cells, which apparently regulate the degree of response of the immune system.

The clinical symptoms of food allergy sometimes vary with levels of estrogen and/or progesterone. Both girls and boys may change their reactivity to allergens at puberty.[9] Symptoms may occur during women's menstrual cycles, appearing more frequently at ovulation and just prior to and at the onset of the menstrual period. In addition, women's allergic responses may change during pregnancy and at menopause. Men may experience a change in their allergic reactivity in their mid-thirties.

Anecdotal reports suggest that levels of other hormones, particularly thyroid hormones, may influence the degree of reactivity of the immune system and result in food allergy or intolerance. Although the effect of thyroid hormone levels on the clinical course of allergy is not being studied at present, future research could show that this factor influences adverse reactions to foods in individuals with dysfunctional thyroid.[10]

Stress

Many allergy sufferers notice that their symptoms appear, or worsen, during periods of stress. This effect may be due to the release of stress hormones that affect the degree of responsiveness of the immune system.[11]

Frequency of Exposure

The foods most likely to be allergenic are often those eaten frequently. Although it might appear that frequent exposure to the allergen explains the sensitivity, a more likely explanation is early sensitization (during infancy) to foods contained in the family diet. Definitive clinical trials on this topic have yet to be undertaken.

What is Food Intolerance?

Food intolerance can be defined as an adverse reaction to food that results in clinical symptoms but is not caused by a reaction of the immune system. The physiological mechanisms responsible for these reactions can be diverse and complex, and many are poorly understood.[12]

Examples of substances involved in non-immune mechanisms of food intolerance are:

- Lactose[13]
- Other disaccharides[14]
- Biogenic amines (e.g., histamine[15] and tyramine[16])
- Artificial colors, especially tartrazine
- Salicylates[17]
- Preservatives such as benzoates, butylated hydroxyanisole (BHA), butylated hydroxytoluene (BHT), and sulfites
- Monosodium glutamate (MSG), and other artificial flavorings.

These chemicals are discussed in Part III of this book.

References

1.   Botey, J., Roger, A., Eseverri, J.L., Marin, A., Pena, M. Immunoallergic techniques for the diagnosis of food allergy. In: *Food Allergy in Infancy: Proceedings of the International Symposium*, Palma de Mallorca, Spain, December 1991. 91-100.

2.   Joneja, J.M.V., Bielory, L. *Understanding Allergy, Sensitivity and Immunity: A Comprehensive Guide*. Rutgers University Press, New Jersey, 1990. (Reprinted 1994).

3.   Willoughby, D.A. (Ed), *Inflammation - Mediators and Mechanisms*. Brit. Med. Bulletin 1987 43(2):247-477.

4.   Goldman, A. Cow milk sensitivity; A review. In: *Food and Immunology*. Symposium of the Swedish Nutrition Foundation XIII. Almqvist and Wiksell, Uppsala, 1977. 99-104.

5.   Bellanti, J.A. Developmental Aspects of Food in Infancy and Childhood. In: *Food Allergy*. Immunology and Allergy Clinics of North America. November 1991. 885-891.

6.   Befus, D., Pearce, F., and Bienenstock, J. Intestinal mast cells in pathology and host resistance. In: Brostoff, J., and Challacombe, S.J. (Eds). *Food Allergy and Intolerance*. Baillière Tindall, London, 1987. 88-102.

7.   Brostoff, J. Personal communication, June 1993.

8.   Pearson, D.J., and Rix, K.J.B. Psychological effects of food allergy. In: Brostoff, J., and Challacombe, S.J. (Eds). *Food Allergy and Intolerance*. Baillière Tindall, London, 1987. 688-708.

9.   Grossman, C.J. Interaction between the gonadal steroids and the immune system. Science 1985 227:257-259.

10.   Filteau, S.M. and Woodward, B. Thyroid hormones and the immune system. Ph.D. thesis, Department of Nutritional Sciences, University of Guelph, Ontario, Canada, N1G 2W1, 1987.

11.   Zwilling, B. Stress affects disease outcomes. ASM News 1992 58(1):23-25.

12.   Furukawa, C.T. Nonimmunologic food reactions that can be confused with allergy. Immunology and Allergy Clinics of North America. November 1991 11(4):815-829.

13.   Littman, A. Lactase deficiency: Diagnosis and management. Hospital Practice 1987 22:111-124.

14. Gray, G. Intestinal disaccharidase deficiencies and glucose-galactose malabsorption. In: Stanbury, J.B., Fredickson, D.S., Goldstein, J.S. and Brown, M.S. (Eds), *The Metabolic Basis of Inherited Disease*, 5th Edition. McGraw-Hill, New York, 1983. 1729-1742.

15. Falus, A. *Histamine and Inflammation*. R.G. Landes Company, Austin, Texas, 1994.

16. Shulman, K.I., Walker, S.E., MacKenzie, S., *et al*. Dietary restrictions, tyramine, and the use of monoamine oxidase inhibitors. J. Clin. Psychopharmacol. 1989 9:397-402.

17. Winkelmann, R.K. Food sensitivity and urticaria or vasculitis. In: Brostoff, J., and Challacombe, S.J. (Eds). *Food Allergy and Intolerance*. Baillière Tindall, London, 1987. 602-617.

2

Adverse Reactions To Food Additives

The legal definition of a food additive, according to the Canadian Food and Drug Regulations,[1] is: "Any substance, including any source of radiation, the use of which results, or may reasonably be expected to result, in it or its byproducts becoming a part of or affecting the characteristics of a food."

Ingredients that are not considered to be food additives include nutritive materials such as salt, sugar, and starch because they are "used, recognized or commonly sold as an article or ingredient of food".

Food additives are used as preservatives, as coloring agents, and to provide taste, odor and texture in manufactured foods. They include dyes such as tartrazine and erythrosine; preservatives such as sulfites, benzoates, and sorbates; flavoring agents and flavor enhancers such as monosodium glutamate (MSG); ripening agents such as ethylene; antioxidants such as butylated hydroxyanisole (BHA), butylated hydroxytoluene (BHT), and sodium nitrite; emulsifiers such as lecithin and polysorbate; texturizers such as calcium chloride; humectants such as glycerine and propylene glycol; and thickeners and stabilizers such as gum tragacanth and agar-agar.

Source and Use of Food Additives

All additives approved for use in foods have been designated as safe by government regulated agencies. In the United States, foods thus designated are included on the GRAS (Generally Recognized as Safe) list. However, according to a 1984 report from the US National Research Council, toxicity data are not available for 80% of the 49,000 chemicals used commercially in foods, drugs, cosmetics, and other common products.[2] The report also indicated that data are inadequate or nonexistent for 80% of the 8,600 allowed food additives.

Because chemical additives are now used extensively in manufactured foods, they present complex problems for persons with food sensitivities. The chemicals themselves are diverse in composition, and different types may be used in the same food. Some additives are derived from natural sources by complex chemical processes, whereas others are synthesized from inorganic sources. For most, there is very little understanding of how the chemical causes the adverse clinical effect.

Clinical Reactions to Food Additives

Reactions to food additives include urticaria, angioedema, asthma, rhinitis, headache, and irritable bowel syndrome.[3] Recent research shows that hyperactivity may be associated with sensitivity to food colors, preservatives, and many foods.[4] Sensitivity to monosodium glutamate is associated with symptoms that can resemble myocardial infarction, including tightness and pain in the chest which radiates to the arms, palpitations, and faintness.[3]

Clinical studies based on oral challenges provide clear evidence that some additives produce a variety of symptoms in the sensitive individual. However, most of these reactions show no evidence of antibodies of any class, including IgE, nor of sensitized lymphocytes, therefore failing to indicate involvement of the immune system.[5] Possibilities to explain the effect of additives are:[3] the release of non-specific inflammatory mediators by mechanisms not mediated by the immune system; direct action on the effector organs; and pharmacological actions, such as sub-toxic effects. A few of the physiological mechanisms responsible for the clinical symptoms are partially understood, such as that of erythrosine, which alters the membrane permeability of neurons in animals, causing the release of neurotransmitters at the neuromuscular junction.[6] This action could be related to behavior disorders in humans.

Only a few additives are considered to be consistently associated with adverse reactions to foods,[7] and clinical practitioners disagree about the reactivity of these substances. Unless definitive laboratory results are available, many clinicians do not acknowledge the role of food components and additives in people's symptoms, and believe that avoidance of foods based on unsubstantiated evidence places an unnecessary burden on the food-sensitive person. Extensive food restrictions are often discouraged, therefore, on nutritional, social, economic, and ethical grounds. Although sensitivity to additives is not a life threatening situation in most cases, it can have a major effect on the quality of life. On this basis, therefore, measures to identify the offending substances are usually justified, unless such investigations impose nutritional or other risks that outweigh the inconvenience of the reactions.

Identifying Sensitivity to Food Additives

Saifer and Saifer[8] use a number of anecdotal markers to identify the person exhibiting signs of sensitivity to food additives. These investigators indicate that one of the first signs of food additive intolerance is development of a sensitivity to alcohol, starting with adverse reactions to red wine and beer and followed by reactions to white wine and distilled spirits. In addition, sensitivity to odors from chemicals such as perfumes, gasoline, cigarette smoke, paint solvents, and household cleaners may indicate sensitivity to ingested chemicals. Since no specific set of symptoms is typically associated with additive intolerance, Saifer and Saifer consider that the probable indicators of chemical food additive intolerance are multi-system reactions, especially central nervous system symptoms such as headache, fatigue, poor concentration, and muscle weakness, together with skin and respiratory symptoms.

Only in a very small number of cases of isolated reactions to additives is the culprit identified. Obtaining diagnostic confirmation that additives are the cause of a person's symptoms is often difficult. At present, the only indicator of food additive intolerance in most cases is elimination and challenge with foods containing the suspected additive(s).[9]

The food additives most frequently implicated in adverse reactions include:[10]

- Tartrazine and other food dyes
- Sulfites
- Nitrates and nitrites
- Benzoates
- Sorbates
- Butylated hydroxyanisole (BHA)
- Butylated hydroxytoluene (BHT)
- Salicylates
- Monosodium glutamate and other glutamates.

Compounds that are similar or closely related to additives sometimes occur naturally in foods, thus posing an additional dilemma for the food-sensitive person. Although an additive may be adequately described on a package label (even though current labeling requirements are sometimes vague in this regard), the same chemical present as a natural ingredient may not be suspected. Examples of physiologically reactive compounds that occur both naturally and as additions in a wide range of foods are benzoates, nitrates, nitrites, and salicylates. (See pages 205, 241, and 187)

Naturally occurring compounds probably produce symptoms by physiological mechanisms similar to those occurring in reactions to food additives. Because these reactions appear not to involve activation of the immune system, they are considered food intolerances, rather than allergy.[3] Reactions to chemicals such as nickel (which is implicated in some cases of dermatitis) and the biogenic amines tyramine, histamine, octopamine, and phenylethylamine (which may be implicated in a variety of clinical conditions, especially migraine and other headaches) are examples of such intolerances.[10]

To further complicate matters, the levels of these naturally occurring compounds tend to differ noticeably from one sample of food to another, depending on the conditions under which the food was grown, the variety of the plant, and sometimes the degree of ripeness.[11]

Once additives and/or naturally occurring compounds have been identified as the cause of intolerance in food-sensitive persons, use of the standardized approach set out in later parts of this book should determine the most likely sources of these substances.

References

1.   Health Protection Dispatch. Food Additives. Health Protection Branch, Health and Welfare Canada, Ottawa, Ontario, K1A 0L2, January 1988.

2.   National Research Council (US), Toxicity testing strategies to determine needs and priorities. National Academy Press, Washington, DC 1984.

3.   Finn, R. Pharmacological action of foods. In: Brostoff, J., and Challacombe, S.J. (Eds), *Food Allergy and Intolerance.* Baillière Tindall, London, 1987. 425-430.

4.   Egger, J. The hyperkinetic syndrome. In: Brostoff, J., and Challacombe, S.J. (Eds), *Food Allergy and Intolerance.* Baillière Tindall, London, 1987. 676-687.

5.   Botey, J., Roger, A, Eseverri, J.L., Marin, A., Pena, M. Immunoallergic techniques for the diagnosis of food allergy. In: *Food Allergy in Infancy: Proceedings of the International Symposium*, Palma de Mallorca, Spain, December 1991, 91-100.

6.   Winter, R. *A Consumer's Dictionary of Food Additives*, Third Edition Crown Publishers, Inc. New York, 1989.

7.   David, T.J. *Food and Food Additive Intolerance in Childhood.* Blackwell Scientific Publications, Oxford, London, 1993.

8.   Saifer, P.L. and Saifer, M. Clinical detection of sensitivity to preservatives and chemicals. In: Brostoff, J., and Challacombe, S.J. (Eds), *Food Allergy and Intolerance.* Baillière Tindall, London, 1987. 416-424.

9.   Wilson, N. And Scott, A. A double-blind assessment of additive intolerance in children using a 12-day challenge period at home. Clin. Exper. Allergy 1989 19(3):267-272.

10.   Metcalfe, D.D., Sampson, H.A., and Simon, R.A. (Eds). *Adverse Reactions to Foods and Food Additives.* Blackwell Scientific Publications, Oxford, London, 1991.

11.   Jorhem, I., and Sundstrom, B. Levels of lead, cadmium, zinc, copper, nickel, chromium, manganese and cobalt in foods on the Swedish market 1983-1990. J. Food Composition and Analysis 1993 6:233-241.

3

Anaphylactic Reactions to Foods

An anaphylactic reaction is a severe reaction of rapid onset that involves most organ systems and that results in circulatory collapse and a drop in blood pressure.[1] The first symptoms usually are burning, itching, or irritation of the lips, the inside of the mouth, and the throat. This reaction may be followed by nausea, vomiting, abdominal pain, and diarrhea as the food enters the digestive system.[2]

Symptoms in Anaphylactic Reactions

Once the food antigen enters the general circulation, the person begins to feel unwell, becomes anxious and warm, develops generalized itching and faintness, and may experience nasal irritation and sneezing. Skin reactions include urticaria, angioedema, and reddening. Chest tightness, bronchospasm, rhinitis, voice hoarseness, and irritated eyes may occur.

In addition, the pulse may be rapid, weak, irregular, and/or difficult to detect. In severe cases this set of symptoms is rapidly followed by loss of consciousness. Death from suffocation (due to edema of the larynx, epiglottis, and pharynx) or from shock and cardiac arrhythmia may occur within minutes of ingestion of the offending food.[1]

The later the onset of symptoms following food ingestion, the less severe the reaction is likely to be.[2] Severe reactions usually occur from within minutes to one hour of food ingestion, although the reaction may be delayed for up to two hours.

Occurrence of Anaphylactic Reactions to Foods

In a significantly high number of anaphylactic reactions to foods, the person is asthmatic, indicating that individuals with asthma are more likely than the general population to experience anaphylactic reactions to foods. This likelihood is increased when the person is receiving desensitization injections or is allergic to wasp and bee venom.[3]

Almost any food can cause an anaphylactic reaction, but the foods most commonly responsible are: peanuts, nuts, shellfish, fish, cow's milk, and eggs. Most studies indicate that 80% of atopic children are allergic to only one or two foods.[1]

Anaphylactic reactions to cow's milk, egg, wheat, and chicken have occurred most often in children under three years of age.[1] Infants and toddlers tend to outgrow early allergies to certain foods, such as milk, egg, wheat, and soy; however, when the onset of food allergy occurs after three years of age, the allergy is less likely to be outgrown.[2] Allergies to certain other foods are less likely to be outgrown and may persist for a person's lifetime. These foods include peanuts, nuts, shellfish, and fish.

In adults, a surprisingly large number of anaphylactic reactions to foods occur in conjunction with factors such as the concomitant intake of alcohol or exercising directly before or after eating the food.[1] Exercise-induced anaphylaxis has been reported to occur most frequently within two hours of ingestion of the allergenic food. Foods known to have been associated with exercise-induced anaphylaxis are celery, shellfish (especially shrimp and oysters), squid, peaches, and wheat.

Foods Implicated in Anaphylactic Reactions

The following list gives examples of foods reported to cause fatal and non-fatal anaphylactic reactions.[1] The list does not include every food capable of inducing an anaphylactic reaction because anaphylactic reactions are individual and no list could include all foods that might be implicated.

Nuts	Seeds	Grains	Vegetables
Peanut	Millet	Wheat	Potato
Pecan	Sunflower	Rice	Celery
Pistachio	Sesame		Pea
Cashew	Cottonseed extract		Pinto bean
Brazil	Annatto (color extract)		Soybean
Piñon	Psyllium		Chick pea
			Corn

Poultry	Fish	Beverages
Chicken	Cod	Chamomile tea
	Halibut	Wine

Fruit	Shellfish	Egg
Orange	Crab	Hen
Tangerine	Shrimp	
Mango	Lobster	
Banana	Limpet	
Kiwi fruit		

Milk Products
Cow's milk (usually in children under 5 years of age)

Avoiding Food-Mediated Anaphylactic Reactions

A person who has shown an anaphylactic reaction to a particular food should avoid all sources of that food. Achieving this goal means making sure that the food does not enter the home and that, as much as possible, all meals are made using basic ingredients. If a manufactured food is used, all ingredients in the food must be known.

When eating outside the home, the person must make sure that all ingredients used in preparing the meal are known. Becoming familiar with terms used on food labels and enquiring about the ingredients used in restaurants is part of this process.

Cross-reactivity among foods in the same botanic or zoological family is uncommon.[1] For example, cross-reactivity between members of the legume family (e.g., peanut, soy, peas, beans, lentils) is very uncommon, and allergic individuals usually demonstrate hypersensitivity to only one or two foods in this group. Thus, when a person is allergic to one food, the restriction of all foods in that family is unjustified. For example, because a person is allergic to peanuts, it is not necessary to exclude all legumes from the diet.[2] Other related foods should be excluded only if separate testing shows that they are further allergens.

The crustaceans are exceptions to this rule, as they seem to exhibit a high degree of antigenic cross-reactivity. Individuals who are allergic to shrimp, lobster, crayfish, or crabs are advised to avoid all shellfish. This form of restriction does not apply to fish, which do not exhibit cross-reactivity; instead, hypersensitivity to bony fish appears to be species specific.[4]

Further Precautions for Persons Who Experience Anaphylactic Reactions

The most important preventive measure for persons known to experience anaphylactic reactions to foods is to take every precaution possible to avoid exposure to the anaphylaxis inducing food.

Persons who have experienced an anaphylactic reaction are usually instructed by their physicians to obtain and keep at hand an Anakit® or Epipen® for use when accidental exposure to the allergen occurs. Obtained by prescription only, these kits contain injectable adrenalin (epinephrine) and an oral antihistamine. The physician advises the person to take the antihistamine and inject the adrenalin at first onset of a reaction and then proceed without delay to the nearest hospital emergency department. It is critical that the person goes to the hospital after injecting the adrenalin, even if the symptoms seem to be disappearing: a secondary phase of the response can prove fatal. Specific instructions for the use of the Anakit® or Epipen® should be obtained from the attending physician.

Anaphylaxis-prone persons are also advised to wear a Medic-Alert® bracelet to expedite appropriate treatment if they become unconscious.

Most experts agree that persons with asthma are at particular risk of a severe or fatal anaphylactic reaction.[2] As a result, taking appropriate precautions is particularly important for these individuals.[56]

References

1.   David, T.J. *Food and Food Additive Intolerance in Childhood.* Blackwell Scientific Publications, Oxford, London, 1993. 399-408.

2.   Settipane, R., and Settipane, G. Anaphylaxis and food allergy. In: Metcalfe, D.D., Sampson, H.A., and Simon, R.A. (Eds) *Food Allergy: Adverse Reactions to Foods and Food Additives.* Blackwell Scientific Publications, Oxford, London, 1991. 150-163.

3.   Lockey, R.F., Benedict, L.M., Turkeltaub, P.C., and Bukantz, S.C. Fatalities from immunotherapy (IT) and skin testing (ST). J. Allergy Clin. Immunol. 1987 79:660-677.

4.   Bernhisel-Broadbent, J., and Sampson, H.A. Oral challenge and *in vitro* study results in fish hypersensitivity patients. J. Allergy Clin. Immunol. 1990 85:(1):270.

5.   Yunginger, J.W., Sweeney, K.G., Sturner, W.Q., Giannandrea, L.A., Teigland, J.D., Bray, M., Benson, P.A., York, J.A., Biedrzycki, L., Squillace, D.L., Helm, R.M. Fatal food-induced anaphylaxis. JAMA 1988 260(10):1450-1452.

6.   Sampson, H.A., Medelson, L., and Rosen, J.P. Fatal and near-fatal anaphylactic reactions to food in children and adolescents. New. Eng. J. Med. 1992 327(6):380-384.

4

Allergenic Cross-reactivity

Allergenic Cross-reactivity Between Botanically Related Plants

Cross-reactivity may be defined as a connection between two or more allergens, whether related or not, that causes them to induce similar clinical reactions. Cross-reactivity among botanically related inhaled allergens such as grass pollens has been known for many years.[1] However, much uncertainty exists about the degree of clinical cross-reactivity among members of botanically related food plants.[2] It is not always valid to assume that, because plants belong to the same family, they are necessarily related antigenically. An allergic reaction to a single species does not automatically lead to allergy to all members of that plant family.

Many people have limited their diets unnecessarily, assuming that an allergy to one member of a botanic family means they will be allergic to all plants from that family.[2] For example, individuals who are allergic to peanuts and soy are frequently advised to avoid all legumes on the assumption that all legumes have similar allergenic potential. However, it is rare for an person to react to all members of the *Leguminosae* (legumes such as peanut, soy, peas, beans, lentils, licorice, carob, and gum arabic). The principle that should guide final dietary restrictions is that each food must be tested separately before it is excluded from the diet.[2]

Allergenic Cross-reactivity Between Unrelated Plant Species

Recent research has demonstrated the presence of a number of cross-reacting antigens in botanically unrelated, allergenic plant species.[1] These allergens may be inhaled or consumed as food.
Common antigens have been demonstrated within each of the following groupings:

1. Birch pollen, hazelnut, potato, and apple[3]
2. Apple, carrot, and celery[4]
3. Birch pollen, nut, apple, and fruit with stones[1]
4. Hazelnut, rye grain, sesame seeds, kiwi, and poppy seeds[1]
5. Birch pollen, mugwort pollen, apple, celery, and carrot[5]
6. Birch pollen, apple, carrot, celery, potato, hazelnut, orange, tomato, and peanut[6]
7. Ragweed pollen, and watermelon[7]
8. Ragweed pollen, melon, and banana[8]
9. Latex, banana, avocado, kiwi fruit, chestnut, soybean, peanut[9], papaya, fig[10]

Hypersensitivity to these plants is an individual idiosyncrasy. Even for species known to have common antigens, research studies have not demonstrated clinical cross-reactivity in most of the persons tested.[2] Persons allergic to one species in an antigenically related group do not necessarily experience an adverse reaction to other species in that group.

Relatedness of Other Food Allergens

Milk

Milks from unrelated animal species have been shown to cross-react frequently.[2] In one study, 22 out of 28 infants with cow's milk allergy were shown to also be allergic to goat's milk.[11] In a more recent study of weanling rats sensitized to cow's milk, 100% showed clinical reactivity to goat's milk. The authors of the study suggest that "goat's milk is not a safe alternative to cow's milk in children with cow's milk allergy."[12]

Eggs

Eggs from a variety of birds (hen, turkey, duck, goose, and seagull) have been reported to cross-react antigenically.[13]

Fish

Allergic reactivity to one species of fin fish does not usually lead to allergy to other fish.[2] Although 55% of children in one clinical study[14] were allergic to both cod and sole, and 35% to both cod and tuna, other studies[15] indicate that allergy to multiple fish species is uncommon. Restricting all fin fish because of an allergy to a single fish species is generally unwarranted. However, in cases where a potentially life threatening anaphylactic reaction to a fish has occurred, the individual is usually advised to avoid contact with all fish in the interests of safety.

Shellfish

In contrast to fin fish allergy, individuals allergic to crustaceans (shellfish) are often allergic to all species, including crab, lobster, shrimp, prawn, and crayfish.[16]

Less clear, however, is the cross-reactivity between crustaceans and molluscs (clam, mussel, oyster, octopus, squid, scallop, snail, and abalone).[15] Although some reports indicate that allergy to both types of shellfish in one individual is rare, the degree of clinical cross-reactivity between these two is not known.[2]

Nuts

Whether a person who is allergic to specific nuts should avoid nuts of all species is an unanswered question.[2] The incidence of cross-reactivity among nuts from unrelated trees is unknown. At present, someone who has experienced an anaphylactic reaction to nuts should be advised to avoid nuts of all types.

The likelihood of persons reacting to tree nuts if they are anaphylactic to peanuts is also unknown.[2] To ensure that inadvertent exposure to peanut is avoided, individuals who are anaphylactic to peanuts should be advised to avoid all tree nuts as well.

References

1. Vocks, E., Borga, A., Sciska, C., Seifert, H.U., Seifert, B., Burow, G., and Borelli, S. Common allergenic structures in hazelnut, rye grain, sesame seeds, kiwi, and poppy seeds. Allergy 1991 48:168-172.

2. David, T.J. *Food and Food Additive Intolerance in Childhood.* Blackwell Scientific Publications, Oxford, London. 1993 447-450.

3. Andersen, K.E., and Lowenstein, H. An investigation of the possible immunological relationship between allergen extracts from birch pollen, hazelnut, potato and apple. Contact Dermatitis 1978 4:72-79.

4. Halmepuro, I., and Lowenstein, H. Immunological investigations of possible structural similarities between pollen antigens and antigens in apple, carrot and celery tuber. Allergy 1985 40:264-272.

5. Vallier, P., Dechamp, C., Valenta, R., Vial, O. and Deviller, P. Purification and characterization of an allergen from celery immunochemically related to an allergen present in several other plant species. Identification as a profilin. Clin. Exper. Allergy 1992 22:774-782.

6. Dreborg, S. Food allergy in pollen-sensitive patients. Ann. Allergy 1988 61:41-46.

7. Enberg, R.N., McCullough, J., Ownby, D.R. Antibody responses in watermelon sensitivity. J. Allergy Clin. Immunol. 1988 82(5):795-800.

8. Anderson, L.B., Dreyfuss, E.M., Logan, J. Melon and banana sensitivity coincident with ragweed pollinosis. J. Allergy 1970 45:310.

9. Hovarec-Burns, D., Ordonez, M., Corrao, M., Enjamuri, S., and Unver, E. Identification of another latex cross-reactive food allergen: peanut. J. Allergy Clin. Immunol. 1995 95(1, Part 2): 150 (Abstract).

10.   Blanco, C. Carillo, T., Castillo, R., et al. Latex allergy : clinical featured and cross-reactivity with fruits. Ann. Allergy 1994:73 :309-314.

11.   Juntunen, K., and Ali-Yrkko, S. Goat's milk for children allergic to cow's milk. Kiel Milchwirt Forschungsber 1983 35:439-440.

12.   Hoffman, K.M., Ho, D., and Sampson, H.A. In vivo allergenic cross-reactivity of cow milk and goat milk. J. Allergy Clin. Immunol. 1995 95(1, Part 2):330 (Abstract).

13.   Langeland, T. A clinical and immunological study of allergy to hen's egg white. VI Occurrence of proteins cross-reacting with allergens in hen's egg white from turkey, duck, goose, sea gull, and in hen egg yolk, and hen and chicken sera and flesh. Allergy 1983 39:399-412.

14.   DeMartino, M., Novembre, E., Galli, L. Allergy to different fish species in cod-allergic children: *in vivo* and *in vitro* studies. J. Allergy Clin. Immunol. 1990 86:909-914.

15.   Bernhisel-Broadbent, J., and Sampson, H.A. Oral challenge and in vitro study results in fish hypersensitive patients. J. Allergy Clin. Immunol. 1990 85:270.

16.   Musmand, J.J., Daul, C.B., and Lehrer, S.B. Crustacea allergy. Clin. Exp. Allergy 1993 23:722-732.

5

The Allergenic Potential of Foods

A question frequently asked is: "To what extent should a known allergen be avoided?" For example, if a person is allergic to soy, should all forms of soy be eliminated from the diet, including hydrolyzed soy protein, lecithin made from soy, fermented soy (soy sauce), and so on?

Few practitioners can answer this question with certainty. As a result, for safety, the allergic person is usually advised to avoid all forms of the food, even though this approach may lead to a great deal of work, social and economic stress, annoyance, and possible nutritional deficiency. Additionally, the person may be continually fearful of ingesting the allergen because of food labels that fail to describe the sources of ingredients in manufactured foods.

The degree to which an allergic individual reacts to a food allergen depends on a number of factors, including the allergenic potency of the food. Most authorities agree that, if a person is only mildly allergic to a food, fewer precautions need be taken in detecting the food as a hidden ingredient than if the food is likely to precipitate a life-threatening anaphylactic reaction.[1]

Peanuts, green peas, tree nuts, shellfish, fin fish, and egg white, plus cow's milk protein in infants, are the foods most likely to cause a severe reaction in the hypersensitive person.[1] If the allergic person has shown signs of an anaphylactic reaction to any of these foods, all sources of that food should be strictly avoided. Any other food that has caused a severe reaction should also be strictly avoided.

Quantity of Food Required to Cause an Allergic Reaction

The amount of food that needs to be ingested to cause an allergic reaction appears to depend on the potency of the allergen and the allergic person's response. In a 1986 report of the Food and Drug Administration (FDA), the Ad Hoc Committee on Hypersensitivity to Food Constituents described allergenic levels of foods as follows:[2]

- The usual amount of food that produces an allergic reaction in a sensitized adult is 20 grams.
- Shrimp allergy will be provoked with 1 to 2 g of shrimp.
- Peanut allergy can be precipitated by as little as 25 mg of peanut.

Despite this attempt at quantification, other reports indicate that inhaling food components (e.g., merely being in a room where fish is being cooked),[3] or handling the food can precipitate a reaction in a highly sensitive individual.[4]

Additives Derived from Potentially Allergenic Foods

In some cases, ingredients in processed and manufactured foods are derived from natural food sources, but the origin of these ingredients is obscure. The following table provides examples of common ingredients and their food origins.[5,6] This table is by no means exhaustive. Highly sensitive individuals should be encouraged to obtain information from food manufacturers concerning hidden sources of particular allergens, and to become familiar with terms on food ingredient labels that indicate the presence of these allergens.

Table 5-1: Food Additives from Potentially Allergenic Foods

Name	Sources	Foods Likely to Contain the Additive	Function in Foods
Lecithin	Egg Egg yolk Soy beans Corn	Boxed breakfast cereals Candy Chocolates Breads, Rolls, Buns Margarine	Antioxidant and emollient composed of: choline, phosphoric acid, fatty acids, and glycerine
Starch	Wheat Potatoes Rice Corn Beans Other plants The plant source is not usually identified on an ingredient label	Thickened or creamed products	Thickening agent in a number of manufactured foods Usually used in its modified form

Table 5-1: Food Additives from Potentially Allergenic Foods

Name	Sources	Foods Likely to Contain the Additive	Function in Foods
Modified starch	Derived from plants (above) and modified with acid to make it more digestible.	Baby foods Non-food products such as dusting and face powders, baby powders and bath salts	Present in foods as: bleached starch, acetylated distarch adipate, distarch phosphate, others with "distarch" in the name
Carotene	Carrots	Margarines Butter Shortening Skimmed milk Buttermilk Cottage cheese Beet juice A number of red colored foods	Coloring agent A source of Vitamin A in enriched foods
Annatto	Extract from the seed of a tropical tree	Dairy products (cheese, butter) Breakfast cereals Baked goods Margarines	Coloring agent (yellow to pink)
Hydrolyzed vegetable protein (HVP) **Hydrolyzed plant protein (HPP)**	Soya beans Peanuts Wheat Corn (Soya beans are the most frequently used source)	Soups Meat based entrees Stews Flavoring and seasoning mixes	Flavor enhancer Plant protein is hydrolyzed (broken down) by enzymes or acids High glutamate and salt content
Xanthan gum	Product of the fermentation of dextrose (derived from corn syrup) by the microorganism *Xanthomonas campestris*	Dairy products Salad dressings May replace starch, sugar and oil in low calorie products Xanthan gum is not digested by the body and passes out mostly unchanged	Thickener, stabilizer, emulsifier, suspending agent Prevents ingredients from separating

Table 5-1: Food Additives from Potentially Allergenic Foods

Name	Sources	Foods Likely to Contain the Additive	Function in Foods
Locust bean gum	Carob seed	Ice cream Sauces Salad dressings Sausages (acts as a binder)	Thickening and stabilizing agent Used to blend ingredients and prevent separation Binding agent Texture modifier
Carrageenan	Algae (seaweed) Irish moss	Milk products Pressure dispensed whipped cream Cheese spreads Ice cream Custards Sherbets Salad dressings Sauces Chocolates Artificially sweetened jams and jellies	Emulsifier (blender) and stabilizer Prevents separation of ingredients Thickening agent, and gelling agent
Malt extract	Germinated barley	Beers Meat and poultry products Ice cream Flavored milks Sour cream Chocolate syrup Candy Cough drops Condiments Salad dressings Breakfast cereals	Flavoring agent

References

1.   David, T.J. Elimination diets In: *Food and Food Additive Intolerance in Childhood.* Blackwell Scientific Publications, Oxford, London, 1993. 441-463.

2.   FDA Ad Hoc Committee on Hypersensitivity to Food Constituents. Report, Washington, DC US Food and Drug Administration, 1986.

3.   Lehrer, S.B., Ibanez, M.D., McCants, M.L., Daul, C.B., and Morgan, J.E. Characterization of water-soluble shrimp allergens released during boiling. J. Allergy Clin. Immunol. 1990 85:1005-1013.

4.   Settipane, R., and Settipane, G.A. Anaphylaxis and food allergy. In: Metcalfe, D.D., Sampson, H.A. and Simon, R.A. (Eds), *Food Allergy: Adverse Reactions to Foods and Food Additives.* Blackwell Scientific Publications, Oxford, London, 1991 150-163.

5.   Winter, R. *A Consumer's Dictionary of Food Additives.* Third edition. Crown Publishers, New York. 1989.

6.   Freydberg, N., and Gortner, W.A. *The Food Additives Book.* Bantam Books, New York 1982.

Table 5-2: Joneja Food Allergen Scale

This table is based on the typical North American diet and compiled from a wide variety of sources.
Foods are listed from the highest to the lowest allergenicity.
People vary in their reactivity to foods and show a different pattern of reactivity depending on their individual characteristics.
Persons following ethnic diets tend to show a different order of allergenicity.
Allergenicity depends on a variety of factors including frequency of exposure to the food.

GRAINS & FLOURS	VEGETABLES	FRUITS	NUTS & SEEDS	MEATS & ALTERNATES	DAIRY
Wheat Triticale Semolina Bulgur Spelt Kamut	Tomato Spinach Celery (raw)	Strawberry Raspberry Orange Fig Mango Watermelon	Peanut Nuts: Hazelnut (filbert)	Egg white Egg yolk	Ice cream Cow's milk: Raw milk Homogenized 1%, 2%, Skim
Corn Oats	Carrot (raw) Green pea Lima bean Broad bean (fava bean) Cabbage (heart)	Apple (raw) Apricot (raw) Peach (raw) Date Cantaloupe Pineapple Raisin Apple (cooked)	Walnut Pecan Brazil nut Almond Sesame seed Cocoa bean Chocolate Coconut Flax seed	Shellfish: - Crab - Lobster - Prawn/shrimp Molluscs: - Clam - Oyster - Scallop	Cheese fermented: Cheddar Camembert Blue Swiss Edam Mozzarella Goat cheese
Rye Barley	Cauliflower Brussels sprouts Green bean	Kiwi Cherry Plum/prune Apricot (cooked)	Cashew Pistachio Macadamia	Fin fish - Cod - Sole Other white fish - Tuna - Salmon	Cottage cheese Cream cheese
Brown rice White rice Wild rice	Avocado Cabbage (outer leaves)	Loganberry Boysenberry	Legumes: Soy Dried peas Lentils Dried beans - Navy - Pinto - Garbanzo		Cream Sour cream
Quinoa	Onion Green onion Garlic	Plantain Banana Grape		Processed meats - Pepperoni - Salami - Bologna - Wieners	Canned milk (evaporated)
Buckwheat (kasha)	Celery (cooked) Green/red peppers	Grapefruit Lemon Lime	Carob Sunflower seed	Ham Bacon	Goat milk Sheep milk
Amaranth	Potato Cucumber Lettuce	Currants (red/ black)	Pumpkin seed	Pork	Processed cheese
Tapioca Cassava	Asparagus Broccoli Beets	Peach (cooked/ canned)	Bean sprouts	Chicken Beef Veal	Soft cheese (Philadelphia)
Sago Arrowroot Millet	Squashes (all types) Carrot (cooked) Parsnip	Cranberry Blackberry Blueberry Pear	Poppy seed	Wild meats - Deer - Elk - Moose - Bear - Buffalo	Yogurt Buttermilk Butter
	Turnip Sweet potato Yam	Rhubarb		Turkey Lamb Rabbit	Clarified butter

Part II

Diagnosis and Detection of Food Allergens and Reactive Chemicals in Foods

_____

6

Food Allergy Tests

Used alone, laboratory tests are of little value in detecting food allergy, and can lead to a misleading diagnosis unless the clinical history is also considered. With few exceptions (namely, eggs, nuts, fish), skin tests and blood tests for food allergens are unreliable or misleading for the following reasons:[1]

- People may have IgE antibodies, but no symptoms.
- Foods can cause non-specific ("irritant") skin reactions.
- The reaction may not be mediated by IgE antibodies.

Only about one-third of the persons with positive skin prick tests or serum-specific IgE show clinical symptoms during food challenge.[2] Nevertheless, routine use of these tests is common.

Skin Tests

The skin test is often the first undertaking in the diagnosis of allergy. This test is designed to identify the type of IgE that is fixed to the skin mast cell. When the allergen bridges two IgE molecules on the surface of the cell, inflammatory mediators are released that cause edema (swelling) and erythema (reddening). This combination of symptoms is known as the "weal and flare reaction."

With this test, the allergen is introduced into the skin in one of three methods: placing a drop of allergen extract onto the surface and pricking the skin underneath with a lancet (prick test); scarifying the skin and depositing a drop of allergen onto the site (scratch test); or injecting the allergen into the skin from a syringe (intradermal test). Although intradermal tests are sometimes slightly more sensitive than prick or scratch tests, they cause more non-specific positive responses and may induce systemic reactions. For the latter reason, many allergists strongly discourage use of the intradermal test to avoid the danger of an anaphylactic reaction.[3]

Blood Tests

Blood tests for allergen-specific IgE or total IgE (RAST, or Radioallergosorbent test) have the same limitations as skin tests in the diagnosis of food allergy. Although the percentage risk of allergy based on IgE levels has been estimated,[4] most authorities agree with Botey *et al.*, who stated that, "Many atopic individuals exhibit an IgE with normal values, so no IgE level, no matter how low, rules out the diagnosis of food allergy."[5]

Attempts to identify other antibodies implicated in food allergy use blood tests such as the FAST (Fluorescent allergosorbent test) and ELISA (Enzyme linked immunosorbent assay) for IgG4. However, these tests are even less reliable in diagnosing food allergy.[2] According to Botey *et al.*, "IgG4 may be high in patients with food allergy, but its detection has no diagnostic value on account of its being found frequently in individuals who tolerate these nutrients, and it might only indicate an increase in intestinal permeability or a sub-clinical sensitivity."[5] Readers who require further details of these tests are directed to reference 5 in this chapter.

Controversial Tests

A number of scientifically unproven tests are becoming popular in the often frustrating search for a diagnosis in adverse reactions to foods. When traditional medicine fails to provide a definitive diagnosis, many people with chronic, recurrent complaints seek alternative care.[6] Many methods have been developed to satisfy the demand for a quick and easy diagnosis, but they lack the scientific testing needed to substantiate their efficacy. Two of the most popular non-invasive tests are electroacupuncture (Vega Test) and biokinesiology.

Vega Test

The Vega Test is a method of electroacupuncture that utilizes "energy waves" to indicate a person's reactivity to a food or other allergen. The allergen to be tested is put in a vial and placed within a circuit that includes a meter to measure the degree of reactivity. By this method, practitioners also attempt to measure the activity of organ systems and endocrine glands.

Biokinesiology

The biokinesiology test is based on the assumption that muscles become weak when influenced by the allergen causing a person's symptoms. In this test, the person holds the allergen, contained in a vial, in one hand while the practitioner tests the strength of the person's other arm in resisting downward pressure. A weakening of resistance is considered indicative of a positive (allergic) reaction. When using this test for an infant, an adult holds the child, who is in contact with the vial containing the allergen (placed inside a sock or other clothing). The muscle strength of the adult's arm is measured.

Other Allergy Tests

A good review and discussion of other types of diagnostic tests, such as subcutaneous, intracutaneous and sublingual provocation and neutralization, cytotoxic testing, autologous urine injections, and immune complex assays can be found in reference 5 for this chapter. A detailed discussion of these techniques is beyond the scope of this book.

Reliable Tests

The only reliable diagnostic test available for detecting food allergy or food intolerance requires the use of an exposure diary, followed by an elimination diet and oral challenge. Botey *et al.* claim that, "The oral provocation test is the 'gold standard' due to the fact that we cannot make the diagnosis only with a skin test or a positive serological reaction, and even in the immediate type allergies both may be negative."[5]

Double Blind Placebo Controlled Food Challenge

Many conservative allergists believe that the only valid challenge test is the double blind placebo controlled food challenge (DBPCFC),[7] in which neither the clinician nor patient knows which food is enclosed within a gelatin capsule - the test food or an unreactive placebo (usually glucose powder). The person's reactions to this challenge are monitored and assessed by the clinician.

There are drawbacks to this method of testing. The drawbacks include environmental factors that may cause a reaction inducing symptoms similar to those induced by the food; the person may react to more than one food; and several small capsules may not deliver enough food to induce a reaction.[8]

Open Food Challenge

An important consideration when evaluating the effectiveness of DBPCFC is that indirect methods may trigger the release of inflammatory mediators from the granules of mast cells, even though these cells may not respond to a disguised food alone. Mast cells are found throughout the gut wall, specifically in the mucosa, neural plexuses, and muscle layers, and are often in close proximity to nerves.[8] One mechanism causing their degranulation is mediated by neuropeptides released from nerve cells. The inflammatory mediators released after such neural stimulation may reach levels sufficiently high to produce symptoms similar to true food allergy.[7]

Studies in rats indicate that mast cell degranulation may be induced through audio-visual stimulation alone. Using Pavlovian conditioning, anaphylactic rats have been induced to respond first to simultaneous exposure to the allergen and an audio-visual stimulus and then to the audio-visual trigger alone.[9] Guinea pigs immunized with a foreign protein antigen and presented with an odor at the same time as the antigen, released histamine when subsequently presented with the odor alone, in the absence of the antigen.[10,11] It is therefore conceivable that degranulation of gut-associated mast cells occurs in humans when exposed to the sight or smell of food without having ingested it. In fact, the audio-visual stimulus may be a requirement for mast cell degranulation in some cases. Thus, disguising the food in a capsule may prevent symptoms from developing because the sight and smell (and possibly the taste) of the food are necessary for the release of the inflammatory mediators. Accordingly, in such a case, open challenge of the food would induce symptoms when a DBPCFC would not.

Diagnosis and Management of Food Allergies and Intolerances

Diagnosis

Elimination and challenge to detect food allergens can be tedious, time consuming, and frustrating for both the allergic person and the clinician. A systematic, scientific approach can reduce these drawbacks. The step-by-step process for detecting allergies and intolerances given in this book uses an exposure diary and elimination and challenge protocols, and represents an approach developed and tested in clinical practice.

Management

Most authorities agree that a restricted diet should not be prescribed before food challenges have been performed.[12] Once the offending foods, food components, or additives have been detected, their avoidance is essential for the person to remain symptom free. However, simply removing the foods from the diet may lead to nutritional deficiencies that, in time, can be more dangerous to the person's health than the original adverse reactions. Management of adverse reactions to foods must both eliminate the antagonistic foods and replace them with nutritional equivalents from alternative sources. Special care must be taken to ensure that the final diet is nutritionally adequate, regardless of the number and type of foods that must be avoided.

Prevention

Overall, the best method of allergy management is to prevent the initial sensitization to the allergen. A number of strategies can be used to protect an infant from becoming sensitized to the most powerful allergens during the early vulnerable period when both the immune and digestive systems are still immature. In many cases, lifelong food allergy may be prevented. Part IV of this book explains how to reduce exposure to potential food allergens at this time.

Note on the "Few Foods" Elimination Diet

Many published protocols for the elimination and challenge test advocate a restricted diet using very few (usually only eight to ten) of the least allergenic foods. This diet is to be followed for 10 to 14 days. In practice, however, people seem to continue the diet for much longer, in the hope that their symptoms will resolve.

When a very restricted diet is prolonged beyond the two week limit, the results are complicated by the following two factors:

- Severe nutritional depletion can lead to suppression of the immune system. Since the cause of an allergy is over-responsiveness of the immune system, prolonging an inadequate diet can achieve apparent resolution of allergy symptoms simply by suppressing the immune response. With subsequent refeeding, the immune system is reactivated and symptoms recur, regardless of the foods introduced. People in this situation often report that they now are sensitive to foods that they previously tolerated.

- Depletion of micronutrients (vitamins and minerals) can have deleterious effects on metabolism, as well as on the immune system. People often report feeling worse after a prolonged restricted diet and refeeding than before the diet.

The underlying message is that a "few foods" diet should *never* be followed for more than two weeks. If the symptoms persist after this period, prolonging the diet will not resolve the problem. Other possibilities for consideration are that an alternative test diet might detect the allergen, or that food is not causing the symptoms.

The Ultimate Goal

Finally, after challenge tests have identified a person's antagonistic foods, a diet is developed that will eliminate the problem foods and supply adequate and balanced nutrition from alternative sources. This may require major adjustments in food choices and lifestyle. The ultimate reward of improved health and quality of life justifies the time and effort required to detect the antagonistic foods and to develop a nutritionally balanced and satisfying diet.

References

1.   Kay, A.B., Lessof, M.H. Allergy: Conventional and alternative concepts. A report of the Royal College of Physicians Committee on Clinical Immunology and Allergy. April 1992. 19.

2.   David, T.J. Skin tests. In: *Food and Food Additive Intolerance in Childhood.* Blackwell Scientific Publications, Oxford, London, 1991. 244-292.

3.   Onorato, J., Merland, N., Terral, C., Michel, F.B., Bousquet, J. Placebo-controlled double-blind food challenge in asthma. J. Allergy Clin. Immunol. 1986 78:1139-1146.

4.   Hamburger, R.N., *et al.* Current status of the clinical and immunologic consequences of a prototype allergic disease prevention program. Ann. Allergy 1983 51:281-290.

5.   Botey, J., Roger, A., Eseverri, J.L., Marin, A., Pena, M. Immunoallergic techniques for the diagnosis of food allergy. In: *Food Allergy in Infancy: Proceedings of the International Symposium*, Palma de Mallorca, Spain, December 1991. 91-100.

6.   Goldberg, G.J., Kaplan, M.S. Controversial concepts and techniques in the diagnosis and management of food allergies. Immunology and Allergy Clinics of North America, November 1991 11(4):863-884.

7.   Bock, S.A., Sampson, H.A., Atkins, F.M., Zeiger, R.S., Lehrer, S., Sachs, M., Bush, R.K., Metcalfe, D.D. Double-blind, placebo-controlled food challenge (DBPCFC) as an office procedure: A manual. J. Allergy Clin. Immunol. 1988 82(6):986-997.

8.   Symposium: Food Allergy and Intolerance: New Direction. Annals RCPSC 1993 26(1):29-32.

9.   MacQueen, G., Marshall, J., Perdue, M., Seigel, G., Bienenstock, J. Pavlovian conditioning of rat mucosal mast cells to secrete mast cell protease II. Science 1989 243:83-85.

10.   Russell, M., Dark, K.A., Cummins, R.W. Learned histamine release. Science 1984 225:733.

11.   Brostoff, J. Mechanisms: An introduction. In: Brostoff, J., and Challacombe, S.J. (Eds), *Food Allergy and Intolerance*. Baillière Tindall, London, 1987. 433-455.

12.   Yunginger, J.W. Proper application of available laboratory tests for adverse reactions to foods and food additives. J. Allergy Clin. Immunol. 1986 78:220-223.

7

Elimination and Challenge Test

Stage 1: Exposure Diary

To keep an exposure diary, the subject records the following, daily for 5 to 7 days:

- All foods, beverages, medications, and supplements ingested
- The approximate quantities of each food by volume (e.g., milliliters, cups, teaspoons) or weight (e.g., grams, ounces)
- The composition of mixed dishes and drinks (an ingredient list)
- The time when each food was eaten
- All symptoms experienced, graded for severity as follows:
  1 = mild   2 = mild to moderate   3 = moderate   4 = severe
- The time of onset of any symptoms
- The duration of any symptoms
- Status on waking in the morning (i.e., whether symptom-free or the type and severity of symptoms)
- Any sleep disturbance during the night, and whether it was due to specific symptoms.

Stage 2: Elimination Test Diet

The formulation of an elimination test diet excluding all suspected allergens and intolerance triggers[1,2] should be based on:

- A detailed medical history
- Analysis of the exposure diary
- The results of any previous allergy tests
- The foods which the person suspects are causing the symptoms.

It is critical that this diet provide alternative sources for the energy and nutrients in excluded foods. The duration of Stage 2 is usually 4 weeks.

Few Foods Elimination Test Diet

Sometimes, it is very difficult to determine which foods should be excluded on a selective elimination diet. When there are multiple symptoms that do not fit into any perceivable pattern of reactivity that would suggest a reaction to food allergens, and there are no indicators of food additive intolerance or sensitivity to natural components of foods, a Few Foods Elimination Diet is useful.[2] Because this diet is not nutritionally complete, it should never be followed for more than fourteen days. Seven to ten days is usually sufficient to show results. This period should never be exceeded for children under seven years of age. A role for foods in the etiology of the symptoms should become apparent if symptoms disappear or improve significantly within this time period. Extending the Few Foods Elimination Diet beyond fourteen days if the symptoms remain unchanged is a fruitless exercise and can be detrimental to health because the immune system may become depressed on this semi-starvation regimen.

There are many "few foods elimination diets" in use and each practitioner tends to favor a particular diet. The Few Foods Elimination Diet documented here includes foods which consistently prove low in allergenicity for the majority of the population, and is the one most often followed. Adjustments must be made for individuals with unusual reactions who might respond adversely to one or more of the foods included.

Details of the diet, with meal plans and recipes for fourteen days, are provided in Part VI.

Expected Results of the Elimination Test Diet

If true allergens have been excluded, the person may feel *worse* on Days 2 to 4 of the Elimination Test Diet. This effect has been suggested to be due to a condition known as "serum sickness"[3] caused by an excess of antibodies.

By Days 5 to 7 of the Elimination Test Diet, if the allergens and intolerance triggers have been avoided, the person should begin to feel better.

Symptoms should recede noticeably by Days 10 to 14 of the diet. If all allergens and antagonistic foods have been excluded, all symptoms should have disappeared by about three weeks.

If the alternative foods are adequate to substitute for the excluded energy and nutrients, no weight loss should be experienced. If the symptoms have not subsided, either allergens or intolerance factors remain in the diet, or foods are not the cause of the symptoms. Regardless of why the symptoms have persisted, the original Elimination Test Diet should not be continued for more than four weeks.

When symptoms still persist after three weeks, the person is instructed to keep a second exposure diary for 5 to 7 days prior to the next clinic appointment, while continuing the elimination diet. Analysis of this diary should indicate whether other foods or food components are contributing to the continuing symptoms.

If the second exposure diary records adverse reactions, further foods can be eliminated, in addition to the original list, for another two weeks.

Following four weeks of food elimination (or six weeks if more foods had to be eliminated for two additional weeks after the initial four), a sequential incremental dose challenge is initiated.

If symptoms persist, specific challenges with food components may reveal adverse reactions to the foods that have been avoided.   These reactions may not be noticeable when the food is eaten continuously.

Stage 3: Challenge

Challenging with a suspect food consists of having the person eat a small amount of the food and, if no reaction occurs, of gradually increasing this dose. The purpose of this sequential incremental dose challenge[4] is to determine the person's sensitivity and limit of tolerance to each of the foods excluded in the Elimination Test Diet. Challenges must use the purest form of foods available.

Challenges should not test any food suspected of having produced a severe or an anaphylactic reaction in the past, except under medical supervision in a center equipped with resuscitation facilities.

The person continues to follow the basic elimination diet during the test.

Test foods are not added back to the diet until *all* the eliminated foods have been separately tested, even those producing no reaction during the challenge. Detailed instructions for challenge of individual food components and additives starts on page 35.

Stage 4: Final Diet

The diet followed after all challenges are completed must exclude the foods and additives for which challenges elicited a positive reaction. As well, the final diet must be nutritionally complete, providing adequate energy and nutrients from non-allergenic sources.

If dose related intolerances are a problem, a four day rotation diet might be beneficial, (see *Rotation Diets*, page 67). There is no consensus on the benefits of rotation diets at present.

Notes

The duration of the initial Elimination Test Diet depends on the type of symptoms being experienced. For example, symptoms that occur only intermittently, at widely spaced intervals (such as migraine headaches), or that may be delayed reactions to foods and additives, may require a longer elimination phase. Gastrointestinal symptoms, on the other hand, usually respond promptly to appropriate dietary measures and improvement can be experienced within 7 to 10 days.

An elimination diet should never be followed for longer than 10 to 14 days if there is any danger of nutritional deficiency (e.g., as with a "few foods" diet).

The key reasons why people do not adhere to elimination test diets are:[5]

- The person has insufficient knowledge to understand the restrictions and why they are necessary
- The diet is too intrusive to be acceptable: either it has too many restrictions or it does not accommodate the person's lifestyle and tastes
- The diet fails to reduce or eradicate the symptoms
- excessive expectations of the diet have not been met (i.e., a cure was expected rather than mere improvement)
- The diet is no longer needed because the symptoms abated spontaneously or, in children, the child outgrew the symptoms.

Cost is rarely an important factor in dietary non-adherence. Most elimination test diets are only followed for a short period of time and the cost of the substitute foods is offset by the savings from those eliminated. Studies show that there is no difference in cost between the regular diet and the elimination test diet except in the cases where expensive elemental food replacements and supplements are needed.[1]

References

1.   David, T.J. Elimination diets. In: *Food and Food Additive Intolerance in Childhood.* Blackwell Scientific Publications, Oxford, London, 1993. 441-463.

2.   Pearson, D.J. Clinical diagnosis in food allergy. Clin. Exper. Allergy 1989 19:83-85.

3.   Brostoff, J. Mechanisms: An introduction. In: Brostoff, J., and Challacombe, S.J. (Eds), *Food Allergy and Intolerance.* Baillière Tindall, London, 1987. 433-455.

4.   Wilson, N., and Scott, A. A double-blind assessment of additive intolerance in children using a 12-day challenge period at home. Clin. Exper. Allergy 1989 19(3):267-272.

5.   Yoder, E.R. Maintaining patient compliance during an elimination diet. In: Breneman, J.C. (Ed) *Handbook of Food Allergies*, 1987, 233-247.

Method: Exposure Diary

Instructions:

1. Keep the exposure diary for seven typical days, including weekdays and weekends. If the symptoms occur infrequently, continue the diary long enough to include two or three episodes.

2. Write down everything you eat, drink, take as medications, and nutritional supplements during the day and the approximate quantities taken. Include details of the ingredients of complex dishes (such as stews, stir-fries, casseroles, desserts) whenever possible.

3. Include the times of eating, drinking, and taking medications and supplements.

4. Record how you feel when you get up in the morning and any symptoms you experience throughout the day.   Include:

    *   The intensity of your symptoms rated on a scale of 0-4
        [0=None; 1=Mild; 2=Mild to Moderate; 3=Moderate to Severe; 4=Severe]
    *   What time they occur and how long they last.

5. If you have to get up during the night, record the reason why (e.g. "went to the bathroom") and how you are feeling at that time. Did your symptoms wake you up?

6. Bring your exposure diary with you when you visit your practitioner.

For children: parents record the above information for the child.

If an allergic infant is being breast-fed, keep separate diaries for the mother and the infant. Record the mother's diet as described above. Record the infant's times of nursing, any solid foods or beverages the infant takes, and the time, duration, and intensity of the infant's reactions.

Sample Food Diary

	Day 1	Day 2	Day 3	Day 4	Day 5	Day 6	Day 7
BREAKFAST							
Symptoms							
Medications							
LUNCH							
Symptoms							
Medications							
DINNER							
Symptoms							
Medications							

Method: Challenge Phase

WARNING: DO NOT test any foods that have ever caused a severe or an anaphylactic reaction. If an adverse reaction occurs at any time during the test, discontinue the food.

Continue to eat your known safe foods, the foods allowed on your elimination test diet, or the Few Foods Test Diet (whichever has been prescribed for you) throughout the challenge test period. Details of quantities of specific foods are given in each food category below.

A checklist for each test is provided for recording all responses starting on page 58. This checklist should be completed as the challenge phase proceeds.

Wait at least 48 hours after an adverse reaction has subsided before testing a new food.

Day 1

Morning - Between Breakfast and Lunch

Eat a small quantity of the test food. Monitor your response. Be aware of any adverse reactions. If you have a reaction, you will experience only your usual symptoms, but they may be more severe than usual.

Wait four hours before eating the test food again.

If you have no adverse reaction:

Afternoon - Between Lunch and Dinner

Eat double the quantity of the test food eaten in the morning. Monitor your response.

Wait four hours.

If you have no adverse reaction:

Evening - After Dinner

Eat double the quantity of the test food eaten in the afternoon.

Day 2

Do not eat any of the test food challenged on Day 1.

Eat only the foods allowed on your elimination diet and any other foods already tested and found to be safe. Monitor your reactions throughout the day. Any adverse response may be due to a delayed reaction to the food tested yesterday. If there is no reaction, the food can be considered safe.

Day 3

If no adverse reactions have occurred, test the next food on your list in the manner described for Day 1.

If results of the Day 1 test are unclear:

Test the same food as on Day 1 again on Day 3 as follows:

At midmorning eat a greater quantity of the test food than eaten at midmorning on Day 1.

Continue to double the quantity every four hours and monitor your reactions as described for Day 1.

Day 4

Day 4 will be a monitoring day for observing delayed reactions as described for Day 2. If there is no evidence of an increased adverse reaction by the end of Day 4, the food can be considered safe.

Continue in a similar fashion until all suspect foods have been tested. The problem food can be tested again after eliminating it for a period of not less than two months for a child under the age of five years; not less than six months for an adult.

Pulse Test

Sometimes an adverse reaction to a food is accompanied by an increase in heart rate. Monitor your pulse while testing each food. Take your pulse before eating, and again 2 minutes, 5 minutes, 10 minutes, and 20 minutes after eating the food. An increase of more than 10 beats above baseline (before eating the food) that may continue to increase over the test period (20 minutes) may indicate an adverse reaction.

Method: Sequence of Testing Foods

Separate components of each food are tested individually. The sequence of testing in each category is very important because each of the tests adds an extra ingredient to the previously tested food. When you start testing one category of food (for example, milk and milk products; grains; vegetables) continue the sequence specified for that particular food until the limit of tolerance has been established. Do not switch between categories.

Quantities given are for an adult. When testing foods for a child between two and five years, use smaller quantities. For an infant below the age of two, refer to the method for *Sequence of Adding Solid Foods for the Allergic Infant* page 263.

Milk and Milk Products

Note: The "test component" is highlighted as each is added in sequence.

Test 1:   Test for **casein proteins**

Test food: White hard cheese. For example: Mozzarella; Swiss; Parmesan.

Use a block of about 5 ounces (for a child under five years use 2-3 ounces).
Cut into seven equal cubes.

Morning: one cube
Afternoon: two cubes
Evening: four cubes

Interpretation of Results of Test 1

If there is no reaction after Day 2 (monitoring day), **casein proteins** are tolerated.

If there is an adverse reaction, casein proteins are not tolerated and Tests 2, 3, 4, 7 and 8 should not be attempted, since all of the foods in these tests contain casein. Test 5 (plain yogurt) can be tried, since some people who do not tolerate casein can tolerate yogurt. A separate test for whey proteins can be attempted, using whey-containing margarine as the test food (Test 6).

Test 2:   Test for casein; **annatto (natural beta-carotene yellow dye); biogenic amines**

Test food: Orange or yellow aged cheese. For example: Aged Cheddar.

Test exactly as described for Test 1 (White cheese). Use a block of about 5 ounces (for a child under five years use 2-3 ounces). Cut into seven equal cubes.

Morning:	one cube
Afternoon:	two cubes
Evening:	four cubes

Interpretation of Results of Test 2

If there is no reaction after Day 2 (monitoring day), **annatto and biogenic amines** are tolerated, in addition to casein proteins.

If there is an adverse reaction, biogenic amines and/or annatto are the offensive foods. If the reaction is to the biogenic amines, a headache is the most common symptom experienced. Annatto is more likely to induce a skin reaction such as hives (urticaria). Each of these components can be tested separately later.

Test 3: Test for casein and **whey proteins**

Test food: Lactase treated milk; 99% lactose free milk (Lactaid milk®) (purchased) OR: Lactaid® drops

Add 15 drops to 1 liter of milk (skim; 1%; 2%; or homogenized). Leave treated milk in the refrigerator for 24 hours before the test to allow the enzyme (lactase) to break down the lactose.

	Adult	**Child**
Morning:	¼ cup	⅛ cup
Afternoon:	½ cup	¼ cup
Evening:	1 cup	½ cup

Interpretation of Results of Test 3

If there is no adverse reaction after Day 2 (monitoring day): casein and **whey proteins** are tolerated. If there is an adverse reaction to Test 3, but not to Test 1: casein proteins are tolerated, but whey proteins are not.

Test 4: Test for casein proteins, whey proteins and **lactose**

Test food: Milk (Skim; OR 1%; OR 2%; OR homogenized milk).

	Adult	**Child**
Morning:	¼ cup	⅛ cup
Afternoon:	½ cup	¼ cup
Evening:	1 cup	½ cup

Interpretation of Results of Test 4

If there is no reaction after Day 2 (monitoring day), milk protein allergy and lactose intolerance have all been ruled out. If gastrointestinal symptoms occur after Test 4, but not after any of the previous tests for milk products, **lactose intolerance** is proven.

> Note: 1 cup of homogenized (3.3% M.F.) milk contains 12.0 grams of lactose.
> 1 cup of 2% milk contains 11.2 grams of lactose.
> 1 cup of 1% milk contains 10.8 grams of lactose.

A person who tolerates ¼ cup of milk will be able to tolerate lactose in food and beverages to a total of about 3 grams. If ½ cup of milk is tolerated, lactose to a level of 6 grams in food and beverages will be safe. If 1 cup of milk is tolerated, lactose to a level of 12 grams in food and beverages will be tolerated.

When a lactose intolerant person exceeds their limit of tolerance, gastrointestinal symptoms of gas, bloating, and sometimes abdominal pain and diarrhea will be experienced.

Test 5: Test for **modified milk components**

Test food: Plain yogurt

> Note: 1 cup of plain yogurt contains 8.4 grams of lactose, however, some lactose intolerant individuals can tolerate yogurt containing "live bacterial culture" since the yogurt bacteria *Lactobacillus bulgaricus* and *Streptococcus thermophilus* can survive for a short time in the bowel and produce enough beta-galactosidase enzyme to eliminate the symptoms of lactose intolerance.

	Adult	**Child**
Morning:	¼ cup	⅛ cup
Afternoon:	½ cup	¼ cup
Evening:	1 cup	½ cup

Test 6:   Test for **whey** in margarine

Test food: Any brand of margarine containing whey **but not** casein or milk solids (read labels).

Spread the following quantities on a rice cake, rice cracker, rye cracker, toast, oatcake, or any food that is tolerated.

	Adult	**Child**
Morning:	½ teaspoon	¼ teaspoon
Afternoon:	1 teaspoon	½ teaspoon
Evening:	2 teaspoons	1 teaspoon

Test 7: Test for **complete milk products and lactose**

Test food: Cottage cheese

Note: 1 cup of cottage cheese contains 7.2 grams of lactose.

	Adult	**Child**
Morning:	¼ cup	⅛ cup
Afternoon:	½ cup	¼ cup
Evening:	1 cup	½ cup

Test 8: Test for **complex milk product** with complete milk proteins and lactose

Test food: Ice cream

Start with pure ice cream, plain vanilla flavor. Test other flavors separately. In the manufacture of ice cream, vanilla is made first, then the lighter colored ice creams, usually ending with chocolate. If the vats are not cleaned adequately between different batches, residues from the previous batches may contaminate the later ones. Chocolate ice cream therefore is likely to contain the greatest number of potential allergens and should be tested only after all other flavors have been shown to be tolerated. This is an important consideration if a person is highly allergic to nuts, because the nut-flavored ice creams are usually made before the chocolate-flavored ones.

	Adult	**Child**
Morning:	¼ cup	⅛ cup
Afternoon:	½ cup	¼ cup
Evening:	1 cup	½ cup

Egg

Yolk and white are tested *separately*. Hard boil the egg and separate the yolk from the white.

Test 1: Egg Yolk

	Adult	**Child**
Morning:	½ yolk	½ teaspoon
Afternoon:	1 yolk	1 teaspoon
Evening:	2 yolks	2 teaspoons

Test 2: Egg White

Test exactly as described for egg yolk.

Interpretation of Results of Egg Challenge

If egg yolk, but not egg white, is tolerated (no adverse reaction to egg yolk), egg yolks separated from the white can be used in baking, making omelets, and other egg containing dishes, but cannot be used in dishes that require egg white only.

Egg Beaters® or other similar products which are made from egg white only (often advised in cholesterol lowering diets) cannot be used.

If the egg white (albumin), is tolerated but not egg yolk, egg whites separated from the yolk can be used in recipes. Egg Beaters®, and other products made from egg white only, can be used.

Yeast (Saccharomyces species: brewer's and baker's yeast)

Use debittered brewer's yeast (available from health food stores)

Morning:	Dissolve ¼ teaspoon or less in warm water. Add to any tolerated beverage such as fruit juice.
Afternoon:	Increase the quantity to ½ teaspoon or less in water and chosen beverage.
Evening:	Increase quantity to 1 teaspoon or less in water and chosen beverage.

Cereal Grains

Each cereal grain is tested in its pure form first, before being tested as an ingredient in baked goods such as breads and crackers. Most grains can be obtained as a "bulk food" so a small quantity suitable for the test can be purchased without incurring the expense of buying a packet of the product.

Wheat

Test 1:   Puffed wheat; or wheat flakes (cooked in water); or Cream of Wheat® (cooked in water).

Allowed fruit juice, Rice Dream® or soya beverage may be added if allowed during the elimination phase of the program.

	Adult	Child
Morning:	¼ cup	⅛ cup
Afternoon:	½ cup	¼ cup
Evening:	1 cup	½ cup

Test 2: Yeast-free wheat cracker or yeast-free soda bread

	Adult	**Child**
Morning:	2 crackers	1 cracker
Afternoon:	4 crackers	2 crackers
Evening:	8 crackers	4 crackers

Test 3: White bread

	Adult	**Child**
Morning:	½ slice	¼ slice
Afternoon:	1 slice	½ slice
Evening:	2 slices	1 slice

Test 4: Whole wheat bread

	Adult	**Child**
Morning:	½ slice	¼ slice
Afternoon:	1 slice	½ slice
Evening:	2 slices	1 slice

Other Grains

Test each grain in its purest form first, followed by baked goods (e.g. bread, crackers) as instructed for wheat challenge.

Oats:	(1) oatmeal (cooked natural oatmeal); (2) oat cake
Rye:	(1) rye flakes (cooked in water as porridge); (2) 100% rye cracker (e.g. RyVita® without wheat); (3) 100% rye bread
Quinoa:	(1) quinoa grain; (2) product made with quinoa flour such as bread or pasta
Buckwheat:	(1) buckwheat groats; (2) buckwheat pancake
Corn:	(1) corn on the cob (cooked) in the following amounts:

	Adult	**Child**
Morning:	¼ cob	⅛ cob
Afternoon:	½ cob	¼ cob
Evening:	1 cob	½ cob

OR	(2) corn niblets (cooked from a frozen package)	

	Adult	**Child**
Morning:	1 tablespoon	1 teaspoon
Afternoon:	2 tablespoons	2 teaspoons
Evening:	4 tablespoons	4 teaspoons

Soya

Test 1: Tofu

Use extra firm tofu, available in the produce department of the supermarket. Cut tofu into small cubes. Deep fry cubes in canola oil. Drain on a paper towel to absorb excess oil.

Morning:	1 cube
Afternoon:	2 cubes
Evening:	4 cubes

Test 2: Soya beverage (without milk ingredients)

	Adult	**Child**
Morning:	¼ cup	⅛ cup
Afternoon:	½ cup	¼ cup
Evening:	1 cup	½ cup

Fruits and Vegetables

Heat can change the allergenicity of some vegetables and fruits. The cooked form is usually less allergenic and thus better tolerated than the raw form. When testing vegetables and fruits, test the cooked form first and follow with the food in its raw state.

Vegetables

Cooking for 2-3 minutes in the microwave or cooking in water until vegetables are limp is often enough to change the structure of the molecules sufficiently for the food to be tolerated. Heat the food thoroughly as the raw uncooked center may cause an adverse reaction. Some people find that they need to cook the food more thoroughly before it is tolerated.

Fruits

The heat generated in the canning process is usually sufficient to change the allergenicity of a fruit. Alternatively, fruits can be poached by boiling them in a little water or cooked further. For example, cook apples into apple sauce without any added ingredient such as sugar.

Orange

Test 1: Canned mandarin orange

	Adult	**Child**
Morning:	2 sections	1 section
Afternoon:	4 sections	2 sections
Evening:	8 sections	4 sections

Alternatively, fresh orange sections can be cooked in the microwave oven or toasted under the grill in a conventional oven.

Test 2: Fresh mandarin orange

	Adult	**Child**
Morning:	2 sections	1 section
Afternoon:	4 sections	2 sections
Evening:	8 sections	4 sections

Test 3: Fresh navel orange

	Adult	**Child**
Morning:	2 sections	1 section
Afternoon:	4 sections	2 sections
Evening:	8 sections	4 sections

Grapefruit

Test cooked or canned first then test fresh grapefruit. Test as described for oranges above.

Grapes

Wash grapes well before testing, preferably with a detergent made for washing foods to remove surface molds. Sulfites used as a preservative will *not* be removed entirely by washing.

	Adult	**Child**
Morning:	2 grapes	1 grape
Afternoon:	4 grapes	2 grapes
Evening:	8 grapes	4 grapes

Tomato

Quantities depend on the size of the tomatoes used for the test. Eat without dressing.

Test 1: Canned or cooked tomato

Morning:	¼ tomato or 2 slices cooked
Afternoon:	½ tomato or 4 slices cooked
Evening:	1 tomato or 8 slices cooked

Test 2: Fresh tomato (raw)

Morning:	¼ tomato or 2 slices
Afternoon:	½ tomato or 4 slices
Evening:	1 tomato or 8 slices

Other Fruits and Vegetables

Test each separately as described above.

Juices

Fruit or vegetable juice can be heated in the microwave or brought to boiling on the stove and cooled before drinking.

Test cooked juice first before the fresh raw product.

Lemon or Lime

Squeeze juice from a fresh fruit into ½ glass of water. Add honey or sugar to taste.

	Adult	**Child**
Morning:	Juice from ¼ fruit	Juice from ⅛ fruit
Afternoon:	Juice from ½ fruit	Juice from ¼ fruit
Evening:	Juice from 1 fruit	Juice from ½ fruit

Other Fruit Juices (apple, orange, etc.)

	Adult	**Child**
Morning:	¼ cup	⅛ cup
Afternoon:	½ cup	¼ cup
Evening:	1 cup	½ cup

Chocolate

Pure Chocolate

Purchase dark, bitter, Baker's chocolate in blocks or chips. Melt in a pan over a low heat. Add honey (if tolerated), sugar (if tolerated) or powdered fruit sugar (fructose) to taste. Pour onto a cookie sheet or baking tray. Place in the fridge to solidify. Break into pieces about one inch square.

Eat one square in the morning, two in the afternoon, four in the evening. If any symptoms occur, stop eating chocolate and record your reactions.

Milk Chocolate (if milk is tolerated)

Melt Baker's chocolate as above. Add honey, fructose, or sugar as tolerated. Add powdered milk (1, 2, or 3 tablespoons depending on the amount of Baker's chocolate in the pan) and stir until mixture is smooth and well mixed. Pour onto a cookie sheet or baking tray and proceed as for Baker's chocolate above.

Purchased Chocolates

Start with preservative-free pure chocolates, without fruit, nuts, or other fillings before trying those with complex ingredients.

Sugars

If a person is allergic to sugar, it is the plant from which the sugar is derived that is the source of the foreign protein. In order to determine which sugar source causes the allergic symptoms, each is challenged separately. The same quantity of sugar is taken in each case. If desired, the sugar can be added to half a cup of warm water.

Morning:	1 teaspoon
Afternoon:	2 teaspoons
Evening:	4 teaspoons

Sugars to be challenged individually:

(1) Maple sugar or maple syrup
(2) Cane sugar
(3) Beet sugar
(4) Corn sugar or corn syrup
(5) Date sugar
(6) Fructose (fruit sugar; sometimes called levulose)
(7) Honey (glucose and fructose).

If a person is allergic to the pollen of the plant from which the honey is derived, eating the honey may cause symptoms, whereas honey from a different plant may be tolerated. For example, alfalfa honey may cause an allergic reaction when clover honey is tolerated.

Alcoholic Beverages

Test in the order specified:

(1)   Distilled alcohol (to test enhanced food allergen uptake)
      Use vodka OR white rum OR gin OR tequila
      Mix with boiled and cooled fruit juice to taste, if desired.
(2)   White wine (to test biogenic amines, particularly histamine)
(3)   Red wine (to test biogenic amines, particularly tyramine)
(4)   Lager, beer, ale (to test fermented grains)
(5)   Cider (to test fermented fruit, usually apple) In most cases similar biogenic amines as in wine are responsible for any adverse reactions.

Spices

Spices are tested by adding appropriate quantities to a tolerated food. Some suggestions for "carrier foods" are provided. If the suggested foods are not tolerated, substitute one that is.

Cinnamon (test for benzoates)

Carrier food: Homemade apple sauce sweetened with honey.
Ingredients: Fresh apple, peeled and sliced
                ¼ cup water
                Honey or other sweetener as tolerated, to taste

Place apples, water, and sweetener in a pan. Heat to boiling. Reduce heat and simmer for a few minutes until apple is soft. Add powdered (ground) spice to hot or cooled apple sauce, as preferred. If apples are not tolerated, substitute pears, or any tolerated fruit and cook as above.

Morning:	¼ teaspoon cinnamon
Afternoon:	½ teaspoon cinnamon
Evening:	1 teaspoon cinnamon

Other spices that are sometimes used in baked goods should be tested in the same way. Substitute the following ground spices separately in place of cinnamon in the above test: nutmeg, anise, allspice, caraway seed.

Curry Spice (mixture)

Carrier food: Cooked tomatoes
Ingredients: Fresh tomato, peeled and diced

Place tomato with any juice into a pan. Add a small amount of water to prevent burning. Bring to a boil, reduce heat and simmer until tomato is soft. Add spice to hot cooked tomato. If tomato is not tolerated, substitute mango or any other tolerated fruit or vegetable.

Morning:	¼ teaspoon spice
Afternoon:	½ teaspoon spice
Evening:	1 teaspoon spice

Individual Spices in Curry

If curry powder is not tolerated, each spice in the mixture can be tested separately. Prepare carrier food as above (tomato, mango, or tolerated fruit or vegetable). Add each of the powdered (ground) spices to be tested *individually*. Do not mix spices until it is known that each spice is tolerated. Test for turmeric, cumin, coriander, cayenne, ginger, clove, mace, and cardamom.

Chili Spice (mixture)

Test as described for curry spice mixture above.

If chili spice is not tolerated, test each spice separately, as described in individual spices in curry above. Test for cayenne, cumin, paprika, and onion powder.

Additives in Manufactured Foods

Testing for food additives is more difficult because in most cases it is not easy to obtain the additive in its pure form, or even to find it as a single additive in a manufactured food. This is because several different chemicals such as flavor and texture modifiers, color, preservatives etc. are usually added together.

Some research studies have attempted to test food additives. The chemicals were added in their pure form to an orange drink containing no additives in the following amounts:

Tartrazine	8.5 mg in 250 mL
Sunset yellow	8.5 mg in 250 mL
Sodium metabisulphite	12.5 mg in 250 mL
Sodium benzoate	55.0 mg in 250 mL

For home challenge tests, it is usually sufficient to test the foods containing additives as they would normally be eaten. Choose a food with a high level of the suspect additive and test that in comparison to a similar food without the additive.

Tartrazine

Kraft® Macaroni and Cheese dinner contains tartrazine. Test this in comparison to a similar homemade meal without tartrazine, using Cheddar cheese which has a similar appearance, but contains the natural yellow color annatto instead.

Benzoates

Cinnamon contains a high level of naturally occurring benzoates. Test apple sauce with cinnamon in the schedule outlined above under "spices". Compare to reactions after eating apple sauce without the spice.

Sulfites

Wine and regular beer contain sulfites. Test these in comparison to a wine or beer without the preservative.

Those beverages which have no added sulfites will usually be labeled "preservative free". In the U.S.A. alcoholic beverages which contain added sulfites will have "sulfite" on the label. Choose a beverage which does not have a reference to "sulfite" on the label.

Test regular (sulfited) dried fruit in comparison to non-sulfited dried fruit which can be obtained in some specialty health food stores.

Nitrates and Nitrites

Test additive-free beef in comparison to a beef steak to which nitrates have been added to preserve color. A butcher will know which meats have nitrates or nitrites added to preserve the red color of meats for display in the store under fluorescent lights.

Monosodium Glutamate (MSG)

MSG can be obtained as a flavor enhancer in some specialty stores. Test food with and without MSG to determine sensitivity. Test with a carrier food as tolerated: (minced chicken, turkey, beef; homemade sauces).

Add MSG powder in increasing doses as follows:

Morning:	¼ teaspoon
Afternoon:	½ teaspoon
Evening:	1 teaspoon

*Source of data: U.S. Department of Agriculture. USDA 8-1

Method: Challenge Test Check List

Instructions

1. Eat the test food in the quantities and frequency as detailed in the method for *Challenge Phase*, or as instructed by the supervisor of your test.

2. Record any reactions you experience in column two.

3. If you experience no reactions after the length of time specified on the Method Sheet or by the supervisor of your test, record a "Pass" and follow the instructions in that column.

4. If an adverse reaction has been recorded, record a "Fail" and follow the instructions in that column.

5. Proceed *exactly as instructed,* and in the *specified sequence* for each selected food category. However, you can test the **food category** (dairy products, grains, fruits) in any order you wish.

6. **For adults:**   Do not add any food back into your diet until *all the eliminated foods have been tested.*

    For infants: Include each tolerated food in the diet as testing proceeds.

7. When introducing foods for the first time to an allergic infant, apply some of the test food to the cheek. Wait twenty minutes and look for reddening at the test site. If a red weal appears at the test site, *do not give any of that food by mouth.* If there is no local reaction on the cheek, apply a little of the food to the outer lip, and again wait for a local reaction. If no reaction occurs on the lip, a small quantity can be given by mouth as instructed.

Challenge Test Checklist

Test Food	Reaction	Pass	Fail
DAIRY PRODUCTS			
1. Casein White hard cheese, e.g. Mozzarella Parmesan Swiss		---------------- Not allergic to casein proteins ---------------- Proceed	---------------- Allergic to casein proteins ---------------- **PROCEED TO TEST 6**
Casein **2. Biogenic amines** **2. Annatto** Orange/yellow aged cheese e.g. Old Cheddar		---------------- Not sensitive to annatto or biogenic amines ---------------- Proceed	---------------- Sensitive to biogenic amines or annatto ---------------- Proceed
Casein **3. Whey** Lactaid® milk (99% lactose free)		---------------- Not allergic to whey or casein proteins: Not allergic to cow's milk protein ---------------- Proceed	---------------- Allergic to whey proteins, but not allergic to casein proteins ---------------- **STOP HERE**
4. Lactose Milk: Homogenized, 2%; 1%, or skim		---------------- Not lactose intolerant Not allergic to cow's milk ---------------- Proceed	---------------- Lactose intolerant Not allergic to cow's milk proteins ---------------- Proceed
5. Modified milk proteins; **partially digested lactose** Yogurt (plain only)		---------------- Not allergic to milk ---------------- Proceed	---------------- Not allergic to milk; lactose intolerance confirmed ---------------- **STOP HERE**

Challenge Test Checklist

Test Food	Reaction	Pass	Fail
6. Whey (without casein) Test only if Test 1 for casein proteins is positive (Failed Test 1) Margarine (containing whey but free from casein and milk solids) Note: May contain a small amount of lactose		--------------- Not allergic to whey proteins --------------- **STOP HERE**	--------------- Allergic to whey proteins --------------- **STOP HERE**
7. Complete milk proteins and lactose Cottage cheese		--------------- Confirmed not allergic to milk; not lactose intolerant --------------- Proceed	--------------- Suspect milk intolerance <u>or</u> lactose intolerance. --------------- **REPEAT TESTS:** (1) lactose intolerance (2) milk allergy
8. Complex milk product with complete milk proteins and lactose Ice cream		--------------- Not allergic to milk; Not lactose intolerant; Not sensitive to food additives; Not sucrose intolerant	--------------- **SUSPECT**: (1) Sucrose intolerance (2) Sensitivity to food additives
EGG			
1. Egg yolk		--------------- Not allergic to egg yolk proteins --------------- Proceed	--------------- Allergic to egg yolk proteins --------------- Proceed

Challenge Test Checklist

Test Food	Reaction	Pass	Fail
2. Egg white		------------- Not allergic to egg white ------------- If a "pass" has been recorded for egg yolk: not allergic to eggs	------------- Allergic to egg white protein ------------- If a "fail" has been recorded for egg yolk also: Allergic to eggs
YEAST			
Yeast *Saccharomyces* (debittered brewer's yeast)			
GRAINS			
Wheat			
Single grain product Cream of Wheat® Puffed wheat Wheat flakes (cooked)		------------- Not allergic to wheat ------------- Proceed	------------- Allergic to wheat ------------- **STOP HERE**
Grain in a yeast-free baked product Graham cracker Wheat-free soda bread Wheat-free flat bread		------------- Not allergic to wheat Not allergic to other ingredients in the product Check label if using a manufactured food ------------- Proceed	------------- Allergic to an ingredient in the product other than wheat Check label if using a manufactured food to identify possible allergens or additives ------------- **STOP HERE**

Challenge Test Checklist

Test Food	Reaction	Pass	Fail
Partial grain in a baked product with yeast White bread		--------------- Not allergic to yeast (*Saccharomyces*) --------------- Proceed	--------------- May be allergic to yeast Carry out the challenge of *Saccharomyces* separately as instructed --------------- **STOP HERE**
Whole grain in a baked product with yeast Whole wheat bread		--------------- Not allergic to wheat Not allergic to yeast ---------------	--------------- Possibly allergic to proteins in wheat bran ---------------
Rye			
Single grain Rye flakes (cooked)		--------------- Not allergic to rye --------------- Proceed	--------------- Allergic to rye --------------- **STOP HERE**

Whole grain in a yeast-free baked product
100% rye cracker:
  RyVita®
  Wasa®
		----------- 	
		Not allergic to rye
		Not allergic to other ingredients in food (read product label)
		-------- 	
		
		Proceed
			--------------- 	
			Possibly allergic to an ingredient in cracker
			Read product label carefully to identify possible allergens or additives
			--------------- 	
			STOP HERE

Whole grain in a baked product with yeast 100% rye bread		--------------- Not allergic to rye Not allergic to yeast ---------------	--------------- Possibly allergic to yeast ---------------

Challenge Test Checklist

Test Food	Reaction	Pass	Fail
Other Grains			

Proceed as instructed for wheat:
Single grain
For example:
   White rice
   Brown rice
   Oatmeal
   Niblets corn
   Millet grain
   Buckwheat groats
   Quinoa grain
   Amaranth grain
   Other			

Single grain in a yeast-free baked product
For example:
   Brown rice cracker
   Scottish oat cake
   Popcorn
   Other			

Single grain in a baked product with yeast
For example:
   Rice bread
   Oat bread
   Corn bread
   Other			

FRUIT			
Orange			
Juice; heated Heat to boiling and cool Heat in microwave and cool Pasteurized juice			
Juice; raw Fresh squeezed Reconstituted from frozen			

Challenge Test Checklist

Test Food	Reaction	Pass	Fail
Canned mandarin orange **Cooked mandarin orange** Segments heated in the microwave or toasted under a grill until thoroughly cooked			
Fresh mandarin orange			
Cooked navel orange Segments heated in microwave or toasted under a grill until thoroughly cooked			
Fresh navel orange			
Apple			
Juice; heated Cooked (heat in microwave or bring to boiling) and cool			
Juice Reconstituted from frozen Fresh pressed			
Cooked apple Apple sauce Baked apple			
Fresh apple Golden Delicious			
Fresh apple Other varieties			

Challenge Test Checklist

Test Food	Reaction	Pass	Fail

Proceed as above with any other fruit
For example:
    Banana
    Pear
    Peach
    Apricot
    Nectarine
    Kiwi
    Pineapple			

VEGETABLES			
Tomato*			
Cooked tomato **Canned tomato**			
Raw tomato			

Proceed as above with any other vegetable
For example:
    Spinach
    Celery
    Carrot
    Green pea
    Avocado
    Green bean			

Cooked or canned in water or vegetable juice			
Raw			
SPICES			
Cinnamon			
Nutmeg			
Anise			
Curry spice mixture			
Chili spice mixture			
Other			

Challenge Test Checklist

Test Food	Reaction	Pass	Fail
SOYA			
Tofu Cooked cubes			
Soya beverage			
Soya sauce without wheat (Tamari®)			
Soya sauce with wheat			
CHOCOLATE			
Dark Baker's chocolate Sweetened with honey or sugar			
Dark Baker's chocolate With milk powder and sweetener			
Purchased chocolates Without preservatives or fillers			
ALCOHOL			

Distilled alcohol
  (uncolored)
  Vodka
  Gin
  White rum
  Tequila			

White (grape) wine			
Red (grape) wine			
Beer, ale, or lager (Fermented grain)			
Cider (Fermented apple)			
ADDITIVES			
Tartrazine			
Benzoates			

Challenge Test Checklist

Test Food	Reaction	Pass	Fail
Sulfites			
Nitrates / nitrites			
MSG			
OTHER FOODS			

*The author acknowledges that tomatoes are classified as fruits; however, the author has chosen to place tomato in the vegetable category in this book as most people associate tomatoes with vegetables.

8

Rotation Diets

A number of published articles and books indicate that people who are mildly intolerant to foods may benefit from a diet that spaces the antagonistic foods, so that no one food is eaten too frequently. Theoretically, if the foods that cause a reaction are not allowed to "build up" in the body, a person's "limit of tolerance" is not exceeded and symptoms either do not occur or are kept to a minimum.

Four day,[1] five day,[2] seven day,[3] and even thirty-one day rotations[4] have been advised. Since two to four days is the approximate gastrointestinal transit time, a four day rotation is considered to be the most effective schedule. After four days, the amount of a specific food in the body is considered to be sufficiently low so that eating it again will not increase the level to a reactive threshold.[1]

There have been no well designed, controlled studies to prove whether rotation diets are of any real value. Rotation diets as a management strategy for food allergy and intolerance are considered by most authorities to be controversial and of little or no benefit.[5,6] Furthermore, following a strict rotation diet can be very tedious, time consuming, and can pose nutritional risks unless the foods are balanced very carefully and appropriate substitutes are included.

Since some practitioners and their patients request a trial on a rotation diet, a sample four day rotation diet is included here. This diet should prove nutritionally sound and provide enough variety to be acceptable when the appropriate adjustments are made for individual intolerances.

References

1.   Butkus, G., Davis, J., and Martin, S. Food Intolerances. In: *Applied Nutrition and Diet Therapy*. W.B. Saunders, Philadelphia, London, Toronto, 1988. 686-691.

2.   Mandell, E. *Dr. Mandell's Five-Day Allergy Relief System*. Pocket Books, New York, 1979.

3.   Rowe, A.H., and Rowe, A. *Food Allergy in its Manifestations and Control and the Elimination Diets*. Charles C. Thomas, Springfield, 1972.

4.   Monro, J. Food families and rotation diets. In: Brostoff, J., and Challacombe, S.J. (Eds), *Food Allergy and Intolerance*. Baillière Tindall, London, 1987. 303-343.

5.   David, T.J. Elimination diets. In: *Food and Food Additive Intolerance in Childhood*. Blackwell Scientific Publications, Oxford, London, 1993. 441-463.

6.   Olejer, V.L. Food hypersensitivity. In: Queen, P.M., and Lang, C.E. (Eds), *Handbook of Pediatric Nutrition*. Aspen Publications, Gaithersburg, MD, 1993. 206-231.

Method: Use of The Rotation Diet Table

Instructions

1. Cross out all the foods to which you react adversely.

2. With the foods that are left, construct your own personal rotation schedule. Make sure there are at lease two foods each day in each food category (except for seeds and sweeteners). Move foods from one day to another to achieve this.

3. If you do not have sufficient tolerated foods to make a four day rotation for every food category, use a two day rotation for the food groups that are limited. Do not eat any one food every day.

4. Milk and milk products have not been included in this rotation, because a person either tolerates them or is allergic to them. If you are allergic to milk and milk products, you must eliminate all these products from the Rotation Diet. If you tolerate milk, any milk and milk products can be eaten every day without fear of causing an adverse reaction. This will make any rotation diet more nutritionally complete.

5. Make sure that the foods you eat every day follow the Canada Food Guide as closely as possible. Ensure that you have adequate daily servings of grains, meat and alternates, fruits, vegetables, and dairy products (if you tolerate dairy products).

6. Try to avoid eating foods on the same day that cross-react antigenically. If you cannot avoid eating cross-reacting foods on the same day, try to avoid eating them at the same meal. The most important foods which cross-react are:

   Group 1: Apple, hazelnut, potato, rye, carrot, celery
   Group 2: Hazelnut, rye, sesame seed, kiwi, poppy seed
   Group 3: Melon, banana
   Group 4: Banana, avocado, kiwi fruit, chestnut, soy bean, peanut (these foods cross react with latex)

Recipes and Meal Planning

When planning meals, assemble recipes that include the allowed foods for each day of the rotation.

The Rotation Diet Table has been constructed so that a few favorite recipes can be accommodated. For example:

Pasta Sauce without Meat and Tomato (Day 1):

Sauté the following in olive oil and clarified butter: 4-5 chopped green onions, 10-12 black olives, chopped cucumber, herbs, salt and pepper to taste. Add 1-2 cans of water packed tuna. Sprinkle with blanched chopped almonds.

Hummus (Day 2):

Cooked or canned chickpeas (garbanzo beans), sesame tahini, garlic, lemon juice, herbs. Blend until smooth.

Avocado Dip (Day 3):

Mashed avocado, grated onion, pureed or chopped tomato, olive oil.

Bread and Pastry Mixes (Day 3):

Good 'n Easy®, tapioca flour, soy flour, cream of tartar.

Ham & Lentil Soup (Day 4)

Rice-stuffed Cabbage Rolls (Day 4)

Sample Four Day Rotation Diet

Food Category	Day 1	Day 2	Day 3	Day 4
Grains	Wheat Arrowroot Buckwheat	Oats Amaranth Corn	Rye Millet Tapioca	Barley Quinoa Rice

Vegetables	Roots:
	  Turnip
	  Rutabaga
	  Potato
	  Carrot
	  Parsnip
	  Radish
	  Beets
	Cucumber
	Asparagus
	Olives
	Green onion
		Green leafy:
		  Spinach
		  Chard
		  Kale
		  Lettuce
		Green and red
		peppers
		Squashes (all
		  types)
		Mushroom
		Corn
		Garlic
			Legume:
			  Green pea
			  Green bean
			  Yellow bean
			  Lima bean
			  Fava bean
			Tomato
			Sweet potato
			Bean sprouts
			Onion
			Avocado
			Eggplant
			(aubergine)
				Brassicas:
				  Cabbage
				  Broccoli
				  Cauliflower
				  Brussels
				  sprouts
				Chinese
				  cabbages
				Yam
				Alfalfa sprouts
				Celery

Fruits	Apricot Peach Nectarine Plum Prune Rhubarb Grape Raisin	Orange Grapefruit Lemon Lime Papaya (pawpaw) Fig Date Banana	Apple Pear Mango Star fruit Berries Cherry Currants	Watermelon Cantaloupe Other melons Pineapple Fig Passion fruit Kiwi fruit
Meat and Poultry	Chicken Egg Quail Moose	Beef Veal Lamb Goat	Turkey Goose Duck Venison	Pork Ham Bacon Rabbit
Fish	Tuna Trout Pike	Snapper Halibut Perch	Salmon Mackerel Orange roughy	Cod Sole Turbot
Seeds	Sunflower	Sesame Caraway	Pumpkin Poppy	Flax Anise
Legumes Dried peas and beans	Peanut Kidney bean	Chickpea Pinto bean	Soy Mung bean Carob	Lentils Navy bean
Sweeteners	Beet sugar	Honey	Cane sugar	Maple sugar
Nuts	Brazil nut Almond	Cashew Macadamia	Walnut Pecan Coconut	Hazelnut Pistachio

Part III

Specific Food Restrictions

9

Important Nutrients in Common Allergens

Table 9-1 and Table 9-2 Summary list the major micronutrients that are excluded when the most allergenic foods are eliminated from the diet. Suggestions are provided in Table 9-3 for alternative food sources of each of the excluded micronutrients.

These tables are provided so that any elimination diet that excludes these important nutrient sources can be designed so that complete nutrition can be provided from nutritionally equivalent food sources.

Table 9-1: Important Nutrients in Common Allergens

Milk and Dairy Products	Calcium
	Phosphorus
	Pantothenic
	  acid
	Potassium
		Vitamin D*
		Vitamin B12
		Riboflavin
			Smaller amounts:
			  Vitamin A*
			  Vitamin E

Egg	Vitamin D*
	Vitamin B12
	Pantothenic
	  acid
	Selenium
		Folacin
		Riboflavin
		Biotin
		Iron
			Smaller amounts:
			  Vitamin A
			  Vitamin E
			  Vitamin B6
			  Zinc

Peanuts	Niacin
	Vitamin E
	Manganese
	Chromium
	Pantothenic acid
	Magnesium
			Smaller amounts:
			  Potassium
			  Vitamin B6
			  Folacin
			  Phosphorus
			  Copper
			  Biotin

Soybean	Thiamin Riboflavin Vitamin B6 Phosphorus Magnesium	Iron Folacin Calcium Zinc	

Fish and Shellfish	Niacin
	Vitamin B6
	Vitamin B12
	Vitamin E
	Phosphorus
	Selenium
	Calcium (in shellfish and fish bones)
			Smaller amounts:
			  Vitamin A
			  Potassium
			  Magnesium
			  Iron
			  Zinc

Wheat	Thiamin*
	Riboflavin*
	Niacin*
	Iron*
	Selenium
		Chromium	Smaller amounts:
			  Magnesium
			  Folacin
			  Phosphorus
			  Molybdenum

Rice	Thiamin* Riboflavin*	Niacin* Iron*	
Corn	Thiamin* Riboflavin* Niacin*	Iron* Chromium	

* Usually added as fortification to the food product

Table 9-2 Summary: Important Nutrients in Common Allergens

	Milk	Egg	Peanut	Soy	Fish	Wheat	Rice	Corn
Vitamins								
A	✓	✓			✓			
B6		✓	✓	✓	✓			
B12	✓	✓			✓			
D	✓	✓						
E	✓	✓	✓		✓			
Biotin		✓	✓					
Pantothenic acid	✓	✓	✓					
Folacin		✓	✓	✓		✓		
Riboflavin (B2)	✓	✓		✓		✓	✓	✓
Niacin			✓		✓	✓	✓	✓
Thiamin (B1)				✓		✓	✓	✓
Minerals								
Calcium	✓			✓	✓			
Phosphorus	✓		✓	✓	✓	✓		
Iron		✓		✓	✓	✓	✓	✓
Zinc		✓		✓	✓			
Magnesium			✓	✓	✓	✓		
Selenium		✓			✓	✓		
Potassium	✓		✓		✓			
Molybdenum						✓		
Chromium			✓			✓		✓
Copper			✓					
Manganese			✓					

Table 9-3: Alternative Sources of Nutrients

NUTRIENT	ALTERNATIVE SOURCES
Vitamins	
A	Liver, fish liver oils, dark green and yellow vegetables, tomato, apricots, cantaloupe (rock melon), mango, papaya (pawpaw)
D	Liver, fish liver oils, action of sunlight on skin
E (alpha tocopherol)	Liver, legumes, green leafy vegetables, tomato, whole grains, vegetable oils
B1 (thiamin)	Meats, especially pork; dried and green peas, legumes, whole grains, nutritional yeast
B2 (riboflavin)	Organ meats, legumes, green vegetables, whole grains, nutritional yeast
B3 (niacin)	Organ meats, poultry, beef, legumes, whole grains, nutritional yeast
B6 (pyridoxine)	Meats, especially organ meats; legumes, whole grains, green vegetables, carrots, potato, cauliflower, banana, prunes, avocado, sunflower seeds, nutritional yeast
B12 (cobalamin)	Meats, especially organ meats
Biotin	Organ meats, nutritional yeast, mushrooms, banana, grapefruit, watermelon, strawberries
Pantothenic acid	Organ meats, chicken, beef, fresh vegetables, whole grains, nutritional yeast
Folacin	Organ meats, legumes, green leafy vegetables, asparagus, beets, broccoli, avocado, oranges, banana, strawberries, whole grains, nutritional yeast
Minerals	
Calcium	Amaranth, baked beans, rhubarb, green leafy vegetables, broccoli, dates, molasses
Phosphorus	Meats, poultry, legumes, whole grains, seeds, green peas, artichokes, potato, Brussels sprouts
Iron	Meats, liver, legumes, raisins, dried apricots, prunes, pumpkin, asparagus, broccoli, chard, green peas, spinach, molasses
Zinc	Meat, liver, green leafy vegetables, beets, green peas, oranges, strawberries, prunes, chocolate syrup
Magnesium	Legumes, whole grains, meat, poultry, dark green vegetables
Selenium	Whole grains, meat, broccoli, onions, tomato
Potassium	Meats, oranges, banana, dried fruits, cantaloupe (rock melon), honeydew melon, nectarine, papaya (pawpaw), tomato, avocado, dark greens, sweet potato, winter squash, potato, molasses
Molybdenum	Meat, legumes, whole grains, green vegetables (especially spinach), lettuce, Brussels sprouts, carrots, squash, tomatoes, apple juice
Chromium	Vegetable oils, meats, liver, nutritional yeast, whole grains
Copper	Liver, meat, whole grains, green leafy vegetables, broccoli, potato, pears, banana, apple juice
Manganese	Sunflower seeds, whole grains, legumes, nutritional yeast, green beans, broccoli, cranberries, grapes, pineapple

References

Lurie, D.G., Holden, J.M., Schubert, A., Wolf, W.R., and Miller-Ihli, N.J. The copper content on foods based on a critical evaluation of published analytical data. J. Food Comp. Anal. 1989 2(4):298.

Levels of trace elements in food commodity groups. J. Am. Diet. Assoc. 1987 87(12):1646.

Concentration of boron, calcium, copper, iron, magnesium, manganese, molybdenum and zinc in various foods. J. Am. Diet. Assoc. 1991 91(5):560-561.

Krause, M.V., and Mahan, L.K. *Food, Nutrition and Diet Therapy.* W.B. Saunders, Philadelphia, 1984.

Nutrient Values of Some Common Foods. Health and Welfare Canada. Revised 1988.

Burtis, G., Davis, J., and Martin, S. *Applied Nutrition and Diet Therapy.* W.B. Saunders, Philadelphia, 1988.

Koerner, C.B. and Sampson, H.A. Diets and Nutrition. In: Metcalfe, D.D., Sampson, H.A. and Simon, R.A. (Eds), *Food Allergy: Adverse Reactions to Foods and Food Additives.* Blackwell Scientific Publications, Oxford, London, 1991. 332-354.

Nutritionist III and Nutritionist IV Software. N-Squared Computing, Salem, OR. Source: US Department of Agriculture data files.

Action Towards Healthy Eating: Canada's Guidelines for Healthy Eating and Recommended Strategies for Implementation. Supply and Services Canada, Ottawa, 1990.

10

Milk Allergy and Lactose Intolerance

An adverse reaction to milk and dairy products is not uncommon and results in a variety of symptoms.[1] The most frequent reactions are skin rashes[1,2] and gastrointestinal symptoms such as abdominal bloating, pain, gas, diarrhea, and nausea.[1,2,3] Occasionally, upper respiratory tract symptoms and asthma may be caused or exacerbated when milk or dairy products are ingested.[2]

Occult blood loss associated with cow's milk allergy can be a cause of iron deficiency anaemia in children.[3] Another effect of cow's milk that is currently being investigated in children is an inability to fall asleep and restless, disturbed sleep.[4,5] In an infant, failure to thrive may be a result of manifestations of milk allergy causing intestinal inflammation and malabsorption of nutrients.[1,2,6]

The diagnosis of milk allergy is not a simple matter.[7] Often, any adverse reaction experienced after drinking milk is ascribed to "milk allergy." However, when the symptoms are localized in the gastrointestinal tract, the problem may be lactose intolerance, not milk allergy.[1,8]

Causes of Milk Allergy and Lactose Intolerance

Milk allergy is caused by an immune reaction to milk proteins. More than 30 milk proteins are identifiable, (see *Table 10-1: Levels of Individual Proteins in Cow's Milk*, page 80). Any number of these may trigger an immune response.[9]

Lactose intolerance is due to an inability to produce sufficient lactase, or beta-galactosidase, the enzyme which splits lactose into its constituent monosaccharides, glucose and galactose.

Milk Allergy

Biological Mechanisms

Milk allergy results when the immune system produces antibodies against milk allergens. The allergenicity of individual milk proteins has been studied using skin tests and oral challenges.[1] Although casein proteins produced the highest number of positive skin tests in children with milk allergy, beta-lactoglobulin produced the highest number of positive oral challenges.[10] Most milk allergic persons, whether children or adults, react to more than one milk protein.[2]

The heat stability of individual milk proteins varies. Serum proteins and beta-casein are the most heat labile, whereas beta-lactoglobulin and alpha-lactalbumin are the most heat stable.[2]

Antibodies produced against milk proteins may be IgE, IgM, IgG, or sometimes IgA.[11] Complexing of the milk protein antigen with its homologous antibody leads to the release of inflammatory mediators which act directly to cause tissue inflammation in the digestive tract, the skin, or the respiratory tract. Symptoms typical of allergy result. Milk allergy is much more common in infants and young children than in adults.[1,6]

Table 10-1: Levels of Individual Proteins in Cow's Milk[9]

Protein	Level (g/liter)
Caseins	24 - 28
Alpha-caseins	15 - 19
Alphas1	12 - 15
Alphas2	3 - 4
Beta-caseins	9 - 11
Kappa-caseins	3 - 4
Gamma-caseins	1 - 2
Whey proteins	5 - 7
Beta-lactoglobulin	2 - 4
Alpha-lactoglobulin	1 - 1.5
Proteose peptones	0.6 - 1.8
Serum proteins	
Albumin	0.1 - 0.4
Immunoglobulins	0.6 - 1.0

Table 10-1: Levels of Individual Proteins in Cow's Milk[9]

Protein	Level (g/liter)
Other Proteins[4] Present in Small Quantities	
Lactoferrin	
Lactoperoxidase	
Alkaline Phosphatase	
Catalase	

Management of Milk Allergy

Milk allergy is treated by the dietary elimination of milk, foods containing milk, and products made from milk. Liquid and evaporated milks, fermented milks (yogurt, buttermilk), cream, all cheeses (hard cheeses, cottage cheese, cream cheese), ice cream, and ice milk are excluded from this diet. Also excluded are foods containing milk solids, such as butter and margarine containing whey, and foods containing individual components of milk such as casein, whey, lactoglobulin, or hydrolysates of these proteins.

Nutritional Substitutes

Milk provides protein, calcium, and Vitamin D (added after pasteurization), all of which are obtainable from sources other than milk products.[6] Protein is readily available from meat, fish, or combinations of legumes, nuts, grains, and vegetables. Obtaining adequate dietary protein does not depend on ingesting milk.

The situation with calcium is different, however, as milk is the most abundant and readily available source of calcium in the North American diet, with 250 mL (one cup) providing 290 mg of calcium. Alternative sources of dietary calcium include the following:

- Canned fish such as sardines, tuna, and salmon, eaten with the bones (the calcium is in the bones; the canning process softens them, making them more easily digested)
- Green leafy vegetables such as arugula, kale, beet and turnip greens, collards, mustard greens, and broccoli; however, the calcium in vegetables is not as readily available as from animal sources
- Some nuts and legumes that contain moderate levels of calcium.

Refer to the method for *Non-dairy Sources of Calcium*, page 102.

When all milk and dairy products are removed from the diet, it can be difficult to obtain sufficient calcium from these alternative sources on a regular basis. A supplement is then necessary. Calcium gluconate and calcium citrate malate are the most well absorbed and well utilized forms of calcium,[12] and thus are superior to calcium carbonate as a source of the mineral.[13] The use of an antacid containing calcium (e.g., Tums®) is not recommended, because it neutralizes the gastric acid needed for protein digestion. In addition, the antacid produces an alkaline environment that may reduce the uptake of minerals such as iron, zinc, and copper, and of calcium itself, all of which require an acidic medium for efficient absorption.

Heating or boiling milk will not make it non-allergenic, although many of the proteins may be denatured, reducing their allergenicity somewhat. Milk as an ingredient in cooked products is sometimes tolerated, even though unheated milk is not.   Some milk-allergic persons can tolerate canned milk (e.g., evaporated milk) that has been extensively heated. However, some allergenic milk proteins are heat stable and may cause a reaction even after cooking.

Similarly, cow's milk in infant formulas remains allergenic and induces an allergic reaction in milk allergic infants. Only formulas such as Alimentum®, Nutramigen®, and Pregestimil®, which contain extensively hydrolyzed casein (i.e., broken down into small peptides and individual amino acids) are usually tolerated by the milk-allergic infant.

Soy based formulas may be tolerated by milk-allergic infants. Approximately 50% of infants with milk allergy seem to also develop an allergy to soy, thus requiring casein hydrolysate formulas (see *Composition of Infant Formulae*, page 264).

Substitutes in Meals and Recipes

Most milk substitutes are not nutritionally equivalent to milk, but substitute for milk in appearance, flavor, and texture. Because some of these products contain potentially allergenic ingredients such as soy or nuts, they should not be used without first establishing that the milk allergic person is not allergic to these alternatives.

Soy Milk

Soy milk is an acceptable substitute for milk on breakfast cereals and in many recipes. Some highly allergic individuals may not tolerate soybeans or soy products. Soy products and soybeans should be introduced with caution.

Most liquid soy milk sold today can be substituted directly for milk without dilution. If the taste of soy milk is unpalatable, the addition of lime juice may make it more acceptable.

Mocha Mix®

Some consumers find this non-dairy soy product superior in taste to other milk substitutes.

Rice Dream®

This milk substitute is made from brown rice and safflower oil, and makes an acceptable alternative to milk on cereals and in baking.

Meat stock, vegetable bouillon, fruit juice, vegetable oil mixed with water, or water may be added to recipes when only a small amount of milk is needed. When making puddings from rice, tapioca, or semolina, fruit juice can be used instead of milk. Potato water can be used instead of milk in making breads.

Coconut Milk

Coconut milk can be substituted in some recipes in the same quantity as milk.

Nut Milks

Nut milks are made by combining ground nuts or coconut with water (250 mL nut meal plus 500 mL water) and mixing in a blender until smooth. Nut milks may be used in recipes in the same quantity as milk.

Whey-free Margarine

Also called milk-free margarine, these products have no added milk solids and may be used instead of butter.

Non-dairy Creamers

Made of vegetable oil, these products (e.g., Coffee Rich®) can be used in tea and coffee.

Non-dairy Toppings

Vegetable oil product toppings can be used instead of whipped cream in desserts.

Soy Bean Curd or Cake (Tofu)

Tofu can be substituted for cheese in many recipes. Fresh soybean curd may be substituted for cottage cheese. Care must be taken as some products (e.g., "tofu cheese") contain milk solids.

Lactose Intolerance

Lactose intolerance does not involve a response by the immune system and no antibodies are produced. In this condition, the enzyme *lactase* is insufficient to break down the quantity of lactose consumed at any one time.[14] Lactase is produced by the brush border cells of the small intestine. When these cells are damaged, for example, as a result of inflammation (in gastrointestinal infections, or food allergy), or as a congenital characteristic, the sugar remains undigested in the intestine. Microbial enzymes metabolize lactose, resulting in a variety of organic acids (e.g., lactic and propionic acids) and gases such as hydrogen. Because an osmotic imbalance results from the excess sugar and excess acid, water is drawn into the digestive tract to correct the problem, which results in diarrhea. The symptoms of pain, bloating, and gas are due to bacterial fermentation of lactose.

results in diarrhea. The symptoms of pain, bloating, and gas are due to bacterial fermentation of lactose.

Incidence of Lactase Deficiency

A number of ethnic groups such as the Asian and black African races, and people of the Mediterranean region, lose the ability to produce lactase, starting at about five years of age. Lactose intolerance among these groups may be as high as 80% of the population. In contrast, only about 20% of people of northern European origin lose the ability to produce lactase.[8,14]

Lactase deficiency is uncommon in infants, because lactose is the principal sugar in human milk and infants require lactase to digest their mother's milk. However, a secondary lactase deficiency can develop in an infant following a bacterial or viral infection of the digestive tract. Inflammation damages the brush border cells in the lining of the small intestine which produce the enzyme. The infant is unable to tolerate lactose until the infection subsides and the intestinal mucosa recovers.

Distinguishing Between Milk Allergy and Lactose Intolerance

It is frequently difficult to distinguish milk allergy from lactose intolerance on the basis of clinical symptoms alone,[8] because some of the symptoms, such as abdominal pain, diarrhea, vomiting, gas and bloating, are common to both conditions. However, milk allergy will sometimes cause symptoms in the upper respiratory tract (e.g., a stuffy, runny nose, or pain, itching, and serous drainage from the ears) or skin reactions (e.g., eczema or hives) that are not seen with lactose intolerance.

Since secondary lactase deficiency is a consequence of inflammation in the digestive tract, the intestinal inflammation caused by milk allergy sometimes results in lactase deficiency. Thus, both milk allergy and lactose intolerance can exist concomitantly. Because milk is the only source of lactose in the normal diet, eliminating milk from the diet cures both conditions, without identifying the cause of the symptoms.

Despite these difficulties, it is important to determine which of these conditions is causing the problem, because milk and dairy products are a significant source of nutrients, especially for infants and young children, and should not be eliminated unless absolutely necessary. Furthermore, it is not easy to completely eliminate milk from the diet, because it is contained in many different foods (e.g., baked goods, soups, salad dressings, gravies, desserts) and avoiding these foods can make meal planning very challenging.

Diagnosis

Allergy tests such as skin tests, and blood tests such as RAST, are not reliable methods for diagnosing milk allergy. The most reliable method is to remove all milk and dairy products from the diet for two or three weeks to see if symptoms subside. If the symptoms disappear, appropriate challenge tests are used to determine the source of the symptoms, (see the methods for *Challenge Phase,* page 41, and *Sequence of Testing Foods,* page 43).

Laboratory Tests for Lactose Intolerance

There are a number of tests to diagnose lactose intolerance[14].

The Fecal Reducing Substance Test is perhaps the most reliable. This test detects the presence of a reducing substance in feces when lactose has not been broken down by lactase.

The Hydrogen Breath Test[14] is a more common test for lactose intolerance. In this test, the patient ingests a quantity of lactose and, after a prescribed interval, a breath sample is analyzed for the presence of hydrogen. If hydrogen is detected, it indicates that bacteria in the digestive tract have acted on undigested lactose and produced hydrogen as one of their metabolic byproducts. Unfortunately, this test is not specific for lactase deficiency, because any sugar remaining in the digestive tract will be metabolized by bacteria, resulting in production of hydrogen. Undigested sucrose, maltose, or a starch will give a similar result.

The level of glucose in the blood after consuming a lactose-containing drink is sometimes used as a test for possible lactase deficiency. An increase in blood glucose indicates that lactose has been broken down into glucose and galactose, the levels of which rise in the blood when the body is producing an adequate amount of lactase.

However, because it is often possible to assume lactose intolerance if a person remains free from symptoms after consuming milk treated with a commercial lactase enzyme (e.g., Lactaid®), but suffers gastrointestinal symptoms after drinking milk containing a normal level of lactose, these tests are not usually considered necessary.

Treatment

As outlined earlier, the only treatment for milk allergy is the complete dietary exclusion of cow's milk. Some people find they can tolerate milk from other animals, such as goats, but 70 to 80% of people allergic to cow's milk are also allergic to goat's milk proteins. A milk substitute is usually necessary.[15]

Lactase deficiency is easier to manage than milk allergy, because the lactose in milk can be broken down by adding a commercial form of lactase (sold as Lactaid®) to the milk before consumption. Lactase splits lactose into its two component sugars - glucose and galactose - which the body can absorb and use without harm (except in the very rare disorder galactosaemia, apparent in early infancy, in which the individual cannot metabolize galactose). It is difficult to avoid lactose in prepared foods, however, because anything containing milk or milk solids is likely also to contain lactose. Some people find that they can eat lactose containing foods with ease if they take Lactaid® tablets before eating.

When lactose intolerance has been diagnosed, the degree of lactase deficiency can be assessed by taking increasing quantities of lactose in a variety of dairy products (Table 10-2). Most lactase deficient individuals can process the lactose in one glass of milk, but taking several types of milk and dairy products in a 24-hour period would exceed their enzyme's capacity to break down lactose, and digestive tract symptoms would result. For more information on lactose intolerance and determining an individual's degree of tolerance of lactose, see the method for *Disaccharide Intolerance,* page 273.

Table 10-2: Lactose Content of Foods[16]

>35 g Lactose/100 g	g/100 g
Nonfat dry milk	50.0 - 52.3
Buttermilk powder	49.0 - 50.0
Condensed whey	38.5 - 39.0
Dry whole milk	35.9 - 38.4
10 - 35 g Lactose/100 g	**g/100 g**
Sweetened condensed milk	10.0 - 16.3
Evaporated milk (whole and skim)	9.7 - 11.0
American cheese, pasteurized, processed	1.8 - 14.2
3 - 10 g Lactose/100 g	**g/100 g**
Velveeta Cheese Food®	9.3
Ice cream	3.1 - 8.4
Ice milk	7.6
Yogurt, low fat	1.9 - 7.7
Human milk	6.2 - 7.5
Skim milk	4.3 - 5.7
1% milk	4.8 - 5.5
2% milk	3.7 - 5.3
American ("Jack") cheese	1.6 - 5.2
Whole cow's milk	3.7 - 5.1
Ricotta cheese	0.2 - 5.1
Buttermilk	3.6 - 5.0
Chocolate milk	4.1 - 4.9
Goat's milk	4.1 - 4.7
Yogurt, whole milk	4.1 - 4.7
Sour cream	3.4 - 4.3
Feta cheese	4.1
Light cream (half-and half) 10.5% milk fat	3.7 - 4.0

Table 10-2: Lactose Content of Foods[16]

3 - 10 g Lactose/100 g	g/100 g
Parmesan cheese	2.9 - 3.7
Romano cheese	0.0 - 3.6
Cottage cheese, 2% milk fat	3.6
Cottage cheese, uncreamed	0.0 - 3.6
Swiss cheese	0.0 - 3.4
Cottage cheese, creamed	0.6 - 3.3
Mozzarella, part-skim cheese (15% milk fat)	0.0 - 3.1
Whipping cream (35% milk fat)	2.8 - 3.0
<3 g Lactose/100 g	**g/100 g**
Cream cheese (e.g. Philadelphia®)	0.4 - 2.9
Neufchatel cheese	0.4 - 2.9
Brick cheese	0.0 - 2.8
Cottage cheese, 1% milk fat	2.7
Blue cheese	0.0 - 2.5
Colby cheese	0.0 - 2.5
Provolone cheese	0.0 - 2.1
Cheddar cheese	0.0 - 2.1
Gouda cheese	0.0 - 2.1
Orange sherbet	0.6 - 2.1
Roquefort cheese	0.0 - 2.0
Brie cheese	0.0 - 2.0
Camembert cheese	0.0 - 1.8
Edam cheese	0.0 - 1.4
Butter	0.8 - 1.0
Lactaid® milk*	0.0 - 0.025

* Information supplied by the manufacturer

References

1. David, T.J. Cow's milk intolerance. In: *Food and Food Additive Intolerance in Childhood*. Blackwell Scientific Publications, Oxford, London, 1993. 27-84.

2. Bahna, S.L., and Heiner, D.C. *Allergies to Milk*. Grune and Stratton, New York, 1980

3. Wilson, N.W., and Hamburger, R.N. Allergy to cow's milk in the first year of life and its prevention. Ann. Allergy 1988 61:323-327.

4. Kahn, A., Rebuffat, E., Blum, D. Difficulty in initiating and maintaining sleep associated with cow's milk allergy in infants. Sleep 1987 10(2):116-121.

5. Kahn, A., Mozin, M.J. Rebuffat, E., Sottiaux, M., Muller, M.F. Milk intolerance in children with persistent sleeplessness: A double-blind cross-over evaluation. Pediatrics 1989 84(4):595-603.

6. Perkin, J.E. Major food allergens and principles of dietary management. In: Perkin, J.E. (Ed), *Food Allergies and Adverse Reactions*. Aspen Publications, Gaithersburg, MD, 1990. 51-67.

7. Bahna, S.L. The diagnostic dilemma of milk allergy. Ann. Allergy 1989 63:475-476.

8. Weyman-Daum, M. Milk-free, lactose-free, and lactose-restricted diets. In: Chiaramonte, L.T, Schneider, A.T., Lifschitz, F. (Eds), *Food Allergy: A Practical Approach to Diagnosis and Management*. Marcel Dekker, New York, 1988. 401-420.

9. Swaisgood, H.E. Characteristics of edible fluids of animal origin: milk. In: Fenneman, O.R. (Ed), *Food Chemistry*, 2nd Edition. Marcel Dekker, New York, 1985. 791-827.

10. Yunginger, J.W. Food antigens. In: Metcalfe, D.D., Sampson, H.A., and Simon, R.A. (Eds), *Food Allergy: Adverse Reactions to Foods and Food Additives*. Blackwell Scientific Publications, Oxford, London, 1991. 36-51.

11. Bahna, S.L. Milk Allergy. In: Chiaramonte, L.T., Schneider, A.T., Lifschitz, F. (Eds), *Food Allergy: A Practical Approach to Diagnosis and Management*. Marcel Dekker, New York, 1988. 107-116.

12. Dawson-Hughes, B., Dallal, G.E., Krall, E.A., Sadowski, L., *et al.* A controlled trial of the effect of calcium supplementation on bone density in post-menopausal women. New Eng. J. Med. 1990 323:878-883.

13. Hearney, R.P., Recker, R.R. and Hinders, S.M. Variability of calcium absorption. Am. J. Clin. Nutr. 1988 47:262-264.

14. Littman, A. Lactase deficiency: Diagnosis and management. Hospital Practice 1987 22:111-124.

15. Hill, L.W. Immunologic relationships between cow's milk and goat's milk. J. Pediat. 1993 15:157-162.

16. Scrimshaw, N., Murray, E. Lactose content of milk and milk products. In: *The Acceptability of Milk and Milk Products in Populations with a High Prevalence of Lactose Intolerance*. Am. J. Clin. Nutr. (Suppl.) 1988 48:1099-1104.

Method: Milk-free Diet

Components of milk and dairy products to be avoided include:

Milk	Cheese	Cream
Condensed milk	Cottage cheese	Sour cream
Evaporated milk	Cream cheese	Casein
Milk solids	Feta	Sodium caseinate
Milk powder	Ricotta	Potassium caseinate
Yogurt	Quark®	Whey
Butter	Sherbet	Lactoglobulin
Buttermilk	Ice cream	Lactose
Curd		

Lactic acid, lactate, and lactylate do not contain milk and do not need to be eliminated. The nutrients in milk can be replaced by a variety of foods, and there are a number of choices for milk in recipes.

Nutritional Substitutes

There are alternative sources of all the nutrients that milk provides.

Calcium

The method for *Non-dairy Sources of Calcium*, page 102, includes an extensive list of calcium-rich foods free of milk and dairy products. The method also includes information about calcium requirements and supplements.

Vitamin D

The body makes its own Vitamin D when exposed to sunlight. This exposure is our main source of Vitamin D. In addition, egg yolk and fish, particularly fish liver oils, are good sources of Vitamin D. There are small quantities of Vitamin D in carrots, pumpkins, sweet potatoes, apricots, cantaloupe (rock melon), squash, broccoli, spinach, and other dark leafy greens.

Protein

The protein ordinarily obtained from milk and dairy products such as cheese and yogurt can easily be obtained from other foods. Such foods include poultry, fish, nuts, legumes, and a combination of whole grains and vegetables.

Feeding the Milk Allergic Infant

Cow's milk proteins in the mother's diet can be passed into her breast milk and cause an allergic reaction in her infant. If the breast-fed infant is allergic to cow's milk protein, the elimination of all milk and dairy products from the mother's diet should be beneficial. If the elimination of milk and milk products only partially eases the infant's distress, carefully kept exposure diaries by the mother may isolate other possible dietary or medication irritants.

If the infant is lactose intolerant, a milk-free diet for the mother *will not help.* The lactose content of mother's milk will remain stable at about 6%, regardless of whether or not the mother consumes milk and dairy products. For management of lactose intolerance in a breast-fed infant, see *Lactose Intolerance* page 83.

Infant formulas that are milk-free can be given to a milk allergic infant.

If the infant tolerates soy, a soy-based formula may be tolerated, such as: Isomil® (Ross), Nursoy® (Wyeth), or Prosobee® (Mead Johnson).

If the infant tolerates neither milk or soy proteins, a casein hydrolysate formula such as Nutramagin® (Mead Johnson), Pregestimil® (Mead Johnson), or Alimentum® (Ross), may be tolerated.

This eating plan is designed to remove all milk and milk products from the diet.

Milk-free Diet

Type of Food	Foods Allowed	Foods Restricted

Milk and Dairy	Substitutes:
	  Soy Milk
	  Soy infant formula
	  Hydrolysate formula
	  Rice Dream®
	  Coconut milk
	  Nut milk
	  Milk-free margarine
	  Clarified butter
	  Milk-free soy bean cake
	Non-dairy creamers:
	  Coffee Rich®
		Avoid all milk and milk
		  products

Vegetables	All vegetables and their juices
	  except those listed opposite
		Prepared as:
		  Creamed
		  Scalloped
		  Mashed with milk
		  Breaded or battered
		  Butter or margarine added
		Instant potatoes

Legumes	All plain legumes
	Milk-free tofu
	Peanut butter
		Prepared with:
		  Milk
		  Cheese

Milk-free Diet

Type of Food	Foods Allowed	Foods Restricted
Fruit	All pure fruits and pure fruit juices	None
Breads and Cereals	Breads and baked goods made without milk or milk products French or Italian bread Some whole wheat bread Some rye bread Soda crackers Bagels Pasta Plain cooked or ready to eat cereals All plain grains, flours and starches	Baked products made with milk or milk products Cereals containing milk or milk solids Commercial baking mixes

Meat, Poultry, and Fish	All fresh or frozen meat, poultry or fish
	Kosher processed meats (may be called "parve" or "pareve")
	Other processed meats made without milk or milk products
	Meat, poultry and fish canned without milk or milk products
		Commercially prepared as:
		  Breaded
		  Battered
		  Creamed

Eggs	Plain, boiled, fried or poached
	Omelette or scrambled made without milk or cheese
		Prepared with:
		  Milk
		  Cheese

Nuts and Seeds	All plain nuts and seeds	Prepared with milk or milk products
Spices and Herbs	All	None
Sweeteners	All, except those listed opposite Sugar Twin®	Sugar substitutes containing lactose

Fats and Oils	Clarified butter
	Pure vegetable oils
	Milk-free margarine:
	  Fleischmann's® low sodium, no salt margarine
	  Parkay Diet Spread®
	Real mayonnaise
	Shortening
	Lard
	Meat dripping
	Gravy made without milk
		Butter
		Margarine containing whey or milk
		Salad dressings with milk or milk products

Method: Lactose Restricted Diet

Phase I   Restriction of all lactose. Phase I should be followed until the diarrhea improves. Liberalization of these restrictions will determine each individual's limit of tolerance for lactose.

Phase II   Lactose tolerance is determined by introducing dairy products and milk.

Phase I - Restriction of Lactose

Type of Food	Foods Allowed	Foods Restricted

Milk and Dairy	Cheeses:
	    Brie
	    Camembert
	    Cheddar
	    Cream
	    Gruyere
	    Limburger
	    Monterey Jack
	    Mozzarella
	    Port au Salut
	Non-dairy creamers:
	    Coffee Rich®
	99% lactose-free milk
		Avoid all except those listed opposite

Breads and Cereals	Breads and baked goods without milk or milk products French or Italian bread Some whole wheat bread Some rye bread Soda crackers Bagels Pasta Plain cooked or ready-to-eat cereals All plain grains	Baked goods made with milk or milk products Cereals containing milk or milk solids

Vegetables	All pure vegetables and their juices, except those listed opposite	Commercially prepared as:
		    Creamed
		    Scalloped
		    Mashed with milk
		    Breaded or battered
		    Butter or margarine added
		Instant potatoes

Fruit	All	None

Phase I - Restriction of Lactose

Type of Food	Foods Allowed	Foods Restricted

Meat, Poultry and Fish	All fresh or frozen meat, poultry or fish
	Kosher processed meats (may be called "parve" or "pareve")
	Other processed meats made without milk or milk products
	Meat, poultry and fish canned without milk or milk products
		Commercially prepared as:
		  Breaded
		  Battered
		  Creamed

Eggs	Plain boiled, fried or poached
	Omelette or scrambled without milk or cheese
		Prepared with:
		  Milk
		  Cheese

Legumes	All plain legumes
	Peanut butter
		Prepared with:
		  Milk
		  Cheese

Nuts and Seeds	All plain nuts and seeds	Prepared with milk or milk products

Fats and Oils	Pure vegetable oils
	Milk-free margarine:
	  Fleischmann's® low sodium, no salt margarine
	  Parkay Diet Spread®
	Real mayonnaise
	Shortening
	Lard
	Meat dripping
	Gravy made without milk
		Butter
		Margarine containing whey or milk
		Salad dressings with milk or milk products

Spices and Herbs	All	None
Sweeteners	All, except those listed opposite Sugar Twin®	Sugar substitutes containing lactose

Table 10-3: Levels of Lactose in Normal Serving Sizes of Common Foods and Beverages

Product	Serving Size	Lactose (Grams)
Sweetened condensed milk	125 mL (½ cup)	15
Evaporated milk	125 mL (½ cup)	12
Whole milk	250 mL (1 cup)	11
2% milk	250 mL (1 cup)	11
1% milk	250 mL (1 cup)	11
Skim milk	250 mL (1 cup)	11
Buttermilk	250 mL (1 cup)	10
Ice milk	125 mL (½ cup)	9
Ice cream	125 mL (½ cup)	6
Half and half light cream	125 mL (½ cup)	5
Yogurt, low fat	250 mL (1 cup)	5
Sour cream	125 mL (½ cup)	4
Cottage cheese, creamed	125 mL (½ cup)	3
Whipping cream	125 mL (½ cup)	3
Cottage cheese, uncreamed	125 mL (½ cup)	2
Sherbet, orange	125 mL (½ cup)	2
American (Jack) cheese	30 g (1 oz)	2
Swiss cheese	30 g (1 oz)	1
Blue cheese	30 g (1 oz)	1
Cheddar cheese	30 g (1 oz)	1
Parmesan cheese	30 g (1 oz)	1
Cream cheese (e.g. Philadelphia®)	30 g (1 oz)	1
Lactaid® milk	125 mL (½ cup)	0.025
Butter	5 mL (1 tsp)	trace

Source: American Dietetic Association

Feeding the Lactose Intolerant Infant

Infant formulas that are lactose-free can be given to a lactose intolerant infant.

If the infant is not allergic to milk, the milk based formula Alactamil® (Mead Johnson), which is free from lactose and sucrose, is suitable.

If the infant is allergic to cow's milk proteins, but tolerates soy, the soy-based formula Prosobee® (Mead Johnson), which is sucrose-free, is suitable.

If the infant is allergic to both cow's milk and soy proteins, a casein hydrolysate formula such as Nutramigen® (Mead Johnson) or Pregestimil® (Mead Johnson) may be tolerated. Both are free from lactose and sucrose.

A breast-fed infant will ingest significant quantities of lactose in mother's milk. The lactose composition of mother's milk will remain constant, regardless of whether or not mother consumes milk and dairy products. If the lactose intolerance is secondary to a gastrointestinal tract infection or other condition that is expected to be transient, some authorities advise continuing breast-feeding and expect the diarrhea to gradually diminish as the underlying inflammation disappears.

Alternatively, the mother can pump her breast milk and treat the milk with Lactaid® drops (4 drops per 250 mL milk), and allow the enzyme to act for 24 hours in the fridge. The infant can be fed the lactose-free milk the next day. This is continued until the diarrhea abates, when the infant can be gradually put back to the breast.

Lactose Restrictions

It is necessary only to avoid lactose. The other components of milk are tolerated. Foods, medications, and beverages containing milk and milk solids all contain lactose.

Products labeled as containing lactose, milk, milk solids, milk powder, cheese and cheese flavor, curd, whey, cream, and butter and margarine containing milk solids should be avoided.

Products containing lactic acid, lactalbumin, lactate and casein, do not contain lactose and can be consumed.

Acidophilus milk is milk to which *Lactobacillus acidophilus* has been added. These bacteria do not digest the lactose enough for the milk to be tolerated by people with a lactose intolerance.

Substitutes

Adding the enzyme lactase (commercially available as Lactaid®) to liquid milk, and allowing the enzyme to act for a minimum of 24 hours in the refrigerator, will make it digestible, and no substitutes are then necessary. The amount of the enzyme that needs to be added will depend on the degree of lactase deficiency. Instructions are provided with the product. Usually, 15 drops in one liter of milk will render it 99% lactose free; 10 drops reduces the lactose to 90%; 5 drops will provide a milk that is 70% lactose free.

Lactaid® tablets may be taken before eating or drinking lactose containing products and may be sufficient to break down the amount of lactose consumed in the following meal.

Lactaid milk® or Lacteeze milk® are 99% lactose free and are available in the dairy section of grocery stores. These are tolerated by lactose deficient individuals, but are more expensive than regular milk.

Some cheeses may be tolerated, since most of the lactose is removed with the whey during their manufacture.

Fermented milks such as yogurt and buttermilk may be tolerated, because the level of lactose in these products is reduced (but not completely eliminated) by bacterial enzymes. Treating the products with Lactaid® as described above may render it acceptable for the severely lactose intolerant individual.

Phase II - Determining Lactose Tolerance Levels

A lactose intolerance is dose related. Usually some level of the enzyme lactase is produced and a certain amount of lactose can be processed. It is important to establish how much lactose can be broken down at one time (Step 1) and how much lactose can be processed over the day (Step 2).

Step 1:

Day 1

Morning: Eat a portion of food containing 1 gram of lactose (e.g., 1 oz or 2 tbsp cream cheese). If there are no symptoms of intolerance, double the amount of lactose the next day.

Day 2

Morning: Eat a portion of food containing 2 grams of lactose (e.g., 2 ounces or ¼ cup cream cheese or ½ cup of uncreamed cottage cheese). If there are no symptoms of intolerance, increase the amount of lactose on Day 3.

Day 3

Morning: Eat a portion of food containing 5 grams of lactose (e.g., 1 cup of low fat yogurt). If there are no symptoms of intolerance, increase the amount of lactose on Day 4.

Day 4

Morning: Eat a portion of food containing 10 grams lactose (e.g., 1 cup of regular 2% milk).

Step 2:

To establish how much lactose may be tolerated over the day, go back to the amount last tolerated. (For example, on Day 2, 2 grams of lactose were tolerated, but on Day 3, there was bloating, cramping, and diarrhea following one cup of yogurt).

Day 1

Morning: Eat a portion of food containing the amount of lactose tolerated in Step 1 (e.g., 2 grams of lactose).

Afternoon: Repeat the morning procedure. If there are no symptoms of intolerance, increase the number of servings on Day 2.

Day 2

Morning: Eat a portion of food containing the amount of lactose tolerated in Step 1. Repeat the process in the afternoon and evening.

Method: Calcium

Calcium Absorption

The percentage of the calcium contained in foods that is actually absorbed, used, and retained by the body is variable depending on age, level of calcium intake, type of food eaten, and other nutrients eaten at the same time. An average adult will absorb approximately 20-40% of the calcium in their diet. This is increased during growth, pregnancy, and lactation, and reduced during aging. In general, the lower the intake, the more calcium is retained by the body (i.e. less calcium is excreted when intake is low).

In order to efficiently absorb calcium, an adequate level of Vitamin D in the body is necessary. Vitamin D is obtained from some foods (milk, liver, egg yolk) but the best source is the action of sunlight (UV light) on the skin.

A diet high in phosphorous and protein (a traditional high-protein North American diet) tends to reduce the amount of calcium retained in the body.

Calcium Supplements

Calcium carbonate provides 625-750 mg elemental calcium per 2.5 mL (½ teaspoon). However, calcium gluconate, calcium citrate, and the Krebs cycle derivatives (citrate, fumarate, malate, succinate, and glutarate) appear to be more efficiently utilized supplements than calcium carbonate. In addition, some research studies indicate that they may interfere less with the absorption of iron and other trace elements than calcium carbonate alone. For young children, a liquid calcium supplement is preferable. Liquid Calcium Sandoz® or Calcium Stanley® are available at most drug stores.

Supplements should contain allowed ingredients only.

Calcium and Vitamin D Supplements

A calcium supplement is recommended with a milk-free diet.   Authorities differ in their recommendations regarding the amount of calcium required daily for different age groups. Table 10-4 indicates the Canadian Recommended Daily Allowances (RNI) for calcium.

Table 10-5 indicates the amount of calcium and Vitamin D required per day for each age group according to the latest Dietary Reference Intakes (Adequate Intake [AI]).

Vitamin D is usually provided by skin exposure to sunlight. A daily multivitamin/mineral supplement will usually provide 100% of the daily requirement of Vitamin D.

References

Burtis, G, David, J., and Martin, S. *Applied Nutrition and Diet Therapy.* W.B. Saunders Co., Philadelphia, 1988.
Calcium: You Never Outgrow The Need. Dairy Bureau of Canada Nutrition Communications, 1990.

Auto-nutritionist III software. Salem, OR, 1990. Based on USDA data.

Nutrient Value of Some Common Foods. Health and Welfare Canada, Ottawa, 1988.

Dawson-Hughes, B., Dallal, G.E., Krall, E.A., Sadowski, L., *et al.* A controlled trial of the effect of calcium supplementation on bone density in post-menopausal women. New Eng. J. Med. 1990 323:878-883.

Hearney, R.P., Recker, R.R., and Hinders, S.M. Variability of calcium absorption. Am. J. Clin. Nutr. 1988 47:262-264.
Health and Welfare Canada Nutrition Recommendations, 1990

Miller, D.D. Calcium in the diet: Food sources, recommended intakes, and nutritional bioavailability. Adv. Food Nutr. Res. 1989 33:103-156.

Table 10-4: Daily Calcium Requirements
Canadian Recommended Daily Allowances (RNI)

Category	Age	Calcium (mg)
Infants	0 - 4 months 5 - 12 months	250* 400
Children	1 year 2 - 3 years 4 - 6 years	500 550 600
Males	7 - 9 years 10 - 12 years 13 - 15 years 16 - 18 years 19 - 24 years 25 - 49 years 50 - 74 years 75+ years	700 900 1100 900 800 800 800 800
Females	7 - 9 years 10 - 12 years 13 - 15 years 16 - 18 years 19 - 24 years 25 - 49 years 50 - 74 years 75+ years	700 1100 1100 700 700 700 800 800
Pregnancy (additional) 1st trimester 2nd trimester 3rd trimester		 500 500 500
Lactation (additional)		500

* source of calcium is mother's milk

Source of Data

Health and Welfare Canada Nutrition Recommendations 1990.

Table 10-5: Dietary Reference Intake Values for Calcium and Vitamin D[2]

Life Stage Group [a] Male and Female	Calcium AI (mg/day)	Vitamin D AI (mcg/day) [b] [c]
0 to 6 months	210	5
6 to 12 months	270	5
1 through 3 years	500	5
4 through 8 years	800	5
9 through 13 years	1300	5
14 through 18 years	1300	5
19 through 30 years	1000	5
31 through 50 years	1000	5
51 through 70 years	1200	10
> 70 years	1200	15

Pregnancy
  18 years and under
  19 through 50 years
	1300
	1000
		55

Lactation
  18 years and under
  19 through 50 years
	1300
	1000
		55

a) Female only for pregnancy and lactation values
b) As cholecalciferol (1 microgram [mcg] = 40 IU Vitamin D)
c) In the absence of adequate exposure to sunlight

Source of Data

Institute of Medicine, National Academy of Sciences, Office of News and Public Information, 2101 Constitution Avenue, NW, Washington, D.C. 20418 August 13, 1997

Table 10-6: Non-Dairy Sources of Calcium

Food	Portion	
	Metric	**Imperial**
>300 mg Calcium		
Arugula (rocket kale)	170 g	1 cup
Sardine, with bones, canned	85 g	3 oz
Wheat flour, artificially enriched	125 g	1 cup
250 - 300 mg Calcium		
Sockeye salmon, with bones, canned	½ can (213 g can)	½ can (7.5 oz. can)
200 - 250 mg Calcium		
Pink salmon, with bones, canned	½ can (213 g can)	½ can (7.5 oz. can)
150 - 200 mg Calcium		
Amaranth (cooked grain): uncooked wt.	100 g	1⅓ cup (cooked)
Baked beans, canned	267 g	1 cup
Kale, frozen, cooked	130 g	1 cup
Rhubarb, frozen, cooked*	127 g	½ cup
Soy beans, cooked	182 g	1 cup
White beans, cooked	189 g	1 cup
100 - 150 mg Calcium		
Almonds	38 g	¼ cup
Chili con carne with beans	269 g	1 cup
Dandelion greens, cooked*	105 g	1 cup
Molasses, cane, blackstrap	20 g	1 tbsp
Scallops	90 g	7 medium
Shrimp, meat only	90 g	28 medium
Spinach, cooked*	95 g	½ cup
50 - 100 mg Calcium		
Beet greens, cooked*	76 g	½ cup
Brazil nuts	37 g	¼ cup
Broccoli spears, cooked	82 g	½ cup
Chili con carne with beans	250 mL	1 cup
Chinese cabbage (bok choy)*	76 g	1 cup
Garbanzo beans (chickpeas) (cooked)	173 g	1 cup
Hazelnuts, chopped	28 g	20 nuts
Orange, raw	131 g	1 medium
50 - 100 mg Calcium		
Orange sections	180 g	1 cup
Oysters	90 g	9 small
Red kidney beans, cooked	250 mL	1 cup
Tofu (8 x 6 x 2 cm = deck of cards)	89 g	3 oz.

Table 10-6: Non-Dairy Sources of Calcium

Food	Portion	
	Metric	**Imperial**
15 - 50 mg Calcium		
Breads		
Cracked wheat (22 mg Ca)	1 slice	1 slice
Mixed grain (27 mg Ca)	1 slice	1 slice
Rye, light (19 mg Ca)	1 slice	1 slice
White (24 mg Ca)	1 slice	1 slice
Whole wheat 100% (25 mg Ca)	1 slice	1 slice
Whole wheat 60% (23 mg Ca)	1 slice	1 slice
White bun, hamburger or hot dog (37-44 mg Ca)	1	1
Pita, whole wheat, 16.5 cm diam. (49 mg Ca)	1	1
Tortilla, corn (42 mg Ca)	1	1
Nuts and Seeds		
Peanuts, oil roasted	39 g	¼ cup
Sesame seeds	20 g	2 cups
Sunflower seeds, kernel	38 g	¼ cup
Soy milk, liquid	254 g	1 cup
Fruit		
Fig, dried, uncooked	19 g	1
Grapefruit, raw	150 g	1 large
Kiwi	91 g	1 large
Pear, raw	169 g	1 medium
Raisins	44 g	¼ cup
Cereals		
All-Bran®	45 g	½ cup
Bran Buds®	44 g	½ cup
Bran Flakes and Raisins	43 g	¾ cup
Bran 100%	35 g	½ cup
Corn Bran	30 g	¾ cup
Cheerios®	24 g	1 cup
Oatmeal, cooked	186 g	¾ cup
Granola, homemade	64 g	½ cup
Shredded Wheat® (10 mg Ca)	1 biscuit	2 cups
Shreddies®	44 g	¾ cup

Table 10-6: Non-Dairy Sources of Calcium

Food	Portion	
	Metric	**Imperial**
15 - 50 mg Calcium		
Vegetables		
Asparagus, cooked, 5 spears	75 g	1 serving
Beans, green or yellow, cooked	72 g	½ cup
Brussels sprouts*	83 g	½ cup
Cabbage, raw, shredded*	74 g	1 cup
Cabbage, cooked, shredded*	80 g	½ cup
Carrot, raw, medium	72 g	1 medium
Carrot, cooked	83 g	½ cup
Cauliflower, raw or cooked	95 g	½ cup
Celery, diced, raw	64 g	½ cup
Lentils	209 g	1 cup
Lima beans, cooked	199 g	1 cup
Olives, black	20 g	5 large
Olives, green	28 g	7 medium
Onions, cooked	111 g	½ cup
Parsley, raw, chopped	12 g	3 tbsp
Parsnip, cooked	83 g	½ cup
Peas, boiled	85 g	½ cup
Spinach, raw, chopped*	30 g	½ cup
Turnip, cooked	62 g	½ cup
Sauerkraut*	125 g	½ cup
Tomatoes, canned	135 g	½ cup
Other		
Egg, whole, cooked	50 g	1 large
Brown sugar	18 g	2 tbsp
Chocolate	30 g	1 square
Maple syrup	21 g	1 tbsp

* Contains oxalic acid, which impairs calcium absorption. Although the calcium is present in the food at the given level, the actual amount absorbed is significantly less.

11

Egg Allergy

The major proteins responsible for egg allergy are present in egg white and are ovalbumin, conalbumin (ovotransferrin), and ovomucoid.[1] Some proteins in egg yolk may also induce the production of IgE antibodies, and antigenic cross-reactivity may occur between egg yolk and egg white proteins. In addition, proteins in eggs from different bird species sometimes cross-react antigenically.[1]

Cooking denatures many egg proteins, so that cooked eggs may be tolerated in cases where raw egg causes an allergic reaction. Some egg proteins, especially ovomucoid, are heat stable and persons allergic to this component react to both cooked egg and raw egg.[1]

In most cases of egg allergy, IgE antibodies are produced specifically to egg proteins, which differ from the proteins in chicken flesh. It should be noted that livetins, which are proteins found in egg yolk, are derived from the blood of the hen. Thus, IgE antibodies to these proteins can result in allergy to both egg and chicken.[1]

Foods Containing Eggs

Avoidance of egg as an individual food in a meal (e.g., scrambled, boiled, fried, or as an omelette) is relatively easy. However, eggs are frequently included as an ingredient in prepared foods, and as such may not be easily recognized. Both the practitioner and allergy sufferer need to be aware of the foods traditionally made with eggs.[2] As well, they need to read food labels and become familiar with terms indicating the presence of egg protein.[3] Egg proteins must be avoided to exclude egg from the diet.

Protein Composition of Eggs

On average, 56 to 61% of the weight of a chicken egg is the white, 27 to 32% is yolk, and the rest is shell.[4]

Egg white proteins include:[2]

- Ovalbumin
- Conalbumin
- Ovomucoid
- Ovomucin
- Lysozyme
- Trace amounts of other proteins, including:

   Catalase
   Ovoflavoprotein
   Ficin inhibitor
   Ovoglycoprotein
   G2 and G3 globulins
   Ovomacroglobulin
   Ribonuclease
   Ovoinhibitor
   Avidin

Egg yolk proteins include:[2]

- Lipovitellin
- Phosvitin
- Low density lipoproteins
- Livetins

References

1.   Yunginger, J.W. Food Antigens. In: Metcalfe, D.D, Sampson, H.A. and Simon, R.A. (Eds), *Food Allergy: Adverse Reactions to Foods and Food Additives.* Blackwell Scientific Publications, Oxford, London, 1991. 36-51.

2.   Powrie, W.D. and Nakai, S. Characteristics of edible fluids of animal origin: eggs. In: Fennema, O.R. (Ed), *Food Chemistry*, 2nd Edition. Marcel Dekker, New York, 1985. 829-855.

3.   *Mayo Clinic Diet Manual: A Handbook of Nutrition Practices.* 7th Edition. Mosby, St. Louis, Baltimore, 1994. 102-103.

4.   Perkin, J.E. (Ed). *Food Allergies and Adverse Reactions.* Aspen Publishers, Gaithersburg, MD, 1990. 253-256.

Method: Egg-free Diet

All products containing egg or components of egg must be avoided, including:

Albumin	Mayonnaise
Egg	Most commercial baking powder
Egg powder	Ovalbumin
Egg protein	Ovoglobulin
Egg white	Ovomucin
Egg from all other poultry	Ovomucoid
(e.g., duck)	Ovovitellin
Egg yolk	Pasteurized egg
Frozen egg	Simplesse® (a fat substitute)
Globulin	Vitellin
Livetin	

Other sources of egg include: eggnog, omelette, custard, soufflé, quiche, egg noodles, angel food cake, Caesar salad, some salad dressings, sauces such as Hollandaise, Bearnaise, and Newburg, battered foods such as fritters, pancakes, and waffles, egg whirl and wonton soup, candy made with egg such as nougat and divinity, candy brushed with egg white to give it a shine, some ice creams, cream pies, meringue pies, meringues, pavlova, and some packaged dessert mixes.

Eggs are frequently used as a garnish and as a binding agent in meat loaves, sausages, etc. Egg may be used as a clarifier in consommé, soft drinks (root beer) or beer and wine.

Several non-food items may also contain egg. Including:
- Egg shampoo
- Sensitized photographic film
- Printed natural fabrics which have not been washed
- Some fur garments
- Vaccinations should be discussed with your doctor as traces of egg may be present in some live vaccines.

Egg Replacers

The commercial low cholesterol product Egg Beaters® is not egg-free. Suitable egg replacers such as Jolly Joan Egg Replacer® or Ener-G Foods Egg Replacer® are available in specialty shops.

Eggs in Recipes

Eggs have various purposes in recipes:
- Leavening agent
- Binding agent
- Source of liquid
- Glaze on baked goods.

Substitute for Egg as a Leavening Agent:

1 tbsp allergen-free baking powder + 2 tbsp liquid* = 1 egg
2 tbsp flour + ½ tbsp shortening + ½ tsp allergen-free baking powder + 2 tbsp liquid* = 1 egg
*Liquid can be any liquid that is appropriate for that recipe (water, vinegar, fruit juice, broth, etc.).

Some recipes call for only one egg and quite a large proportion of baking powder, e.g. 2 tsp of baking powder or 1½ tsp baking soda. Try these recipes without egg, and add 1 tbsp of vinegar instead of the egg.

Substitutes for Egg as a Binder

Combine ⅓ cup water and 3-4 tsp brown flax seeds. Bring to a boil on high heat, then simmer on low heat for 5-7 minutes until a slightly thickened gel begins to form. Strain the flax out of the liquid and use the gel in the recipes. This recipe makes enough substitute for 1 egg. Increase quantities as needed.

Mix ⅓ cup ground flax seed in 1 cup water. Bring mixture to a boil. Simmer for 3 minutes. Refrigerate. 1 tbsp of the mixture replaces 1 egg.
⅓ cup extra water + 1 tbsp arrowroot powder + 2 tsp guar gum = 1 egg
2 ounces tofu = 1 egg

Substitutes for Egg as a Liquid

⅓ cup apple juice = 1 egg
4 tbsp puréed apricot = 1 egg
1 tbsp vinegar = 1 egg

Substitute for Egg as a Glaze

Glazes are cosmetic and not strictly necessary, but a sugar or gelatin glaze can replace an egg glaze. If it is established that egg yolk is tolerated but not egg white, egg yolks separated from the whites can be used as long as egg white does not cause an anaphylactic reaction. If egg white has caused anaphylaxis in the past, do not use egg yolk, because the small amount of egg white which will adhere to the yolk might be sufficient to cause a reaction.

Feeding the Egg Allergic Infant

Egg proteins in the mother's diet can pass into the breast milk and cause a reaction in the egg allergic infant. If the breast-fed infant is allergic to egg protein, the elimination of all eggs and egg containing products from the mother's diet should be beneficial. If egg elimination only partially eases the infant's distress, exposure diaries carefully kept by the mother may isolate other possible dietary or medication irritants.

Egg-free Diet

Type of Food	Foods Allowed	Foods Restricted

Milk and Dairy	Milk, cream, yogurt
	Ice cream and frozen yogurt
	  made without egg
	Cheese
		Eggnog and other milk drinks
		  made with egg
		Frozen desserts containing
		  egg

Breads and Cereals	Bread, buns, and baked
	  goods made without egg
	French or Italian bread
	Soda crackers
	Plain cooked grains
	Plain oatmeal
	Regular Cream of Wheat®
	Ready to eat cereals made
	  without egg
	Egg-free pasta
	Egg-free baking mixes:
	  Kingsmill®, Ener-G®
		Commercial or homemade
		  baked goods made with egg
		
		Instant oatmeal
		Instant Cream of Wheat®
		
		All baking mixes containing
		  egg or baking powder

Vegetables	All pure vegetables and their
	  juices
		Vegetable dishes made with
		  egg
		Salads containing egg or with
		  dressings containing egg

Fruit	All pure fruits and fruit juices	None

Meat, Poultry, and Fish	All fresh, frozen or canned
	  meat, poultry and fish prepared
	  without egg
		Meat, poultry and fish dishes
		  made with egg
		Sausages, loaves, croquettes
		  made with egg
		Check labels on processed
		  meats

Eggs	None	All
Legumes	All pure legumes Plain tofu Plain peanut butter	Legume dishes containing egg
Nuts and Seeds	All plain nuts and seeds	Glazed or in baked goods made with egg

Egg-free Diet

Type of Food	Foods Allowed	Foods Restricted
Fats and Oils	Butter, cream, margarine, shortening Pure vegetable oils Lard and meat drippings Gravy	Salad dressings that list egg in any form as an ingredient Real mayonnaise
Spices and Herbs	All	None
Sweeteners	All	None

12

Grain Allergy

Although the carbohydrate content of grains is much higher than the protein content, it is the proteins which cause the immune system response in an allergic reaction.[1] Wheat is the grain most commonly reported to cause allergic reactions; it is also the one most common in the Western diet. Allergy to other grains (e.g., oats, rye, barley, corn, or rice) is less common.[1]

Proteins in Wheat

Protein makes up about 12% of the dry wheat kernel.[2] Wheat proteins are roughly divided into the following four classes:

- Gliadins
- Glutenins
- Albumins
- Globulins

Gliadins and glutenins form the gluten complex. Gliadins contain as many as 40 to 60 distinct components; glutenins contain at least 15. The molecular size of the protein components in wheat is 10 to 40 kilodaltons,[2] the size considered optimal for triggering a Type I hypersensitivity reaction. Other cereal grains contain similar mixtures of proteins which theoretically could trigger a hypersensitivity reaction.

Allergy to Wheat Proteins

No single protein or class of proteins seems to be responsible for wheat allergy. Hoffman showed that persons allergic to wheat tended to react to the albumins and globulins, rather than the gliadins and glutenins.[3] On the other hand, other studies demonstrated immune responses to gliadins[4] and globulins;[5] however, in spite of this immune reactivity (demonstrated by RAST in most cases), some subjects showed no clinical evidence of wheat allergy.[1]

Symptoms of Grain Allergy

The most common manifestations of cereal grain allergy are asthma, rhinitis, and conjunctivitis, resulting from flour or grain dust in work environments.[6]

Grains and Celiac Disease

Individuals with gluten sensitive enteropathy (celiac disease or sprue) react to the alpha-gliadin fraction of gluten. Although a variety of mechanisms involving immune reactions have been proposed as the primary trigger in the etiology of celiac disease, there is no definitive evidence that it is due to an allergy.[7]

Symptoms of celiac disease are diarrhea, weight loss, malabsorption (especially of fat), signs of iron or folate deficiency, sometimes rickets, and indications of other vitamin and mineral deficiencies. Occasionally the condition is accompanied by an itchy rash (dermatitis herpetiformis).[7]

Celiac disease is diagnosed by a jejunal biopsy that reveals villus atrophy (flattened, short, or absent villi) and other abnormal morphology of the lining of the jejunum. The diagnosis should always be confirmed by laboratory data, so that treatment is not undertaken inappropriately. Treatment is lifelong and consists of the strict avoidance of all grains that contain gluten, namely, wheat, rye, oats, and barley.[7]

It is important to realize that not all wheat intolerance, grain intolerance, or even gluten intolerance, is due to celiac disease.[7]

Symptoms Associated with Wheat Allergy

Wheat has been reported to be the provoking allergen in a number of different allergic conditions. Symptoms of abdominal pain and loose stools commencing within 12 to 72 hours after eating wheat are the most frequently reported manifestations of wheat allergy. In children, this pattern often accompanies an allergy to cow's milk proteins.[8]

Ingested and inhaled wheat flour has been demonstrated to cause asthma in both adults and children, and is one of numerous food and environmental allergens implicated in the etiology of eczema. Wheat allergy also may provoke urticaria and angioedema. An anaphylactic reaction to wheat has been reported in a young infant,[9] and exercise-induced anaphylaxis after eating wheat has been reported several times.[10]

Allergy to Other Cereal Grains

The incidence of allergy to other cereal grains and the degree of cross reactivity among cereal grains is unknown.[8] Allergy to oats, rye, or barley is uncommon, and therefore restricting these grains is rarely necessary except for the treatment of celiac disease. Corn allergy is rare,[11] but has been documented in a number of reports, mainly in childhood. Allergy to rice appears to be equally uncommon.[11] If allergy to any grain is suspected, elimination and challenge should be carried out to confirm the suspicion and determine the specific grain causing the adverse reaction.

Grain Restricted Diets in the Management of Allergy

Wheat-free Diet

In Western countries, avoidance of wheat is one of the more difficult diets to manage because wheat is a principal ingredient in many commonly eaten foods. Breads, cereals, crackers, cookies, muffins, pasta, snack foods, luncheon meats, sausages, candies, desserts, cakes, pies, pancakes, waffles, and many other wheat containing products are the basis of the "convenience foods" used in the fast-paced Western lifestyle. These products supply the nutrients occurring naturally in wheat, as well as those added in the fortification of wheat flour, namely; thiamin, riboflavin, niacin, and iron.

Wheat is likely to be present in foods containing:[11]

Bran	Modified starch
Couscous	Semolina
Cracker crumbs	Starch
Durum	Vegetable starch
Enriched flour	Vegetable gum
Farina	Vital gluten
Flour	Wheat bran
Gelatinized starch	Wheat gluten
Gluten	Wheat starch
Graham flour	Wheat germ
High gluten flour	Whole wheat flour
High protein flour	

Hydrolyzed plant protein (HPP), hydrolyzed vegetable protein (HVP), and monosodium glutamate (MSG) may be made from wheat. However, because the hydrolysis process breaks down the protein to a form that is unlikely to be allergenic, avoiding these products is not considered necessary.

If rye, oats, barley, corn, and rice are tolerated, baked products, cereals, and pastas using these grains can be used in place of those using wheat. In addition, unusual grains and flours such as millet, quinoa, amaranth, buckwheat, tapioca, sago, arrowroot, soy, lentil, pea, and bean, as well as nuts and seeds, may be used in interesting combinations to make baked products and cereals.

Corn-free Diet

Corn is a difficult allergen to avoid in the Western diet because so many prepared foods contain corn in the form of corn starch, corn syrup, or their derivatives. Corn products are likely to occur in cereals, baked goods, snack foods, syrups, canned fruits, beverages, jams, jellies, cookies, luncheon meats, candies, other convenience foods, and infant formulas.

Corn oil is not usually allergenic, unless the product is contaminated during its manufacture by protein from the grain. Because corn protein is an extremely rare cause of anaphylaxis and because the quantity likely to be present is very small, it is not usually necessary to restrict corn oil as an ingredient in foods.

Elimination of corn does not lead to nutritional deficiencies as long as the usual intake of corn itself is small. However, if the usual diet contains many convenience foods, alternative corn-free products will be needed for adequate nutrition.

Corn is likely to be present in foods containing:

Baking powder	Grits
Caramel corn	Hominy
Corn flour	Maize
Corn starch	Modified starch
Corn	Popcorn
Corn syrup solids	Starch
Corn alcohol	Vegetable gum
Corn sweetener	Vegetable protein
Cornflakes	Vegetable paste
Cornmeal	Vegetable starch
Food starch	

Hydrolyzed plant protein (HPP), hydrolyzed vegetable protein (HVP), and textured vegetable protein (TVP) may be made from corn. However, as with similar products derived from wheat, the hydrolysis process breaks down the protein to the point where it is unlikely to be allergenic. As a result, it is usually considered unnecessary to exclude these products from a corn restricted diet.

References

1.   Taylor, S.L., Lemansk, R.F., Bush, R.K., and Busse, W.W. Food allergens: structure and immunologic properties. Ann. Allergy 1987 59(Part II):93-99.

2.   Haard, N.F. Characteristics of edible plant tissues. In: Fennema, O.R. (Ed). *Food Chemistry*. 2nd Edition. Marcel Dekker, New York, 1985. 857-911.

3.   Hoffman, D.R. The specifics of human IgE antibodies combining with cereal grains. Immunochemistry 1975 12:535.

4.   Goldstein, G.B., Heiner, D.C., and Rose, B. Studies of reagins to alpha-gliadin in a patient with wheat hypersensitivity. J. Allergy 1969 44:37.

5.   Sutton, R., Hill, D.J., and Baldo, B.A. Immunoglobulin E antibodies to ingested flour components: studies with sera from subjects with asthma and eczema. Clin. Allergy 1982 12:63.

6.   O'Hollaren, M.T. Occupational asthma due to high molecular weight allergens. Immunology and Allergy Clinics of North America 1992 12(4):795-817.

7.   O'Mahony, S.., and Ferguson, A. Gluten-sensitive enteropathy (celiac disease). In: Metcalfe, D.D., Sampson, H.A., and Simon, R.A. (Eds), *Food Allergy: Adverse Reactions to Foods and Food Additives*. Blackwell Scientific Publications, Oxford, London, 1991. 186-198.

8.   David, T.J. Wheat, rye, barley and oat intolerance. In: *Food and Food Additive Intolerance in Childhood*. Blackwell Scientific Publications, Oxford, London, 1993. 149-153.

9.   Rudd, P., Manual, P., and Walker-Smith, J. Anaphylactic shock in an infant after feeding with a wheat rusk. A transient phenomenon. Postgrad. Med. J. 1981 57:794-795.

10.   Armentia, A., Martin-Santos, J.M., Blanco, M., Carratero, L., Puyo, M., and Barber, D. Exercise-induced anaphylactic reaction to grain flours. Ann. Allergy 1990 65:149-151.

11.   Koerner, C.D., and Sampson, H.A. Diets and nutrition. In: Metcalfe, D.D., Sampson, H.A. and Simon, R.D. (Eds), *Food Allergy: Adverse Reactions to Foods and Food Additives*. Blackwell Scientific Publications, Oxford, London, 1991. 332-354.

Method: Restricted Grain Diet

Restricted Grains and Flours

Wheat	Wheat germ	Oats
Wheat bran	Wheat berries	Oatmeal
Wheatena	Durum	Barley
Spelt	Farina	Corn
Triticale	Couscous	Cornmeal
Semolina	Kamut	(See below for details of
Bulgur	Rye	corn products)
Cracked wheat		

Restricted Flours, Breads, and Crackers Made from Any of the Above Grains, Including:

Any bread made from restricted grain	Cracked wheat flour
White bread	Bran (unless from allowed grains)
Whole wheat bread	Wheat germ
Bread crumbs	Crackers made from restricted grain
60% wheat bread	Cracker meal
Sourdough bread	Graham crackers
All purpose flour	Matzoh
Gluten flour	Starch made from restricted grain
Enriched flour	Cream of Wheat®
Graham flour	Rye bread
Phosphated flour	Rye crackers
Protein flour	Oat bread
Durum flour	Oat flour
Pastry flour	Barley flour
Self-rising flour	Mixed grain flours, cereals, and mixes

Restricted Corn Products, Including:

Corn sugar*	Masa harina
Corn dextrose*	Nachos
Corn syrup*	Popcorn
Cornmeal	Sorbitol*
Corn flour	Tacos
Grits	Tamales
Hominy	Tortillas
Maize	Vegetable gum*

*Sugar, syrup, and sugar alcohols derived from grains are usually considered to be non-allergenic. However, if they are contaminated with a small amount of protein, they may cause an allergic reaction in extremely sensitive individuals. It is wise to avoid them until the limit of tolerance is known.

Products that May Contain Corn

Commercial baking powder.
Breads, cookies, cereals, desserts may contain cornstarch.
Commercial gravies and sauces may be thickened with corn starch.

Products that May Contain the Restricted Grains as a Hidden Ingredient

Any product containing bread or bread
  crumbs
Any product labeled "gluten
  enriched"
Bouillon cubes
Breaded meat or fish
Cereal coffee substitutes
  (e.g. Postum®)
Commercial baking powder
Croquettes
Grain derived alcoholic beverages
Ice cream cones
Icing sugar
Luncheon meats
Malted milk
Meat loaf
    Meat or fish in batter

Mustard pickles
Paté
Patties
Pie fillings
Pies
Root beer
Sausages
Some canned soups
Some cheese spreads or "cheese foods"
Some soy sauces
Some salad dressings
Spreads
Stuffing
Wieners
Thickened soups or gravies

Miscellaneous Restricted Products (May Be Derived from Wheat)

Malt
Malt vinegar
Sprouts from any restricted grain
Beer, ale, lager, porter
Malt flavoring
Bourbon, vodka, and gin may contain
  corn

Sprouted wheat
Monosodium glutamate (MSG)
Hydrolyzed vegetable protein (HVP)
Hydrolyzed plant protein (HPP)

Oils From Restricted Grains

Pure oils are non-allergenic. However, if the oil is not completely pure, it may contain a small amount of the grain protein as a contaminant, and it may cause an allergic reaction in the extremely sensitive individual. Therefore, it is wise to avoid oils of the restricted grains until the limit of tolerance is known.

Allowed Grains and Flours:

Amaranth grain and flour	Potato starch and flour
Arrowroot starch and flour	Quinoa grain and flour
Buckwheat groats and flour	Rice flour
Chickpea (garbanzo) flour (Besan)	Sago flour
Millet flour (Bajri)	Soy flour
Nut meal or flour (any type)	Tapioca starch and flour

Feeding the Grain Allergic Infant

Proteins from grains in the mother's diet can pass into the breast milk and cause symptoms in the infant who is allergic to specific grains.

If the breast-fed infant is allergic to the grains to which people are most frequently allergic, elimination of the common grains from the mother's diet should be beneficial. If removing these grains only partially eases the infant's distress, exposure diaries carefully kept by the mother may isolate other possible dietary or medication irritants.

Restricted Grain Diet

Type of Food	Foods Allowed	Foods Restricted
Milk and Dairy	All milk, buttermilk, cream, yogurt, aged cheese, cottage cheese	Instant cocoa Chocolate mixes Malted milk Cheese sauces, spreads, and foods containing restricted grains
Breads, Cereals, and Substitutes	Flours, grains and starches made with: 　Amaranth flour 　Arrowroot starch or flour 　Buckwheat groats and flour 　Chickpea (garbanzo) flour (Besan) 　Kasha 　Lentil or pea flour 　Millet flour (Bajri) 　Nut meal and flour (all types) 　Potato flour 　Quinoa flour 　Rice starch and flour 　Sago flour 　Seed meal and flour (not from restricted grains) 　Soy flour 　Tapioca starch and flour Breads and baked goods: 　Any made from allowed flours and starches 　Rice bread 　Rice and soy bread 　Breads, muffins, cookies, pancakes, waffles, and cakes made with allowed grains Crackers and snacks: 　Rice cakes, plain, with seeds or with other allowed grains 　Rice crackers 　Potato chips	All starches except from allowed grains All bran except from allowed grains All corn products (see list) Barley flour Bulgur Couscous Durum Farina "Gluten enriched" Graham Kamut Malt Matzoh Oat flour and meal Rye flour Semolina Spelt Triticale Wheat flour, berries Wheatena Any item made from restricted flours Bread crumbs Cracker meal Graham crackers Matzoh All containing restricted grains

Restricted Grain Diet

Type of Food	Foods Allowed	Foods Restricted

	Cereals:
	  Cream of Rice®
	  Rice Krispies®
	  Puffed Rice
	  Puffed Millet
	  Kenmei Rice Bran®
	  Puffed Amaranth
	  Any grain on allowed list
	
	Pasta:
	  Soy pasta
	  Buckwheat pasta
	  Mung bean pasta
	  Rice noodles and pasta
	  Brown rice pasta
	  Wild rice pasta
		All cereals containing
		  restricted grains
		
		Pasta made with restricted
		  grains

Vegetables	All prepared with allowed
	  ingredients
	All vegetable juices
	Sprouted grains and seeds
	  not on restricted list
		Vegetables prepared with a
		  dressing or garnish containing
		  restricted grain
		Sprouted restricted grains

Fruit	All pure fruits and fruit juices	Commercial pie fillings All fruit dishes containing restricted grains

Meat, Poultry, and Fish	All plain, fresh, frozen, or
	  canned meat, poultry, or fish
	Those prepared with allowed
	  grain crumbs or batters
	Plain deli meats such as
	  roast beet, smoked turkey,
	  chicken, ham, without MSG,
	  HPP or HVP or grains in any
	  form
		Meats which may contain
		restricted grain:
		  Battered/breaded
		  Croquettes
		  Luncheon meats
		  Meat loaves
		  Patties
		  Sausages
		  Spreads, paté
		  Stuffing
		  Wieners
		  Processed meats
		  containing HVP, HPP, or MSG

Eggs	All prepared with allowed
	  grains
		Egg dishes containing
		  restricted grains

Restricted Grain Diet

Type of Food	Foods Allowed	Foods Restricted
Legumes	All prepared with allowed ingredients Plain tofu Peanut butter	Legume dishes containing restricted grains
Nuts and Seeds	All plain seeds and nuts	Snack nuts and seeds with HVP**, HPP** or MSG**, or restricted grain products
Fats and Oils	Butter Margarine made with allowed grains All pure vegetable, nut, seed and fish oils, including olive, sunflower, safflower, canola, avocado, soy, peanut, sesame, mustard and walnut oils Lard and meat drippings Peanut and other pure nut and seed butters	Margarine made with restricted grains Wheat germ oil Corn oil Salad dressings and sauces made with restricted grains Gravy thickened with wheat
Spices and Herbs	All plain spices and herbs	Seasoning mixes containing restricted grains, HVP**, HPP**, MSG**, or malt
Sweeteners	Sugar, honey, molasses, maple syrup Jams, jellies and preserves prepared with allowed grain sugar Baking chocolate and pure cocoa powder	All sweets containing restricted grains or of unknown origin Icing sugar* Corn sugar* Corn dextrose* Corn syrup* Sorbitol* Marshmallows

*Sugar, syrup and sugar alcohols derived from grains are usually considered to be non-allergenic. However, if they are contaminated with a small amount of protein, they may cause an allergic reaction in extremely sensitive individuals. It is wise to avoid them until the limit of tolerance is known.

**Avoid these products unless the source is known not to be wheat.

Method: Wheat-free Diet

This eating plan is designed to remove all wheat and products made with wheat from the diet of people who have a wheat allergy. This diet is not suitable for persons with celiac disease.

Restricted Grains and Flours

Bulgur	Spelt
Couscous	Triticale
Cracked wheat	Wheat berries
Durum	Wheat germ
Farina	Wheat bran
Kamut	Wheat
Semolina	Wheatena

Restricted Flours, Breads, Cereals and Crackers Made from Wheat, Including:

60% wheat bread	Graham flour
All purpose flour	Matzoh
Bran (unless from allowed grains)	Pastry flour
Bread crumbs	Phosphated flour
Cracked wheat flour	Protein flour
Cracker meal	Self-rising flour
Crackers made from wheat	Sourdough bread
Cream of Wheat®	Starch (unless labeled "corn starch" only)
Durum flour	Wheat germ
Enriched flour	White bread
Gluten flour	Whole wheat bread
Graham crackers	

Products that May Contain Wheat as a Hidden Ingredient

Any product containing bread or bread crumbs	Ice cream cones
	Icing sugar
Any product labeled "gluten enriched"	Luncheon meats
	Meat loaf
Bouillon cubes	Mustard pickles
Breaded meat or fish	Paté
Cereal coffee substitutes	Patties
Commercial baking powder	Pie fillings
Commercial sauces and gravies	Pies
Croquettes	Sausages

Some canned soups (read labels)
Some corn starch
Some cheese spreads or "cheese foods"
Some soy sauces

Some salad dressings
Spreads
Stuffing
"Thickened" soups or gravies
Wieners

Miscellaneous Products (May Be Derived from Wheat)

Sprouted wheat
Monosodium glutamate (MSG)
Hydrolyzed vegetable protein (HVP)
Hydrolyzed plant protein (HPP)
Malt

Wheat Germ Oil

Pure oils are non-allergenic; however, if the oil is not completely pure, it may contain a small amount of the grain protein as a contaminant. Therefore, it is wise to avoid wheat germ oil until the limit of tolerance is known.

Allowed grains	**Allowed flours and products**
Rice (all types)	Rice flour
Rye	Potato flour and starch
Oats	Soy flour
Barley	Lentil flour (Besan)
Corn	Millet flour (Bajri)
Millet	Sago flour
Buckwheat	Rye flour
Kasha	Oatmeal and oat flour
Amaranth	Barley flour
Quinoa	Arrowroot flour and starch
Tapioca	Tapioca flour and starch
Sago	Amaranth flour
Rye	Buckwheat flour
	Nut meal or flour (any type)
	Seed meal or flour (all types)
	Corn flour or meal
	Corn starch (wheat-free; read labels)

Feeding the Wheat Allergic Infant

Proteins from wheat in the mother's diet can pass into the breast milk and cause allergy symptoms in the wheat allergic infant.

If the breast-fed infant is allergic to wheat protein, the elimination of all wheat and wheat containing products from the mother's diet should be beneficial. If wheat elimination only partially eases the infant's distress, exposure diaries carefully kept by the mother may isolate other possible dietary or medication irritants.

Wheat-free Diet

Type of Food	Foods Allowed	Foods Restricted
Milk and Dairy	All milk, buttermilk, cream, yogurt, aged cheese, cottage cheese	Instant cocoa Chocolate mixes Malted milk Cheese sauces, spreads, and foods containing wheat
Breads, Cereals, and Substitutes	Flours, grains, and starches made with: 　Amaranth 　Arrowroot 　Barley 　Buckwheat 　Corn 　Lentil or pea flour 　Kasha 　Nut meal and flour (all types) 　Oats 　Quinoa 　Rice (all types) 　Rye 　Sago 　Seed meal and flour (all types) 　Soy flour 　Tapioca	Bulgur Couscous Cracked wheat Durum Farina "Gluten enriched" Graham Kamut Malt* Matzoh Semolina Spelt Starch* Triticale Wheat Wheatena Wheat bran and germ Wheat berries
	Breads and baked goods: 　Any made from allowed flours and starches 　Rice bread 　Rice and soy bread 　Breads, muffins, cookies, pancakes, waffles, and cakes made with allowed grains	Any item made from restricted flours or starches Bread crumbs Cracker meal Graham crackers Matzoh

Wheat-free Diet

Type of Food	Foods Allowed	Foods Restricted
	Crackers and snacks: Corn Chips Corn nachos Corn taco chips Potato chips Rice cakes, plain, with seeds or with other allowed grains Rice crackers	All containing wheat
	Cereals: Any grain on allowed list Barley, rye and corn Corn Flakes Cream of Rice® Rice Krispies® Puffed Rice Puffed Millet Kenmei Rice Bran® Puffed Amaranth Any grain on allowed list	All cereals containing wheat
	Pasta: Soy pasta Buckwheat pasta Mung bean pasta Rice noodles and pasta Brown rice pasta Wild rice pasta Corn pasta	Pasta made with wheat flour
Vegetables	All prepared with allowed ingredients All vegetable juices All pure fresh, frozen or canned vegetables	Vegetables prepared with a dressing or garnish containing wheat Sprouted wheat
Fruit	All pure fruits and fruit juices	Commercial pie fillings All fruit dishes containing wheat

Wheat-free Diet

Type of Food	Foods Allowed	Foods Restricted
Meat, Poultry, and Fish	All plain, fresh, frozen or canned meat, poultry, or fish Those prepared without wheat or bread crumbs or wheat batters	Meats which may contain restricted grain: Battered/breaded Croquettes Luncheon meats Meat loaves Patties Sausages Spreads, paté Stuffing Wieners Processed meats containing HVP* HPP* or MSG*
Eggs	All prepared without wheat	Egg dishes containing wheat
Legumes	All prepared without wheat Plain tofu Peanut butter	Legume dishes containing wheat
Nuts and Seeds	All plain seeds and nuts	Snack nuts and seeds with HVP*, HPP* or MSG*, or restricted grain products
Fats and Oils	Butter and cream Margarine, shortening All pure vegetable, nut, seed and fish oils Lard and meat drippings Peanut and other pure nut and seed butters Homemade gravy with thickener other than wheat	Wheat germ oil Salad dressings and sauces made with wheat Gravy thickened with wheat flour or starch
Spices and Herbs	All plain spices and herbs	Seasoning mixes containing wheat, HVP*, HPP*, MSG*, or malt*
Sweets and Sweeteners	Sugar, honey, molasses, maple syrup Jams, jellies and preserves prepared without wheat Baking chocolate and pure cocoa powder	All sweets containing wheat or of unknown origin Icing sugar* Candy* Marshmallows*

* Avoid these products unless the source is known not to be wheat.

13

Peanut Allergy

Peanuts are legumes. Peanuts and soy are the most allergenic of the family *Leguminosae*, which contains over 30 species, including fresh and dried peas, fresh and dried beans, all types of lentils, soya beans, carob, and licorice. Research studies indicate that symptomatic reactivity to more than one member of the legume family is rare.[1] Because a person is allergic to peanut and/or soy, it does not follow, therefore, that the person will also be allergic to other members of this family.[1] Reactions to peanut, soy, and other legumes are managed as separate allergies.

Peanuts are one of the most frequently cited causes of life threatening anaphylactic reactions. Once a person has had an anaphylactic reaction to peanuts, extreme caution must be exercised to avoid all sources of peanut.

Peanuts are unrelated botanically to nuts that grow on trees. Most people experience no difficulties eating a variety of tree nuts, such as walnuts, pecans, Brazil nuts, almonds, cashew nuts, hazelnuts, and macadamia nuts. However, because tree nuts also are highly allergenic foods, any difficulties encountered are often strong allergic reactions, including anaphylaxis. An allergy to nuts should be distinguished from an allergy to peanut or other legumes; otherwise the diet can become stressful and cumbersome if all traces of peanuts are avoided, as well as all traces of other nuts.

WARNING

Sometimes no differentiation is made in marketing peanuts and other nuts, and the two are sold together in "nut mixtures". A less obvious problem is the contamination that can occur in the processing or marketing of nuts and nut containing products. Utensils used to handle "bulk nuts" may have been previously used with peanuts without intervening cleaning. In the manufacture of candies, confectioneries, and ice creams, cross contamination occurs between nuts and peanuts. As a result, persons with severe peanut allergy should be advised to avoid any product containing any type of "nuts" because of the danger of encountering peanuts inadvertently.

"Mandalona" nut is one of the names given to a manufactured product made from de-flavored, de-colored peanut meal that is pressed into molds, re-flavored and colored, and sold as a substitute for tree nuts such as almonds, pecans, and walnuts[1] Persons with peanut allergy must be warned about such products. One manufacturer of such a peanut product is Nu-nuts Flavored Nuts Co., Division of Seabrook Blanching Corp., Tyrone, PA, USA.

Symptoms of Peanut Allergy

Symptoms reported to be due to peanut allergy include urticaria, angioedema, wheezing, asthma, vomiting, rhinorrhea, itching, nausea, allergic conjunctivitis, and anaphylaxis.[2] Contact dermatitis and urticaria from direct peanut contact have also been reported. As it is uncommon to lose reactivity to peanuts, the allergy is considered to be lifelong.[3]

Studies have indicated that peanut allergic adults can tolerate pure peanut oil without clinical reactions.[4] In fact, this is true of any pure vegetable oil for persons allergic to the particular source of the oil. The allergic reactivity occurs to the protein but not to the oil. However, because traces of the protein may contaminate the oil, individuals who are anaphylactic to peanut, or to any another plant, should be cautioned to avoid oil derived from the allergenic plant.

References

1.   Koerner, C.B., and Sampson, H. Diets and nutrition. In: Metcalfe, D.D., Sampson, H.A., and Simon, R.A. (Eds), *Food Allergy: Adverse Reactions to Foods and Food Additives.* Blackwell Scientific Publications, Oxford, London, 1991. 332-354.

2.   Kemp, A.S., Mellis, C.M., Barnett, D., Sharota, E., Simpson, J. Skin test, RAST and clinical reactions to peanut allergens in children. Clin. Allergy 1985 15:73-78.

3.   David, T.J. Soya intolerance. In: *Food and Food Additive Intolerance in Childhood.* Blackwell Scientific Publications, Oxford, London, 1993. 107-116.

4.   Taylor, S.L., Busse, W.W., Sachs, M.I., Parker, J.L., Yunginger, J.W. Peanut oil is not allergenic to peanut-sensitive individuals. J. Allergy Clin. Immunol. 1981 68:372-375.

Method: Peanut-free Diet

Symptoms of Peanut Allergy

The most common symptoms of peanut allergy include: hives, tissue swelling, wheezing, asthma, vomiting, runny nose, itching, nausea, and eye irritation.

> **Peanuts are one of the most frequently cited causes of life threatening anaphylactic reactions. If a person has been diagnosed as anaphylactic to peanuts, extreme caution must be exercised in avoiding all sources of peanut. Reactivity to peanuts is usually lifelong.**

Ingredients Indicating the Presence of Peanuts

Peanut protein	Mixed nuts
Hydrolyzed peanut protein	Mandalona nuts
Peanut oil	Artificial nuts
Peanut butter	Goober peas
Peanut flour	Goober nuts

Examples of Products that May Contain Peanut

Marzipan (almond paste)	Baked goods
Chili	Cookies
Egg rolls	Candies
Chinese dishes	Chocolate bars
Thai dishes	Prepared and frozen desserts
Satay sauces	Vegetable oil
Prepared soups (especially dried packaged soup mixes)	Hydrogenated vegetable oil
	Vegetable oil shortening

Peanut Oil

Pure peanut oil is non-allergenic and will not cause an allergic reaction. However, there is a good chance that the oil is contaminated with peanut protein in its manufacture, so peanut allergic persons, especially those who have experienced an anaphylactic reaction, are advised to avoid peanut oil also.

Feeding the Peanut Allergic Infant

Protein from peanuts in the mother's diet can pass into the breast milk and cause allergic symptoms in the breast-fed infant.

If the breast-fed infant is allergic to peanut protein, the elimination of all peanut and peanut containing products from the mother's diet should be beneficial. If peanut elimination only partially eases the infant's distress, exposure diaries carefully kept by the mother may isolate other possible dietary or medication irritants.

Peanut-free Diet

Type of Food	Foods Allowed	Foods Restricted
Milk and Dairy	Milk, cream, plain yogurt, and ice cream made with allowed foods Plain cheese Sour cream, Quark® Dips made with allowed ingredients	Ice cream, etc. with added oils or nuts of undisclosed origin Read labels of cheese foods (slices, dips and spreads) carefully
Breads and Cereals	Any breads, buns, or baked goods made without peanut oil or products, and baked goods which are free from peanut and peanut oil Plain cooked grains Plain oatmeal Regular Cream of Wheat® Ready to eat cereals without added oil or nuts, such as Shreddies®, corn flakes, homemade granola without peanut Dried pasta	Commercial or homemade baked goods made with peanut oil or peanuts, or made with undisclosed sources of "nuts", oil, or shortening Baking mixes Ready-to-eat cereals with added oils and nuts, such as granola
Vegetables	All pure vegetables and their juices	Vegetable dishes made with sauces with peanut, or unknown ingredients and oils Salads with dressings containing unknown oil or nuts Vegetables canned in undisclosed oils
Fruit	All pure fruit and fruit juices	Fruit dishes made with oil or shortening or nuts of peanut or unknown origin

Peanut-free Diet

Type of Food	Foods Allowed	Foods Restricted
Meat, Poultry, and Fish	All fresh or frozen meat, poultry or fish Fish canned in broth, water or non-peanut oils	Meat, poultry or fish dishes made with peanut or undisclosed nuts or oils Fish canned in undisclosed oils Chinese dishes Thai dishes Egg rolls Commercial chili Vegetarian burgers unless "peanut-free" Peanut protein
Eggs	All	Egg dishes prepared with oils or nuts of unknown sources Egg rolls

Legumes	All pure legumes except peanut
	Tofu
		Peanut and peanut products including:
		  Artificial nuts
		  Goober nuts, goober peas
		  Hydrolyzed peanut protein
		  Mandalona nuts
		  Mixed nuts
		  Peanut butter
		  Peanut flour
		  Peanut oil
		  Peanut protein
		Legume dishes containing peanut or oils or nuts of undisclosed source

Nuts and Seeds	All packaged plain, pure nuts and seeds All pure nut and seed oils and their butters, such as sesame tahini, almond butter, almond paste, cashew butter	Mixed nuts Mandalona nuts Artificial nuts Nuts or oils of undisclosed origin Goober nuts, goober peas

Peanut-free Diet

Type of Food	Foods Allowed	Foods Restricted
Fats and Oils	Butter, cream Pure vegetable, nut, or seed oil with source provided (except peanut) Lard and meat drippings Gravy made with meat drippings	Peanut oil Salad dressings that list "oil" without revealing source Margarine, unless source of all oils is revealed and margarine is peanut-free
Spices and Herbs	All pure herbs and spices Blends of herbs, spices, without added oils	Seasoning packets with undisclosed oils Vegetables such as garlic or sun-dried tomato packed in oil, unless source of oil is disclosed
Sweets and Sweeteners	Plain sugar, honey, molasses, maple syrup Corn syrup Pure baking chocolate Cocoa Artificial sweeteners Homemade cookies and candies with allowed ingredients	The following, unless sources are revealed and are peanut-free: Other chocolate Chocolate bars Marzipan (almond paste) Cookies and candies

14

Soy Protein Allergy

Soy is a legume. Soy and peanuts are the most allergenic of the family *Leguminosae*, which contains over 30 species, including fresh and dried peas, fresh and dried beans, all types of lentils, soya beans, carob, and licorice. Research studies indicate that symptomatic reactivity to more than one member of the legume family is rare.[1] Because a person is allergic to peanut and/or soy, it does not follow, therefore, that the person will also be allergic to other members of this family.[1] Reactions to peanut, soy, and other legumes are managed as separate allergies.

Symptoms of Soy Allergy

Soy is a rare cause of anaphylaxis, but can cause symptoms such as asthma, rhinitis, urticaria, angioedema, and gastrointestinal disturbances.[1] Up to 43% of infants who are allergic to cow's milk are thought to develop an allergy to soy when given soy-based infant formulas,[2] (see *Composition of Infant Formulae,* page 264 for a discussion of soy-based infant formulas). Like cow's milk, soy is a frequent contributor to dermatitis (eczema) in atopic children.

Allergy to soy protein is similar to allergy to cow's milk protein in many ways.[3] In infants, soy allergy can cause loose stools and diarrhea, vomiting, abdominal discomfort, irritability, crying, intestinal blood loss, anaemia, and failure to thrive.[3] Respiratory symptoms include coughing, wheezing, asthma, and rhinitis; skin symptoms include urticaria, angioedema, and atopic eczema.

Sources of Soy Protein

Soy protein occurs in a wide range of manufactured foods[4] and infant formulas, and thus is difficult to avoid. As with peanut oil, pure soy oil is not considered allergenic unless contaminated by the protein, which is difficult to detect in the manufactured product. Sometimes the presence of soy in a manufactured food is not immediately obvious. On a food label, soy may be indicated by terms such as "textured vegetable protein" or "hydrolyzed plant protein," or by the use of lecithin, which is often derived from soy. As well, oriental foods such as tempeh, tofu, miso, and bean curd are largely soy, although this may not be obvious to anyone unfamiliar with these foods.[5]

References

1.   Koerner, C.B., and Sampson, H. Diets and nutrition. In: Metcalfe, D.D., Sampson, H.A., and Simon, R.A. (Eds), *Food Allergy: Adverse Reactions to Foods and Food Additives.* Blackwell Scientific Publications, Oxford, London, 1991. 332-354.

1.   David, T.J. Soya intolerance. In: *Food and Food Additive Intolerance in Childhood.* Blackwell Scientific publications, Oxford, London, 1993. 107-116

2.   Hill, D.J., Ford, R.P.K., Shelton, M.J. and Hosking, C.S. A study of 100 infants and young children with cow's milk allergy. Clin. Rev. Allergy 1984 2:125-142.

3.   Visakorpi, J.K. Milk and soybean protein allergy. J. Paediatr. Gastroenterol. Nutr. 1983 2(suppl):S293-S297.

4.   Perkin, J.E. *Food Allergies and Adverse Reactions.* Aspen Publications, Gaithersburg, MD, 1992. 249-252.

5.   Nelson, J.K., Moxness, K.F., Jensen, M.D., and Gastineau, C.F. Food allergy and intolerance. In: *Mayo Clinic Diet Manual*, Seventh Edition. Mosby, St. Louis, 1994.

Method: Soy-free Diet

General Information on Products Containing Soy

Soy beans and soy products have become a major component in manufactured food products in recent years. They occur in many processed foods, infant formulas, breakfast cereals, baked goods, crackers, soups, packaged meals, and sauces.

Although pure soy oil is usually non-allergenic and does not cause a reaction in soy-allergic individuals, it is possible that the oil will be contaminated with soy protein in its manufacture. Therefore, people who are very allergic to soy are advised to avoid soy oil also, although most will tolerate a small amount of the oil without any difficulty.

Most manufactured foods that contain soy will indicate the presence of soy protein on the label. Sometimes the word "soy" or "soya" may not appear, so persons who are soy allergic are advised to become familiar with terms that indicate the likely presence of soy.

Unlabeled products such as bulk foods, unwrapped breads and baked goods may contain soy, especially if flour is an ingredient. People who are allergic to soy are advised not to purchase these products unless the specific ingredients can be determined.

Ingredients that Indicate the Presence of Soy Protein

Emulsifiers*	Soy-based infant formulas
Lecithin*	Soya
Miso	Stabilizers*
Shoyu	Tempeh
Sobee	Tofu
Soy	Unspecified sprouts*
Soy albumin	Vegetable broth*
Soy beans	Vegetable gum*
Soy flour	Vegetable oil*
Soy lecithin	Vegetable paste*
Soy milk	Vegetable protein*
Soy nuts	Vegetable shortening*
Soy oil	Vegetable starch*
Soy protein	Textured vegetable protein (TVP)*
Soy protein isolate	Hydrolyzed vegetable protein (HVP)*
Soy sauce	Hydrolyzed plant protein (HPP)*
Soy sprouts	

*These items may not contain soy, but the source is seldom listed on a food label.

Although pure soy oil is non-allergenic, it is wise to avoid products containing soy oil, especially where it is listed as the main ingredient, such as in soy-based margarine and soy oil-based cooking sprays because of the possibility of the presence of soy protein. Cold-pressed soy oil is likely to contain significant quantities of the protein.

Manufactured Foods that are Likely to Contain Soy Protein as an Ingredient

Bread
Breakfast cereals
Cakes and cake mixes
Canned soup
Cheese substitutes
Chocolates
Commercial fruit products
Cookies and cookie mixes
Crackers
Dessert mixes
Flavored chips
Frozen desserts
Ice cream
Infant pablum

Meat products:
   Cold cuts
   Hamburger
   Meat paste and paté
   Meat pies
   Minced beef
   Sausages
Milk or cream replacers
Other baked goods
Packaged soup mixes
Pancake and waffle mixes
Pastas
Sauces
Vegetable products

Feeding the Soy Allergic Infant

Proteins from soy in the mother's diet can pass into the breast milk and cause a reaction in the soy-allergic infant.

If the breast-fed infant is allergic to soy protein, the elimination of all soy and soy containing products from the mother's diet should be beneficial. If soy elimination only partially eases the infant's distress, exposure diaries carefully kept by the mother may isolate other possible dietary or medication irritants.

Soy-free Diet

Type of Food	Foods Allowed	Foods Restricted
Milk and Dairy	All except those listed opposite	Cheese substitutes Ice cream, frozen desserts, and dessert mixes unless soy-free Milk or cream replacers Soy infant formula Soy milk

Soy-free Diet

Type of Food	Foods Allowed	Foods Restricted
Breads and Cereals	All except those listed opposite	Homemade and commercial breads and baked goods containing soy Soy grits and flour Baking mixes Cereals containing soy (Most infant cereals contain soy)
Vegetables	All pure, fresh, frozen or canned vegetables and their juices	All vegetable dishes made with soy or unknown ingredients Soy or mixed sprouts Salads with sprouts, imitation bacon bits or dressings containing soy Frozen french fries Vegetables that are oiled or polished Commercial vegetable products
Fruit	All pure fresh, frozen, or canned fruits and their juices	Fruit dishes made with soy products Commercial fruit products Fruits that are oiled or polished

Meat, Poultry, and Fish	All fresh or frozen meat, poultry, or fish
	Fish canned in water
		Meat, poultry or fish with soy
		Tuna and other fish canned in oil
		Tofu (soybean curd)
		Meat extenders
		Vegetarian meat replacers (analogs)
		Meat products which may contain soy:
		  Cold cuts
		  Frozen dinners
		  Hamburger
		  Meat paste and paté
		  Meat pies
		  Minced beef
		  Sausages

Eggs	All plain eggs	Egg dishes prepared with soy products

Soy-free Diet

Type of Food	Foods Allowed	Foods Restricted
Legumes	All plain legumes except soy and tofu	All legume dishes containing soy products (see lists, previous pages)
Nuts and Seeds	All packaged plain, pure nuts and seeds All pure nut and seed oils and their butters, e.g., tahini, almond butter Peanuts Peanut butter	Soy nuts or butter Nuts or mixes with soy products Any oils or nuts of undisclosed origin
Fats and Oils	Butter, cream Pure vegetable, nut or seed oil with source provided (except soy) Lard and meat drippings Gravy made with meat drippings Pure olive oil spray Peanut oil	Salad dressings that list "oil" without revealing the source Soy oil Margarine unless sources of all oils are revealed and margarine is soy-free Vegetable oil Other vegetable oil sprays Shortening
Spices, Herbs, and Seasonings	All pure herbs and spices Blends of herbs, spices, without added oils	Seasoning packets with undisclosed oils Sauces containing soy: Barbecue Oriental Soy Worcestershire Imitation bacon bits HVP, HPP, TVP
Sweets and Sweeteners	Plain sugar, honey, molasses, maple syrup Corn syrup Pure baking chocolate Cocoa Artificial sweeteners Pure jams and jellies Homemade cookies and candies with allowed ingredients	The following, unless sources are revealed and are soy-free: Other chocolate Chocolate bars Marzipan (almond paste) Cookies and candies Cake icing

15

Avoidance of Multiple Food Allergens

General Description

Milk and milk products, egg, wheat, corn, soy, peanut, tree nuts, chocolate, fish, and shellfish are the most frequent causes of food allergy. This eating plan is designed to remove all of these foods and their products from the diet for people who appear to be allergic to many foods.

This diet should not be followed unless sensitivity to all the eliminated foods has been proven by challenge. The diet can be used as an elimination diet for up to four weeks after which sensitivity to each food should be determined by sequential incremental dose challenge. For the protocol, see *Challenge Phase*, page 35.

Method: Diet Free From the Ten Most Common Allergens*
*Milk, Egg, Wheat, Corn, Soy, Peanut, Nuts, Chocolate, Fish, and Shellfish

Feeding the Food-Allergic Infant

A casein hydrolysate formula such as Nutramigen® (Mead Johnson) or Pregestimil® (Mead Johnson) may be tolerated. Both are free from restricted foods except for corn syrup solids and modified corn starch.

The casein hydrolysate formula Alimentum® (Ross) does not contain any of the restricted foods. If the breast-fed infant is allergic to one or all of the restricted foods, the elimination of them from the mother's diet should be attempted. Proteins from the mother's diet can be found in the breast milk and may be the source of allergens for the infant. If the removal of the listed foods only partially eases the infant's distress, exposure diaries, carefully kept by the mother, may suggest other possible dietary or medication factors that may be contributing to the infant's symptoms. It is important that the breast-feeding mother following this diet takes supplemental calcium and possibly Vitamin D.

Restricted Foods and Food Products

Each of the foods restricted on this diet can be found in many products and derivatives. It would require extensive lists of foods and their products to cover all possible dietary sources. Reading of food labels is essential to detect the allergen as an ingredient in processed and prepared foods.

The following diet plan is designed to avoid these allergens while providing adequate nutrition from alternate sources. If the wide range of allowed foods are eaten, the only supplements which may be necessary are calcium and possibly Vitamin D.

It is important that only foods listed as allowed are used during this trial.

Diet Free of Milk, Egg, Wheat, Corn, Soy, Peanut, Nuts, Chocolate, Fish, and Shellfish

Type of Food	Foods Allowed
Milk and Dairy	Rice Dream® (made from brown rice and safflower oil) In recipes: substitute fruit or vegetable juice, homemade soup stock, potato water Instead of butter on toast, use pure jelly, jam, honey, or herb flavored olive oil On vegetables and salads, use herbs and homemade salad dressings made with allowed foods
Breads and Cereals	Grains and Flours: Amaranth and amaranth flour Barley and barley flour Buckwheat and buckwheat flour Chickpea or garbanzo flour (Besan) Millet and millet flour (Bajri) Oats and oat flour Potato starch and flour Quinoa and quinoa flour Rice and rice flour Rye flour Sago flour Tapioca, and tapioca starch, and flour Wild rice and wild rice flour
	Breads and Baked Goods: Baked goods and specialty baking mixes containing allowed foods from specialty shops listed at the end of the diet Ener-G® rice, brown rice, or tapioca bread Homemade baked goods with allowed foods

Diet Free of Milk, Egg, Wheat, Corn, Soy, Peanut, Nuts, Chocolate, Fish, and Shellfish

Type of Food	Foods Allowed
	Crackers and Snacks: Potato chips made with allowed oil, such as Nalley 100% Golden Light Chips® Pure rye crisp crackers Rice cakes Rice crackers **Cereals:** Cream of Rice® Kenmei Rice Bran® Oatmeal and oat bran Homemade granola with allowed grains Any of the allowed grains Puffed rice Puffed millet **Pasta:** Brown rice pasta Wild rice pasta Mung bean pasta Rice noodles and pasta
Vegetables	All plain fresh and frozen vegetables and their juices except: corn, soy beans, soy bean sprouts, and mixed sprouts
Fruit	All plain fresh and frozen fruits and their juices
Meat and Poultry	All fresh or frozen, plain meat or poultry Avoid all deli meats
Fish and Shellfish	None
Eggs	Ener-G® Egg Replacer See substitutes for eggs pages 107-108
Legumes	All plain legumes and legume dishes prepared with allowed foods, except soy and peanut
Nuts	None
Seeds	All, including sunflower, sesame, cumin, poppy, pumpkin, flax, caraway, anise
Fats and Oils	Oils: olive, canola, sunflower, safflower Meat drippings and poultry fat Homemade gravy made with allowed foods Tahini (sesame seed butter) Lard
Spices and Herbs	All pure fresh or dried herbs and spices

16

Yeast and Mold Allergy

Occurrence of Yeast and Mold

Yeasts and molds are minute single-celled fungi. They belong to the same biological group as mushrooms, but are smaller. Mold colonies are often seen growing on the surface of moist foods such as bread, jam, and cheese.

Yeasts (*Saccharomyces* species) are used in food production to ferment the nutrient source on which they grow. This property is used in the leavening of bread (by baker's yeast) and the manufacture of beer, wine, and vinegar (by brewer's yeast). When vinegar is distilled, yeast proteins are eliminated; therefore, distilled vinegar is tolerated. Yeast is a source of B vitamins and is present in many multivitamin preparations containing B vitamins.

Allergy to Yeast and Mold

The spores of some mold fungi such as *Aspergillus* and *Cladosporium herbarum* (*Hormodendrum*) are common causes of inhalant allergy, especially for persons with asthma. People sensitive to inhaled fungal spores must avoid all sources of the fungi, such as the moist soil of house plants, and damp rooms, especially basements, where molds grow. Because mold spores are released from damp ground softened by the first thaw of spring, mold allergic persons with asthma may need to limit their time outdoors to avoid inhaling the spores in the air at this time of year.

A small percentage of asthmatic persons sensitive to inhaled fungal spores, and some non-asthmatic persons, develop urticaria (hives) when they eat or drink substances containing yeast or molds.[6,7] Extremely allergic persons can suffer an anaphylactic reaction, with breathing difficulty, hives, angioedema (tissue swelling) especially in the throat, and cardiac symptoms.[8] These people must be particularly careful to avoid all sources of fungi in their diet.

Managing Yeast and Mold Allergy

Management of yeast and/or mold allergy requires the elimination of all foods that might contain yeast or mold. Foods excluded as obvious possibilities are leavened baked products, most cheeses, certain fruits and vegetables, certain beverages, and moldy foods. Some lists of foods to avoid for yeast allergy cite milk because it could be a source of penicillin, an antibiotic derived from fungi belonging to the genus *Penicillium*. In the past, dairy cows were treated with penicillin to protect them from infection; However, this practice has been discontinued because of the danger to penicillin allergic people and milk need not be avoided.

Some diets free from yeast and mold advocate avoiding wheat flour. Modern flour milling does not permit the use of moldy wheat therefore, flour need not be avoided. Nevertheless, all baked goods containing flour leavened with yeast must be avoided. Also, because enriched flours contain vitamins that may be derived from yeast, these products must also be avoided.

Malt is made by fermenting barley or other grains with yeast, and is used to flavor foods such as cereals, candies, and beverages. All sources of malt should be avoided.

All obvious sources of mold, such as moldy jams and jellies, must be avoided. Leftover foods and leftover tea and coffee are potential media for the growth of molds. Only fresh foods and freshly brewed tea and coffee should be consumed. Dried fruit may also be a source of mold.

Extent of Elimination of Yeast and Mold Required

The lengths to which a person must go to avoid all forms of yeast and molds in the diet depends on their level of sensitivity.

After following a yeast and mold free diet for a period of about four weeks, an incremental dose challenge should be carried out to determine whether some yeast derivatives can be taken with impunity.

An example would be malt as a flavoring. It is possible that moderately allergic people will exhibit no adverse effects. Malt is a commonly used flavoring in many baked goods, breakfast cereals and commercially prepared foods, and including malt as an ingredient would allow beneficial liberalization of the diet.

Candida Albicans

Candida albicans is a dimorphic fungus, which means that it grows as a yeast form in a carbohydrate medium and forms hyphae (strands) when the medium is low in nutrients. Thus, it is commonly referred to as a "pseudo-yeast".

The role of *Candida* as a cause of allergy has been much disputed.[9] Positive skin reactions often occur in persons without clinical evidence of *Candida* infection or allergic disease. *Candida* species are extremely common members of the body's resident microflora. Usually they are innocuous, as they are kept in check by other resident microorganisms such as bacteria. However, this balance can be upset, for example, when antibiotics eliminate several species of bacteria or the immune system is not functioning efficiently. In these instances, *Candida* multiply unchecked and soon cause infections such as oral thrush, vaginal moniliasis, and skin eruptions.[10]

Some practitioners believe that repeated imbalances of this sort can lead to chronic *Candida* sensitivity, which in turn can lead to numerous food and chemical sensitivities.[11] A "*Candida* diet" is prescribed to treat this condition, usually excluding foods that contain sugars and more complex carbohydrates.[12] In addition the person is advised to avoid dietary forms of other fungi, which are believed to cross react with *Candida* and produce similar reactions.

Although *Candida* infection or sensitivity may contribute to mold and yeast sensitivity, this connection is not scientifically proven.[13] The instructions in this chapter are for a yeast and mold allergy (Type I hypersensitivity) and should not be used to treat a suspected *Candida* sensitivity.

References

1. Warin, R.P., and Smith, R.J. Challenge test battery in chronic urticaria. Br. J. Dermatol. 1976 94:401-406.

2. James, J., and Warin, R.P. An assessment of the role of *Candida albicans* and food yeasts in chronic urtcaria. Br. J. Dermatol. 1971 84:227-237.

3. Aginder, M., Andrae, M-L., Arrendal, H., et al. Allergy: Which Allergens? Pharmacia AB, Vastra Aros, Sweden, 1985 II:16.

4. Position statement: Executive Committee of the American Academy of Allergy and Immunology. Candidiasis sensitivity syndrome. J. Allergy Clin. Immunol. 1986 78(2):271-273.

5. Yeast Infections: Candidiasis. *The Merck Manual*, 16th Edition, Merck, Sharp and Dohme, 1992. 2422-2423.

6. Crook, W.G. *The Yeast Connection: A Medical Breakthrough*. Professional Books, Jackson, TN 1984.

7. Kroker, G.F. Chronic candidiasis and allergy. In: Brostoff, J., and Challacombe, S.J. (Eds), *Food Allergy and Intolerance*. Balliere Tindall, London, 1987. 850-872.

8. David, T.J. Urticaria and angioedema. In: Adverse Reactions to Foods and Food Additives in Childhood. Blackwell Scientific Publications, Oxford, London, 1993. 339-375.

Method: Yeast and Mold Restricted Diet

Yeasts and molds are widespread in the environment. It is impossible to totally avoid touching, inhaling, and swallowing yeasts and molds. It is important to make a good effort to avoid yeasts and mold in the diet.

Yeast and Mold Restricted Diet

Type of Food	Foods Allowed	Foods Restricted
Milk and Dairy	Butter Buttermilk Cottage cheese Cream Ice cream Panir Plain milk Quark® Ricotta cheese Sherbet Sour cream Yogurt	Fermented cheese of all types (different molds are used in their manufacture) Feta cheese Malted milk Sour milk

Breads and Cereals	Any flour or grain not enriched with vitamins
	Any bread, bun, pita, or pizza dough not leavened with yeast or sourdough starter, or with malt, or with enriched flour
	
	Breakfast cereals without malt and/or enriched with vitamins
	Puffed rice or wheat
	Oats and oatmeal
	All plain grains
	Plain crackers without malt
	Crackers made with wheat flour may be vitamin enriched and should be avoided
	Rice cakes and plain rice crackers without yeast
	Crisp rye crackers without yeast
	Matzoh bread and crackers
	Plain pasta
		Flour or grains enriched with vitamins
		All others, including:
		  Au gratin dishes
		  Bread coating
		  Bread crumbs
		  Bread stuffing
		  Bread pudding
		
		All others

Yeast and Mold Restricted Diet

Type of Food	Foods Allowed	Foods Restricted
Vegetables	All pure fresh, frozen, or canned vegetables and their juices except those listed opposite	Fungi such as mushrooms, truffles, and morels Sauerkraut
Fruit	All pure fresh, frozen, or canned fruits and their juices except those listed opposite	Grapes, raisins, and other dried fruit
Meat, Poultry, and Fish	All fresh, frozen, or canned meat, poultry or fish prepared without bread crumbs	Meat, poultry, and fish dishes made with bread crumbs: Breaded fish Croquettes Fish cakes Hamburger patties not labeled as 100% meat Luncheon meats Sausages
Eggs	All	Any prepared with restricted foods, such as Eggs Benedict with cheese sauce, quiche with cheese, cheese in omelettes, etc
Legumes	All plain legumes	Fermented legumes such as soy sauce
Nuts and Seeds	All plain nuts and seeds	Any nut products containing restricted ingredients (e.g., snacks)
Fats and Oils	Butter, cream, margarine, shortening Pure vegetable oils Salad dressings made with oil and lemon Lard and meat drippings Gravy	Salad dressings with vinegar or fermented products such as soy sauce
Spices and Herbs	All fresh, frozen, or dried herbs, spices	Herb or spice mixes containing restricted foods
Sweeteners	Sugar, honey, molasses Jams, jellies, and sweet syrups (once opened, refrigerate and use quickly)	Malted sweeteners Moldy jam, jelly, and syrups Candies and candied fruits

Yeast and Mold Restricted Diet

Type of Food	Foods Allowed	Foods Restricted
Beverages	Milk and milk drinks without malt Fruit and vegetable juices Carbonated beverages except root beer Freshly brewed coffee Tea made from fresh herbs such as mint Mineral water Distilled alcoholic beverages such as vodka, rum, gin, whiskey	Malted milk drinks and any beverage containing malt Leftover coffee All other tea "Health" drinks made with nutritional yeast Wine, beer, cider, and other fermented alcoholic beverages
Fermented Foods	None	Marmite®, Vegemite® and other manufactured foods containing yeast extract All types of vinegar and all foods containing vinegar, such as pickles, ketchup, relishes, and sauces for meat such as Worcestershire, HP Sauce®, barbecue sauce Soy sauce and other fermented oriental sauces
Vitamins and Medications	Check with your pharmacist for yeast-free vitamin supplements; others are permitted Check with your pharmacist for medications free of penicillin and its derivatives	B vitamins and multivitamin supplements with B vitamins derived from yeast Penicillin and its derivatives All other antibiotics derived from fungi
Miscellaneous		Yeast such as brewer's yeast, baker's yeast, torula yeast, nutritional yeast

17

Biogenic Amines

A number of biogenic amines play roles in regulating the immune, digestive, circulatory, muscular, and other systems. Examples are the vasoactive amines, which alter the permeability and contractibility of blood vessels, thus influencing fluid balance, blood pressure, cardiac performance, and other strategic functions. The synthesis, storage, release, and catabolism of these amines are fine-tuned to achieve specific effects.

A variety of vasoactive amines occurs in foods. Ingestion of a large quantity of any of these amines can lead to the development of symptoms in people who are otherwise non-reactive. Some people have a high level of sensitivity and experience clinical symptoms when they ingest only small quantities of one of these amines. This effect may be due to varying degrees of dysfunction in the enzymes which catabolize these biogenic amines.

These enzymes are part of a family of isoenzymes called the monoamine oxidase system.[1] Suppression of the activity of these enzymes can result from a variety of factors, including an inherited tendency and sometimes, in the case of tyramine, prescribed medications.

The biogenic amines most likely to elicit symptoms are:

- Histamine
- Tyramine
- Octopamine
- Phenylethylamine

Biogenic amines that occasionally elicit symptoms include:

- Serotonin (5-hydroxytryptamine)
- Dopamine
- Epinephrine
- Norepinephrine

Histamine and tyramine are discussed in later chapters in this section of the book.

Phenylethylamine is most often associated with migraine headache. High levels are present in chocolate, a number of fermented cheeses (especially Gouda, Stilton,[2] Cheddar, and cream cheese[3]), and red wine.

Serotonin is present in significant amounts in banana, pineapple, plantain, avocado, plum, tomatoes, and molluscs (e.g., octopus).[2]

Tyramine Sensitivity

People most likely to be sensitive to tyramine are those who:[1]

- are taking monoamine oxidase inhibitors (MAOI),
- suffer from migraine headaches, or
- suffer from chronic urticaria.

For persons who are taking MAOI drugs, a tyramine restricted diet is essential. However, the list of foods that are excluded in the diet recommended for these people is relatively simple, as long as if they have no previous history of tyramine sensitivity.[4]

In contrast, a more restricted diet is advisable for individuals who are experiencing chronic urticaria and/or migraine headaches considered to be the result of tyramine sensitivity. The response to tyramine is dose-dependent, and the amount of tyramine that causes an adverse reaction depends on individual tolerance. Therefore, for these persons, the foods initially restricted are more extensive since foods containing low levels of tyramine are also excluded.[3]

Causes of Sensitivity

Tyramine sensitivity is caused by suppression or relative deficiency of the monoamine oxidase enzyme system that normally breaks down tyramine.[4] When this system is adversely affected for any reason, including the therapeutic use of MAOI drugs, undegraded tyramine causes symptoms.

Medications that are MAOI's include:

Hydrazines (used as antidepressants)

Isocarboxazid (Marplan®)
Phenelzine (Nardil®)

Non-hydrazines

Pargyline (Evtatin®; Eutanyl®)
Tranylcypromine (Parnate®)
Selegiline (Deprenil®; Deprenyl®; Eldepryl®) (used for treatment of Parkinson's disease)

Antibiotic

Isoniazid (anti-tuberculosis)

Note: Only Parnate, Nardil, and Marplan are in common use at present. The requirement for a tyramine restricted diet for persons using other MAOI drugs should be decided by the physician on an individual basis.

Symptoms of Excessive Tyramine

Symptoms indicating excessive tyramine in persons taking MAOI drugs are:[2]

- Hypertension (increased blood pressure)
- Tachycardia (increased heart rate)
- Severe headache, especially migraine

When untreated, hypertension and tachycardia can lead to cardiac failure.

Other symptoms reported to be due to a sensitivity to tyramine are:

- Itchiness
- Hot feeling
- Redness of skin (flushing)
- Sweating
- Chills
- Clamminess
- Lightheadedness
- Hives

Food Sources of Tyramine

Tyramine is present in a number of foods, particularly:

Aged cheeses (especially Camembert and Cheddar)	Other fermented beverages
	Raspberries
Avocados	Red plum
Bananas	Tomato
Beer	Vinegar and pickles
Chicken liver	Wines (especially red)
Eggplant (aubergine)	Yeast extract

References

1.   Zeitz, H.J. Pharmacologic properties of foods. In: Metcalfe, D.D., Sampson, H.A., and Simon, R.A. (Eds), *Food Allergy: Adverse Reactions to Foods and Food Additives*. Blackwell Scientific Publications, Oxford, London, 1991. 311-318.

2.   McCabe, B.J. Dietary tyramine and other pressor amines in MAOI regimens: A review. J. Am. Diet. Assoc. 1986 86:1058-1064.

3.   Moneret-Vautrin, D.A. Food intolerance masquerading as food allergy: False food allergy. In: Brostoff, J., and Challacombe, S.J. (Eds) *Food Allergy and Intolerance*. Baillière Tindall, London, 1987. 836-849.

4.   Shulman, K.I., Walker, S.E., MacKenzie, S., *et al.* Dietary restriction, tyramine and the use of monoamine oxidase inhibitors. J. Clin. Psychopharmacol. 1989 9:397-402.

Method: Tyramine Restricted Diet

Tyramine-containing Foods to Be Avoided When Taking MAOI Drugs

Dairy products

- All fermented cheeses, especially Camembert and cheddar, and including feta. (Allowed cheeses include cottage, ricotta, cream cheese, and Quark®.)

Meats

- Dry fermented sausages such as bologna, pepperoni, and salami
- Yeast and meat extracts such as Bovril®, Oxo®, Marmite® and Vegemite®
- Soups and gravies containing yeast and meat extracts
- Leftover meats, fish or poultry and foods containing them.

Fish

- Smoked or pickled fish or fish roe, smoked salmon, pickled herring, lox, caviar.

Vegetables

- Sauerkraut
- Broad beans (fava beans)
- Any overripe vegetables.

Fruit

- Any overripe fruit.

Beverages

- Red wine.

The following diet removes the above-mentioned foods, but also excludes foods with lower levels of tyramine for people who are sensitive to tyramine for reasons other than taking medications.

Tyramine Restricted Diet

Type of Food	Foods Allowed	Foods Restricted
Milk and Dairy	Plain pasteurized milk Ricotta cheese Plain cream cheese	All other dairy products
Breads and Cereals	Any pure flour or grain Limited amounts of yeast risen breads, including bread, pita, buns, croissants, pizza, English muffins, and crumpets Baking powder leavened products such as biscuits, quick breads, soda bread, scones, and muffins Cookies, pies, etc., made with allowed ingredients	Products made with restricted ingredients Excessive quantities of baked goods with yeast
	Breakfast cereals with allowed foods, including: Puffed rice and wheat Corn flakes Shreddies® Shredded Wheat® Plain oats and oatmeal Plain Cream of Wheat® All plain grains	Others, like muesli and granola with restricted nuts and fruit

	Plain crackers with allowed ingredients:
	  Grissol Melba Toast®
	  RyVita®
	  Rye Krisp®
	  Wasa® Light or Golden Crackers
	All homemade crackers with allowed ingredients
	Plain pasta
	Plain rice and wild rice
	General Foods Minute Rice®
	Rice and pasta dishes with allowed ingredients
		Others with restricted ingredients
		
		All packaged rice and pasta meals with "flavor packets"

Tyramine Restricted Diet

Type of Food	Foods Allowed	Foods Restricted
Vegetables	All pure fresh and frozen vegetables and juices except those listed opposite	Any over-ripe vegetables Any pickled vegetables Avocado Broad beans Green peas Potato Sauerkraut Spinach Sweet potato Tomato All prepared vegetables with restricted ingredients Most commercial salad dressings
Fruit	All pure fresh and frozen fruit and juices, except those listed opposite Fruit dishes made with allowed ingredients	Any over-ripe fruit Banana Plums Prunes Raisins Raspberries Fruit dishes, jams, juices with restricted ingredients

Meat, Poultry, and Fish	All pure, freshly cooked meat, poultry, or fish, except those listed opposite	Any leftover meat, poultry, or fish, and foods containing them
		Dry fermented sausages:
		  Bologna
		  Pepperoni
		  Salami
		Oysters
		Smoked or pickled fish or fish roe (eggs)
		Smoked salmon
		Pickled herring
		Lox
		Caviar

Eggs	All plain eggs	All prepared with restricted foods

Tyramine Restricted Diet

Type of Food	Foods Allowed	Foods Restricted

Legumes	All plain legumes except those listed opposite
	Pure peanut butter
		Soy beans, tofu
		Fermented soy products:
		  Soy sauce
		  Fermented bean curd
		  Soybean paste
		Shrimp paste
		Chili soybean paste

Nuts and Seeds	All plain nuts and seeds except those listed opposite	Walnuts Pecans
Fats and Oils	Pure butter Margarine Pure vegetable oils Homemade salad dressing with allowed ingredients Lard and meat drippings Homemade gravy	Commercial salad dressings with restricted ingredients Commercial gravy
Spices and Herbs	All fresh, frozen, or dried herbs and spices	Seasoning packets Commercial packaged foods labeled with "spices" or "flavoring"
Sweets and Sweeteners	Sugar, honey, molasses Maple syrup, corn syrup Icing sugar Pure jams, jellies, marmalades and conserves made with allowed ingredients Plain artificial sweeteners Homemade sweets with allowed ingredients	Chocolate Cocoa beans Cocoa Spreads with restricted ingredients

Other	Baking powder
	Baking soda
	Cream of Tartar
	Plain gelatin
	Homemade relishes with allowed ingredients
	Small amounts of baker's yeast
		All vinegar
		Flavored gelatin
		Prepared pickles and relishes with vinegar
		Yeast and meat extracts:
		  Bovril®
		  Marmite®
		  Oxo®
		  Vegemite®
		  Brewer's yeast
		  Nutritional yeast

Tyramine Restricted Diet

Type of Food	Foods Allowed	Foods Restricted
Beverages	Plain milk Pure juices of allowed fruits and vegetables Plain and carbonated drinks Tea, herbal tea Coffee	Other dairy drinks Fruit drinks, and cocktails with restricted ingredients Cola drinks Cider Beer, including non-alcoholic beer Wine (especially red) Vermouth
Note:	Some alcoholic drinks tested had no detectable tyramine. These include whiskey, gin, and vodka, but not all brands have been tested. The recommendation is to eliminate all alcoholic beverages to see if symptoms will subside with their removal.	

Histamine Sensitivity

Histamine is an important physiological chemical present in plasma and other tissues. It is manufactured and stored in a number of cells throughout the body, particularly mast cells, which occur most commonly in mucous tissue. Levels of circulating histamine fluctuate throughout the day in a specific type of rhythmic variation.[1]

Physiological Role of Histamine

Histamine plays important regulatory roles in the immune response, the permeability of blood vessels, muscle contraction, and gastric acid secretion. It is a key mediator in inflammation, which is the mechanism by which the immune system protects the body from invasion by infective microorganisms and other threatening events such as trauma.

Histamine is the only proven mediator of pruritus (itching).[1] In addition, by increasing vascular permeability, histamine promotes fluid movement from the blood vessels into the surrounding tissue, thus causing swelling. It can also mediate vasodilation, causing symptoms such as hypotension (decreased blood pressure) and tachycardia (increased pulse rate).[2]

In Type I hypersensitivity (IgE mediated reactions) vast quantities of histamine are released from mast cells to provide one of the most important mediators of the swelling, itching, reddening, and increased vascular permeability that are characteristic symptoms of allergy. Events other than Type I hypersensitivity can also cause the release of histamine from mast cells.[3] Some foods and food additives have been shown to have this effect in the absence of allergy.[4]

Symptoms Associated with Excess Histamine

Symptoms occur when the rate of histamine release increases and the amount of circulating histamine exceeds the capacity of the enzyme systems that catabolize histamine. Excessively high levels of histamine result. Symptoms commonly experienced are:

- urticaria (hives)
- angioedema (swelling), especially of facial tissues
- rhinitis and rhinorrhea (stuffy, runny nose)
- conjunctivitis (irritated, watery, reddened eyes)
- itchiness, especially of eyes, nose, ears, skin.

Histamine has also been implicated as an important mediator in certain types of headaches that are thought to differ from migraine[5] and tend to be located to one side of the head and face.

A histamine restricted diet can prove beneficial in reducing total body histamine in conditions where the cause of symptoms is unknown but their nature suggests that histamine is the principle mediator. Conditions that have responded well are idiopathic urticaria, angioedema, chronic itching, and some headaches.

A limited time trial (four weeks is adequate) of food restrictions is warranted in persons for whom all other treatment modalities have been of little value. A histamine restricted diet for controlling extrinsic histamine is given in *Therapeutic Diets for Angioedema / Urticaria*, (see page 309).

Food Sources of Histamine

Histamine occurs in food as a result of microbial enzymes converting the amino acid histidine (present in all proteins) to histamine. All foods subjected to microbial fermentation in the manufacturing process contain histamine. Included in this category are cheeses, fermented soy products, other fermented foods (e.g., sauerkraut), alcoholic beverages, and vinegars.

Foods exposed to microbial contamination also contain histamine in levels determined by the extent and rate of action of the microbes. Histamine levels reach a reactive level long before any signs of spoilage occur in the food. This characteristic has important implications in fin fish, where bacteria in the gut are particularly active in converting histidine to histamine. The longer the fish remains ungutted, the higher the level of histamine in the flesh.

Some foods such as eggplant (aubergine) and spinach contain high levels of histamine naturally.[6] In addition, a number of food additives such as azo dyes[3] and preservatives mediate the release of histamine.

Some of these chemicals such as benzoates[7] occur naturally in foods, especially fruits, and may have the same effect as the food additive in releasing histamine.

The histamine restricted diet excludes all foods known to contain high levels of histamine or to contain chemicals that can promote the physiological release of histamine.

References

1.   Falus, A. *Histamine and Inflammation*. R.G. Landes Company, Austin, 1994.

2.   Zietz, H.J. Pharmacologic properties of foods. In: Metcalfe, D.D., Sampson, H.A. and Simon, R.A. (Eds), *Food Allergy: Adverse Reactions to Foods and Food Additives*. Blackwell Scientific Publications, Oxford, London, 1991. 311-318.

3.   Finn, R. Pharmacological actions of foods. In: Brostoff, J. And Challacombe, S.J. (Eds), *Food Allergy and Intolerance*. Baillière Tindall, London, 1987. 375-400.

4.   Schachter, M., and Talesnik, J. The release of histamine by egg white in non-sensitized animals. J. Physiol. 1952 118:258-263.

5.   Mansfield, L. The role of food allergy in migraine: A review. Ann. Allergy. 1987 58:313-317.

6.   Feldman, J.M. Histaminuria from histamine-rich foods. Arch. Int. Med. 1983 143:2099-2102.

7.   Jacobsen, D.W. Adverse reactions to benzoates and parabens. In: Metcalfe, D.D., Sampson, H.A., Simon, R.A. (Eds), *Food Allergy: Adverse Reactions to Foods and Food Additives*. Blackwell Scientific Publications, Oxford, London, 1991. 276-287.

Method: Histamine Restricted Diet

This diet excludes all:

- Foods with naturally high levels of histamine
- Fermented foods
- Artificial food coloring, especially tartrazine
- Benzoates including food sources of benzoates, benzoic acid, and sodium benzoate
- Butylated hydroxyanisole (BHA) and butylated hydoxytoluene (BHT)

Histamine Restricted Diet

Type of Food	Foods Allowed	Foods Restricted
Milk and Dairy	Plain milk	All prepared dairy products made with restricted ingredients All cheese All yogurt Buttermilk
Breads and Cereals	Any pure *unbleached* flour or grain Any plain fresh bread, buns, biscuits, pizza dough with allowed ingredients Homemade or purchased baked cookies, pies, etc., made with allowed ingredients	Products made with: Anise Artificial colors Artificial flavors Bleached flour Cheese Chocolate Cinnamon Cloves Cocoa Margarine Preservatives Restricted fruit Some jams, jellies Any food made with or cooked in oils with hydrolyzed lecithin, BHA, BHT Commercial pie, pastry, and fillings Baking mixes Dry dessert mixes
	Breakfast cereals with allowed foods, including: All plain grains Plain oats and oatmeal Plain Cream of Wheat® Puffed rice and wheat	All others

Histamine Restricted Diet

Type of Food	Foods Allowed	Foods Restricted
	Plain crackers with allowed ingredients: Grissol Melba Toast® RyVita® Rye Krisp® Wasa® Light or Golden Crackers	All others
	Plain pasta Plain rice and wild rice General Foods Minute Rice® Rice and pasta dishes with allowed ingredients	All packaged rice and pasta meals All homemade crackers
Vegetables	All pure fresh and frozen vegetables and juices except those listed opposite	Eggplant (Aubergine) Pumpkin Sauerkraut Spinach Tomato All vegetables prepared with restricted ingredients
Fruit	Apple Banana Cantaloupe (rock melon) Figs Grapefruit Grapes Honeydew Kiwi Lemon Lime Mango Pear Rhubarb Watermelon Fruit dishes made with allowed ingredients	Apricot Cherry Cranberry Currant Date Loganberry Nectarine Orange Papaya (pawpaw) Peach Pineapple Prunes Plums Raisins Raspberries Strawberries Fruit dishes, jams, juices, made with restricted ingredients
Meat, Poultry, and Fish	All pure, freshly cooked meat or poultry	All fish and shellfish All processed meat All leftover cooked meat
Eggs	All plain, cooked egg	All prepared with restricted foods Raw egg white (as in some eggnog, hollandaise sauce, milk shakes)

Histamine Restricted Diet

Type of Food	Foods Allowed	Foods Restricted
Legumes	All plain legumes except those listed opposite Pure peanut butter	Soy beans Red beans
Nuts and Seeds	All plain nuts and seeds	All with restricted ingredients
Fats and Oils	Pure butter Pure vegetable oil Homemade salad dressing with allowed ingredients Lard and meat drippings Homemade gravy	All fats and oils with color and/or preservatives Hydrolyzed lecithin Margarine Prepared salad dressings with restricted ingredients Prepared gravy
Spices and Herbs	All fresh, frozen or dried herbs and spices except those listed opposite	Anise Cinnamon Cloves Curry powder Hot paprika (cayenne) Nutmeg Seasoning packets with restricted ingredients Foods labeled "with spices"
Sweeteners	Sugar, honey, molasses Maple syrup, corn syrup Icing sugar Pure jams, jellies, marmalade and conserves made with allowed ingredients Plain artificial sweeteners Homemade sweets with allowed ingredients	Flavored syrups Prepared dessert fillings Prepared icings/frostings Spreads with restricted ingredients Cake decorations Confectionary Commercial candies
Other	Baking powder Baking soda Cream of Tartar Plain gelatin Homemade relishes with allowed ingredients	All chocolate and cocoa Flavored gelatin Mincemeat Prepared relishes and olives Soy sauce Miso Commercial ketchup Gherkin pickles Most commercial salad dressings

Histamine Restricted Diet

Type of Food	Foods Allowed	Foods Restricted
Beverages	Plain milk Pure juices of allowed fruits and vegetables Plain and carbonated mineral water Coffee Alcohol: plain vodka, gin and white rum	Flavored milks Fruit drinks and cocktails with restricted ingredients All other carbonated drinks Flavored coffee All tea All drinks with "flavor" or "spices" Beer, wine, and cider All other alcoholic beverages

Cosmetics

The following may contain benzoates, check labels:

Eye cream

Hair dyes

Hair sprays

Other skin creams

Perfumes

Soups

Sun screens

Vanishing cream

Other cosmetics

Medications and Vitamin Supplements

Tartrazine is in some medications (both prescription and non-prescription), and some vitamin supplements. Essential medications should be tartrazine-free. Pharmacies keep a list of manufacturers who produce tartrazine-free products. Some toiletries and cosmetics may cause contact dermatitis.

18

Nickel Allergy

Nickel Allergy and Foods Containing Nickel

Nickel is a well known cause of contact dermatitis in nickel sensitive persons, inducing a reaction wherever it is in close contact with the skin or a mucous membrane for a period of time. This response is known as a cell-mediated immune reaction (Type IV hypersensitivity reaction).[1] The nickel induces local T-cell lymphocytes to produce cytotoxic cytokines that cause the itching, reddening, and scaling of contact dermatitis.

Food allergy caused by nickel was first suspected when dermatologists noticed that some people exhibited symptoms of dermatitis on skin surfaces that were not in contact with any known allergen. These dermatologists suspected that the allergenic source might be in something ingested and looked for sources of known contact allergens, such as nickel, in commonly eaten foods.[2] They noticed that sometimes the nickel in food is not a natural component but is introduced during processing, for example, from metal containers or cooking and processing utensils.

Management of Nickel Allergy

Clinical studies suggest that some people who are sensitive to nickel benefit from avoiding food sources of nickel. Opinions differ on what constitutes a nickel restricted diet. In one research study, an oral dose of nickel (as nickel sulphate) as low as 0.6 mg produced a positive reaction in some nickel sensitive people.[3] Another report indicated that 2.5 mg of nickel was required to induce a flare-up.[4]

Levels of nickel required to induce a reaction have varied widely in different studies. It is difficult to determine a safe level of dietary nickel for people sensitive to nickel.[5]

The level of nickel in foods varies with the variety of the plant species and with the nickel content of the soil in which the plant was grown. The level of nickel in an aquatic environment[4,6,7] affects the nickel level in seafood. Food processing can increase the nickel in a food product. For example, minute traces of nickel from metal grinders used in milling flour can increase the nickel in flour considerably. Often dietary nickel is not the sole cause of the dermatitis. In these cases, nickel avoidance may improve the situation but does not eradicate the symptoms.

Humans require a minute amount of dietary nickel for essential metabolic processes.[8] For the adult, the US RDA (Recommended Dietary Allowance) for nickel is 50 µg daily. (The Canadian Dietary standard does not include a recommendation for nickel.) The richest sources of dietary nickel are nuts, dried peas and beans, whole grains, and chocolate.

Relationship Between Nickel and Iron

Most ingested nickel remains unabsorbed and is excreted in the feces. Usually less than 10% of the nickel in food is absorbed,[4] but this amount increases in persons deficient in iron and lactating mothers. Nickel and iron use the same transport system to cross the intestinal mucosa, so, if iron is being transported, nickel is excluded. Accordingly, individuals who are sensitive to nickel should be advised to include iron rich foods in their diet.

Nickel Contact Dermatitis and Oral Tolerance

The most common cause of nickel dermatitis is direct contact objects containing nickel.[1,9] Persons who have tested positive for nickel using a patch test (on skin of the forearm or back) should avoid contact with all objects containing the metal.

A recent study indicated that reduction in the severity of contact dermatitis related to nickel, or prevention of symptoms, can be achieved by oral exposure to nickel, for example, in the form of a dental appliance.[10]

According to other studies, oral exposure to nickel can worsen established nickel contact dermatitis initially, but prolonged exposure can reduce the clinical symptoms.[11]

The subject of nickel contact dermatitis, nickel allergy, and achievement of tolerance is confusing from a practical point of view because of the extremely complex series of events that occur in the immune system. Nickel contact dermatitis is mediated by a Type IV hypersensitivity reaction. Nickel allergy is possibly a Type I hypersensitivity.[12] The precise mechanism that allows the immune system to achieve tolerance, especially to foods, is unclear at present.[13]

Nickel Contact Dermatitis

The most common cause of nickel dermatitis is direct contact with nickel-containing objects, such as those listed below:

Bobby pins	Metal pots and pans
Buckles	Metal shoe eyelets
Bullets	Metal pens and clips
Clasps	Metal objects held in mouth
Coins	Needles
Curlers	Paper clips
Dental instruments	Pins
Detergents	Safety pins
Door handles	Screws, etc. in orthopaedic devices
Eyeglass frames	Snap fasteners
Hairpins	Stainless steel cutlery
Hook-and-eye fasteners	Staples
Jewelry	Thimbles
Keys	Wire supports in bras
Knitting needles	Zippers
Medals	

Contact with chromium plated objects should be avoided.

Nail polish with a metal mixing ball in the container should be avoided, as the solvents in the polish can leach out the nickel.

The site of the reactions will be a good indicator of the source of the nickel.

Enamel coated pots and pans, pans with non-stick coating, glass or microwave-safe plastic containers should be used for cooking.

Nickel Allergy

People suspected of having an allergy to nickel that is exacerbated by the ingestion of foods often try a nickel restricted diet for a limited period of time. Usually 4 to 6 weeks is sufficient to determine the effectiveness of the diet.

Relationship of Dietary Nickel to Contact Dermatitis

Clinical studies have indicated that up to half of nickel sensitive persons may benefit from a nickel restricted diet.

The nickel levels in foods, especially acidic foods, will increase when the foods are canned in metal containers. In Table 18-1, common foods are listed in the order of decreasing nickel content, according to composition data from two main sources.[6,7] Because of the variability in nickel content, different analytical reports cite different values and therefore some foods appear twice, at different places in the table.

Table 18-1: Level of Nickel in Common Foods

	Nickel µg per g	Serving Size	Weight	Nickel µg per serving
Dairy Products				
Butter[7]	0.10	1 tsp	5 g	0.50
Cheese[7]	0.10	1 oz	28 g	2.80
Margarine[7]	0.34	1 tsp	5 g	1.70
Milk, skim[7]	< 0.02	½ cup	129 g	< 2.58
Milk, whole[7]	< 0.02	½ cup	129 g	< 2.58
Milk, dried[7]	< 0.09	⅓ cup	25 g	< 2.25
Yogurt[7]	< 0.01	½ cup	122 g	< 1.22
Fruit				
Apples[6,7]	0.009 - 0.07	1 medium	138 g	1.24-9.66
Bananas[6,7]	0.02 - 0.32	1 medium	114 g	2.28-36.48
Black currants[6]	0.16	½ cup	72 g	11.52
Blueberries[6]	0.065	½ cup	77 g	5.01
Currants[7]	0.06	½ cup	72 g	4.32
Fruit juice, canned[7]	< 0.15	½ cup	130 g	< 19.50
Fruit cocktail, canned[7]	0.69	½ cup	130 g	89.70
Fruit juice, bottled[7]	< 0.11	½ cup	130 g	< 14.30
Grapes[7]	0.02	½ cup	135 g	2.70
Orange[7]	0.03	1 medium	131 g	3.93
Pears[6,7]	0.068-0.26	1 medium	169 g	11.49-43.94
Plums[7]	0.12	2 medium	132 g	15.84
Raisins[7]	0.03	¼ cup	44 g	1.32
Raspberries[6]	0.21	½ cup raw	65 g	13.65
Rhubarb[7]	0.13	½ cup raw	65 g	8.45

Table 18-1: Level of Nickel in Common Foods

	Nickel µg per g	Serving Size	Weight	Nickel µg per serving
Strawberries[7]	0.05	½ cup raw	79 g	3.95

Note: The stated level of nickel in **apples** is the mean for several varieties.
All fruit is raw, unless otherwise stated.
Where the same fruit appears with different nickel levels, it indicates different independent analysis reports

Grains				
Bread, white[7]	< 0.06	1 slice	28 g	< 1.68
Bread, whole wheat[6,7]	0.19	1 slice	25 g	4.75
Buckwheat[6,7]	2.0-2.2	½ cup	56 g	112.0-123.20
Flour, white, plain[7]	< 0.06	½ cup	67 g	< 4.02
Flour, whole wheat[7]	0.165	½ cup	64 g	10.56
Flour, white, self-rising[7]	< 0.09	½ cup	67 g	< 6.03
Oatmeal[7]	1.76	½ cup	124 g	218.24
Oats, raw[7]	2.3	½ cup	43 g	98.90
Rice[7]	0.07	½ cup cooked	94 g	6.58
Wheat bran[6]	0.53	1 tbsp	3 g	1.59
Wheat germ[7]	1.0	1 tbsp	7 g	7.00
Sugar and Chocolate				
Chocolate, bitter[6]	2.2	1 oz	28 g	61.60
Milk Chocolate[6]	0.34	1 oz	28 g	9.52
Sugar, brown[7]	< 0.23	1 tbsp	9 g	< 2.07
Sugar, white[7]	< 0.13	1 tbsp	13 g	< 1.69
Meat and Poultry				
Beef kidney[6,7]	0.015-0.25	1 serving	89 g	1.34-22.25
Beef[6,7]	0.011-0.02	1 medium patty, cooked	88 g	0.97-1.76
Chicken[7]	0.11	½ breast, cooked	86 g	9.46

Table 18-1: Level of Nickel in Common Foods

	Nickel µg per g	Serving Size	Weight	Nickel µg per serving
Egg[7]	0.05	1 large	50 g	2.50
Lamb[7]	< 0.09	2 slices	87 g	< 7.83
Liver, beef, lamb, pork[6,7]	0.01-0.1	1 serving	86 g	0.86-8.60
Pork kidney[6]	0.012	1 serving	89 g	1.07
Pork[6,7]	0.01-0.06	2 slices	88 g	0.88-5.28
Fish				
Arctic char[6]	< 0.008	1 serving	93 g	< 0.74
Chilean hake[6]	< 0.01	1 serving	93 g	< 0.93
Cod[6]	0.021	1 serving	88 g	1.85
Fish, unspecified species[7]	0.7	1 serving	92 g	64.40
Fish pastes, unspecified[7]	0.53	1 tbsp	14 g	7.42
Pike/perch[6]	0.01	1 serving	93 g	< 0.93
Trout[6]	0.017	1 serving	93 g	1.58
Whitefish[6]	< 0.01	1 serving	92 g	< 0.92
Vegetables				
Asparagus[6]	0.42	4 spears	60 g	25.20
Beans, frozen and fresh[7]	0.40	½ cup	66 g	26.40
Broccoli[7]	0.28	½ cup cooked	82 g	22.96
Brussels sprouts[7]	0.16	½ cup boiled	83 g	13.28
Cabbage[7]	0.17	½ cup shredded, raw	37 g	6.29
Carrots[6,7]	0.04-0.054	1 medium	72 g	2.88-3.89
Cauliflower[7]	0.30	½ cup pieces cooked	66 g	19.80
Celery[6]	0.06	½ cup diced, raw	64 g	3.84

Table 18-1: Level of Nickel in Common Foods

	Nickel µg per g	Serving Size	Weight	Nickel µg per serving
Chinese cabbage[6]	0.046	½ cup cooked	79 g	3.63
Cucumber[7]	0.04	½ cup sliced	56 g	2.24
Endive[7]	0.31	1 cup raw	60 g	18.60
Green peas[6]	0.076	½ cup, raw	85 g	6.46
Kale[7]	0.20	½ cup cooked	79 g	15.80
Leeks[7]	0.11	½ cup cooked	111 g	12.21
Lettuce[6]	0.27	1 cup raw shredded	60 g	1.62
Mushrooms[7]	0.16	½ cup cooked	83 g	13.28
Onions[7]	0.08	½ cup cooked	111 g	8.88
Peas, canned[7]	0.28	½ cup cooked	90 g	22.68
Potatoes[6,7]	0.048-0.14	1 baked, medium	150 g	7.20-21.0
Spinach[7]	0.52	1 cup chopped, raw	59 g	30.68
Tomatoes[7]	0.07	1 medium	123 g	8.61
Vegetables, canned, mixed[7]	< 0.31	½ cup cooked	86 g	< 26.66
Nuts and Seeds				
Flaxseed[6]	1.9	1 tbsp	12 g	22.80
Peanuts[7]	2.8	¼ cup	39 g	109.20
Poppy seeds[6]	1.2-1.3	1 tsp	3 g	3.60-3.90
Walnuts[7]	3.6	2 tbsp chopped	12 g	43.20
Dried Peas and Beans				
Brown beans[6]	1.7	½ cup cooked, drained	90 g	153.00
Chick peas[6]	1.60	½ cup boiled, drained	87 g	139.20
Dried legumes[7]	1.7	½ cup cooked, drained	95	161.50

Table 18-1: Level of Nickel in Common Foods

	Nickel µg per g	Serving Size	Weight	Nickel µg per serving
Green lentils[6]	3.0	½ cup cooked, drained	105 g	315.00
Soy beans[6]	2.9	½ cup cooked drained	91 g	263.90
Yellow split peas[6]	0.93	½ cup cooked	104 g	96.72
Seasonings				
Curry Powder[7]	1.7	1 tsp	2 g	3.40
Dried Soup Powder[7]	1.10	1 package	39 g	42.90
Herbs mixed[7]	< 2.9	1 tsp	1 g	< 2.90
Mustard powder[7]	< 0.5	1 tsp	2 g	< 1.00
Spices mixed[7]	1.4	1 tsp	2 g	2.80
Stock Cube[7]	0.6	1 cube	5 g	3.00
Beverages and Beverage Powders				
Cocoa powder[7]	9.8	1 tbsp	22 g	215.60
Coffee, instant[7]	1.2	2 tsp	2 g	2.40
Coffee, ground[7]	0.8	2 tsp	2 g	1.60
Soft drink, concentrate, bottled[7]	0.05	½ cup	125 g	6.25
Tea, instant[7]	15.5	2 tsp	2 g	31.00

References

1.   Fisher, A.A. *Contact Dermatitis*. Lea and Febiger, Philadelphia, 1978.

2.   Veien, N. Dietary treatment of nickel dermatitis. Acta Dermatol. Venereol. 1985 <u>65</u>:138-142.

3.   Cronin, E., de Michiel, A., Brown, S.S. Oral nickel challenge in nickel-sensitive women with hand eczema. Ann. Clin. Lab. Sci. 1981 <u>11</u>:91 (abstract).

4.   Veien, N.K. and Menne, T. Nickel contact allergy and a nickel-restricted diet. Seminars in Dermatology 1990 <u>9</u>(3):197-205.

5.   Neilsen, F.H. Ultratrace minerals In: Shils, M.E., and Young, V.R. *Modern Nutrition in Health and Disease*, Seventh Edition, Lea and Febiger, Philadelphia, 1988. 285-286.

6.   Jorhem, L. And Sundström, B. Levels of lead, cadmium, zinc, copper, nickel, chromium, manganese and cobalt in foods on the Swedish market, 1983-1990. J. Food Comp. Anal. 1993 <u>6</u>:233-241.

7.   Booth, J. Nickel in the diet and its role in allergic dermatitis. J. Human Nutr. Dietetics 1990 <u>3</u>:233-243.

8.   Root, E.J. Current perspectives on nickel. Nutrition Today 1990 (May/June):12-15.

9.   Thomson, N.C., Kirkwood, E.M., and Lever, R.S. *Handbook of Clinical Allergy*. Blackwell Scientific Publications, Oxford, London, 1990. 197-200.

10. Van Hoogstraten, I.M.W., Andersen, K.E., Von Blomberg, B.M.E., *et al*. Reduced frequency of nickel allergy upon oral contact at early age. Clin. Exper. Immunol. 1991 <u>85</u>:441-445.

11. Santucci, B., Cristaudo, A., Canmistraci, C., and Picardo, M. Nickel sensitivity: effects of prolonged oral intake of the element. Contact Dermatitis 1988 <u>19</u>:202-205.

12. Estlander, T., Kanerva, L., Tupsela, O., Keskinen, H., and Jolanski, R. Immediate and delayed allergy to nickel with contact urticaria, rhinitis, asthma and contact dermatitis. Clin. Exper. Allergy 1993 <u>23</u>:306-310.

13. Sosroseno, W. A review of the mechanisms of oral tolerance and immunotherapy. J. Roy. Soc. Med. 1995 <u>88</u>(1):14-17.

Method: Nickel Restricted Diet

Avoid all foods canned in metal containers.

Nickel Restricted Diet

Type of Food	Foods Allowed	Foods Restricted

Milk and Dairy	All, including:
	  All cheeses
	  Butter
	  Cream, sour cream
	  Milk and buttermilk
	  Yogurt
		Dairy products made with restricted ingredients, such as raspberry yogurt

Breads and Cereals	Corn and popcorn Rice and rice bran Rye and rye bread White (wheat) bread in moderation White flour in moderation	Buckwheat Multigrain breads Oats and oatmeal Wheat bran Wheat germ Whole wheat bread

	Crackers and snacks:
	  Corn chips and popcorn
	  Corn taco chips
	  Corn nachos
	  Potato chips
	  Pure rye crisp crackers
	  Rice cakes and crackers
	  White flour crackers in moderation
		Crackers, etc. with restricted grains

	Cereals:
	  Corn flakes
	  Corn bran cereal
	  Cream of Rice®
	  Puffed Millet
	  Puffed Rice
	  Rice Krispies®
		Multigrain cereals
		Cereals with restricted grains

	Pasta:
	  Corn pasta
	  Rice vermicelli/noodles
	  White (wheat) pasta in moderation
	  Wild rice pasta
		Canned pasta
		Legume pasta such as mung bean pasta
		Whole wheat pasta

Eggs	All	Egg dishes prepared with restricted ingredients

Nickel Restricted Diet

Type of Food	Foods Allowed	Foods Restricted
Vegetables	All fresh or frozen vegetables and their juices except those listed opposite	Canned vegetables Asparagus Bean sprouts Beans (fresh and frozen) Broccoli Green peas Kale Spinach
Fruit	All fresh or frozen fruits and their juices except those listed opposite	Canned fruit and juice Banana Figs Pear Pineapple Plums, prunes Raspberries

Meat, Poultry, and Fish	Meat from all species
	Chicken, turkey, and all other poultry
	All fish with fins and scales
	Processed meats without cereal fillers/coating
		Canned meat, poultry or fish
		All shellfish, including:
		    Clams
		    Crab
		    Lobster
		    Mussels
		    Oysters
		    Prawns
		    Shrimp
		Processed meats with fillers, extenders, coatings

Legumes	None	All, including:
		    All beans
		    Carob
		    Chickpeas (garbanzos)
		    Green/yellow split peas
		    Lentils
		    Licorice
		    Peanut
		    Soy beans and products such as soy sauce, tofu

Spices and Herbs	All in moderation	None

Nickel Restricted Diet

Type of Food	Foods Allowed	Foods Restricted

Nuts and Seeds	None	All, including:
		   Almond
		   Hazelnut
		   Walnut
		   All other nuts
		   Alfalfa seed
		   Canola seed
		   Flax seed
		   Poppy seed
		   Sesame seed
		   Sunflower seed

Fats and Oils	Butter and cream
	Pure corn and olive oil
	Lard and meat drippings
	Homemade salad dressings
	   with allowed ingredients
	Gravy
		Margarine
		Other oils
		Shortening
		Most commercial salad
		   dressings

Sweets and Sweeteners	All not listed opposite
	White and brown sugar
	Honey, molasses
	Pure jams and jellies made
	   with allowed fruits
	Candy with allowed
	   ingredients (e.g., mints)
		Chocolate and cocoa
		Licorice
		Almond paste (marzipan)
		Any candy or candy bars
		   containing nuts or seeds

Beverages	Plain milk and buttermilk
	Fruit juices and drinks made
	   with allowed fruits
	Regular and herbal tea
	Coffee
	Mineral water
	Carbonated beverages
	Beer, wine and distilled
	   alcoholic beverages
		Chocolate milk
		Canned drinks
		Restricted fruit drinks
		Cereal beverages
		All alcoholic beverages with
		   restricted foods

Other	Vitamin and mineral
	   supplements without nickel
		Vitamin and mineral
		   supplements with nickel

NOTE: The above table is based on a compilation of data from several different sources. It is not possible to provide a reliable scale of the level of nickel in foods, because levels of the metal vary in foods for a number of reasons including: The species or variety of plant from which the food was derived.
- The amount of nickel in the soil in which the plant was grown.
- In the case of fish, the amount of nickel in the water from which the fish was harvested. In the case of flours, how much nickel was introduced into the flour during the process of milling (stone ground flours would avoid this source of metal, but nickel would be present to varying levels in the grain itself, depending on the species and the soil in which it was grown).

19

Tartrazine and Other Food Coloring Agents

Color is one of the most important aspects of food presentation. Unless foods are the right color, they are unacceptable to many people. As a result, various colors are added to manufactured foods to enhance their market appeal and consumption.

In the USA, the Department of Agriculture (FDA) allows ten artificial colors derived from coal tar under the Food Dye and Coloring Act (FD&C).[1] Many other countries including Canada have similar regulations.

Table 19-1: Artificial Food Coloring Agents in General Use (USA)

FDA Name	Common Name	Chemical Class
FD&C Yellow #5	Tartrazine	Pyrazalone
FD&C Yellow #6	Sunset Yellow	Monoazo
FD&C Red #3	Erthyrosine	Xanthine
FD&C Red #4	Ponceau	Monoazo
FD&C Red #40	Allura Red	Monoazo
FD&C Citrus Red #2	Citrus Red #2	Monoazo
Orange B	Orange B	Monoazo
FD&C Blue #1	Brilliant Blue	Triphenylmethane
FD&C Blue #2	Indigotine	Indigoid
FD&C Green #3	Fast Green	Triphenylmethane

Citrus Red #2 is restricted to coloring orange skins in fruit not used for manufacture of food products (such as orange juice).

Orange B is similar in chemical structure to amaranth, which is not allowed in the USA but is permitted for use in Canada. Orange B is restricted to the casings and surfaces of frankfurters and sausages. However, because of health risks, the sole manufacturer in the USA has ceased production of this dye.

In Canada, a number of colors are listed as permitted for use in foods.[2] These include the following natural and artificial food dyes:

Alkanet	Erythrosine*
Allura Red*	Ethyl beta-apo-8' carotenoate
Aluminum metal	Fast Green FCF*
Amaranth	Indigotine*
Annatto	Iron oxide
Anthocyanin	Orchil
Beet red	Paprika
Beta-apo-8'-carotenal	Ponceau SX*
Brilliant blue FCF*	Riboflavin (Vitamin B2)
Canthaxanthine	Saffron
Caramel	Saunderswood
Carbon black	Silver metal
Carotene	Sunset yellow FCF*
Charcoal	Tartrazine*
Chlorophyll	Titanium dioxide
Citrus Red #2*	Turmeric
Cochineal	Xanthophyll

(* Corresponds to FD&C list above)

Most of the colors listed above are considered safe and have not been cited as a cause of adverse reactions.[3] However, tartrazine and some other azo dyes have been implicated in adverse reactions.[4] As a result, regulations in the USA require that tartrazine added to foods or medications be listed separately on the product label. In Canada, at present, this listing is voluntary. Food manufacturers are not required to give the chemical names or common names of the individual artificial colors used in a food product, except for tartrazine in the USA. As a result, colors usually appear on labels as "artificial color" or simply "color".

Table 19-2: Examples of the Use of Colors in Foods[5]

Color Name	Commonly Added to
Annatto	Cheese, butter, baked goods
Beet powder	Frostings, soft drinks
Caramel	Confectionery
Cochineal	Beverages
FD&C Green #3	Mint jelly
FD&C Red #3	Canned fruit cocktail
Titanium oxide	White candy, Italian cheeses
Turmeric	Pickles, sauces

Allergic Conditions Caused by Tartrazine in Sensitive People

Tartrazine (FD&C #5) can cause symptoms of an allergic reaction. Some people who are sensitive to acetylsalicylic acid (ASA, Aspirin®) also experience an adverse reaction to tartrazine. It is unclear whether dietary salicylates, which are naturally present in a large number of foods (primarily fruits and vegetables), also are involved in this cross reactivity. Other azo dyes have also been implicated in adverse reactions.[4]

Mechanism of Action

Evidence indicates that tartrazine may initiate the release of histamine from mast cells. Since tartrazine-induced symptoms are similar to those induced by salicylic acid, tartrazine may have an inhibitory effect on the cyclooxygenase pathway for converting arachidonic acid to prostanoids. This mechanism of action has not been proven.

Symptoms of Tartrazine Sensitivity

Symptoms reported to be caused or exacerbated by tartrazine and other azo dyes are:

Asthma

Urticaria (hives)

Nausea

Migraine headaches

Allergic vasculitis (purpura)

Hyperkinesis (hyperactivity disorder)

Contact dermatitis

At present, there are no double blind placebo controlled trials proving that any of these conditions is caused by tartrazine.[4]

References

1.   Francis, J.F. Pigments and other colorants. In: Fennema, O.R. (Ed) *Food Chemistry*, Second Edition. Marcel Dekker, New York and Basel, 1985. 545-584.

2.   *Additives Pocket Dictionary*. Minister of National Health and Welfare, Health Protection Branch, Department of National Health and Welfare, Ottawa, Canada, K1A 0L2, 1987 (reprinted 1990).

3.   Simon, R.A. Adverse reactions to drug additives. J. Allergy Clin. Immunol. 1984 74:623-630.

4.   Stevenson, D.D. Tartrazine, azo and nonazo dyes. In: Metcalfe, D.D., Sampson, H.A., and Simon, R.A. (Eds), *Food Allergy: Adverse Reactions to Foods and Food Additives*. Blackwell Scientific Publications, Oxford, London, 1991. 267-275.

5.   Lindsay, R.C. Food additives. In: Fennema, O.R. (Ed), *Food Chemistry*, Second Edition. Marcel Dekker, New York and Basel, 1985. 629-687.

Method: Diet Restricted in Tartrazine and Other Food Coloring Agents

Tartrazine in Foods

Although tartrazine is yellow, it is also used to produce other colors such as orange, turquoise, green, maroon, and brown. It is not enough to avoid only yellow colored foods.

Foods Restricted

Any food or medication listing tartrazine as an additive.

Any food described as containing "color" or "artificial color", unless it is specifically labeled "tartrazine-free". This is particularly important for medications.

If it has been established that tartrazine is the only color causing symptoms, General Foods Inc. provides a list of their tartrazine-free products.

Tartrazine in Medications and Supplements

Tartrazine is in some medications (both prescription and non-prescription) and vitamin and mineral supplements.

Essential medications should be tartrazine-free. Pharmacies keep a list of manufacturers who produce tartrazine-free products.

Some toiletries and cosmetics containing colors may cause contact dermatitis.

Caramel

Caramel is made by heating sugar or glucose and adding small quantities of alkali or mineral acid during heating. This process produces the pleasant burnt sugar taste.

Caramel is used as a color and a flavor in many ice creams, baked goods, soft drinks, candies, confectioneries, syrups, and meats.

Some people experience increased bowel movements with soft or liquid stool after eating foods containing caramel. This reaction is thought to be caused by the sulfite ammonia used in the production of caramel.

Tartrazine and Other Food Color Restricted Diet

Type of Food	Foods Allowed	Foods Restricted

Milk and Dairy	Plain milk, buttermilk, cream, sour cream and yogurt
	All plain uncolored cream cheese, cheddar, mozzarella, cottage cheese, Quark®, Parmesan
	Additive-free ice cream
	Butter
		Chocolate flavored milk
		Milkshakes
		Flavored yogurt
		Commercially prepared:
		  Cheese foods
		  Cheese slices
		  Dips
		  Spreads
		Frozen ice cream, sherbet, yogurt, dairy barks, ice milk, dairy treats with color added

Breads and Cereals	Any pure flour or grain Any prepared, additive-free, plain bread, buns, biscuits, pizza dough with allowed ingredients, (bread machines are useful in making additive-free bread products) Homemade or purchased baked cookies, pies, etc, made without additives	Commercial products made with food coloring Commercial icings and frostings Most commercial baked goods Baking mixes

	Breakfast cereals without color added, such as:
	  Homemade granola
	  Oats and oatmeal
	  Plain oat bran
	  Plain Cream of Wheat®
	  Puffed wheat Puffed rice
	  Red River Cereal®
	  Shredded Wheat®
	  Shreddies®
	Some corn flakes
	All plain grains and their flakes
		Commercial breakfast cereals with added color
		
		Flavored instant oatmeal
		
		Flavored instant Cream of Wheat®

	Crackers without color added, such as:
	  Grissol Melba Toast®
	  RyVita Rye Krisp®
	  Wasa Light or Golden Crackers® Homemade crackers
		Crackers with color or flavor added

Tartrazine and Other Food Color Restricted Diet

Type of Food	Foods Allowed	Foods Restricted
	Plain pasta All cereals and pasta dishes without food colors Plain and wild rice General Foods Minute Rice®	Read all labels carefully on all packaged pasta Colored pasta Macaroni and cheese dinners Pasta or rice dinners with color or flavor packets
Vegetables	All pure fresh and frozen vegetables and juices	Vegetable cocktails (V8®) Vegetables in sauces and/or seasoning packets Most pasta sauces unless additive-free Prepared salads with commercial dressing
Fruit	All pure fresh, frozen or canned fruit Pure frozen and canned juices Fruit dishes made without added colors	Fruit cocktail with maraschino cherries Maraschino cherries Prepared fruit drinks, drinks, cocktails, with additives Fruit Rollups® Fruit flavored gelatin (Jell-O®) Fruit dishes and preserves with color
Meat, Poultry, and Fish	All pure fresh, frozen or canned meat, poultry, or fish Processed meat made without added color	Commercially prepared with added color: Fish pastes, fish roe Imitation crab Smoked fish Processed meats with added color Commercial gravies and sauces
Eggs	All	All prepared with ingredients with added color
Legumes	All plain legumes Pure peanut butter without additives	
Nuts and Seeds	All plain nuts and seeds	All with added color

Tartrazine and Other Food Color Restricted Diet

Type of Food	Foods Allowed	Foods Restricted
Fats and Oils	Pure butter Cream Shortening Pure vegetable oils Homemade salad dressings not made with "flavor packages" Lard and meat drippings Homemade gravy	Margarine Commercially prepared salad dressings with added color Commercial sauces and gravies
Spices and Herbs	All pure fresh, frozen, or dried herbs and spices Seasoning salts including turmeric, paprika and saffron	Flavor packets Flavoring extracts
Sweets and Sweeteners	Sugar, honey, molasses Maple syrup, corn syrup Icing sugar Pure jams, jellies, marmalades, and conserves without added color Plain artificial sweeteners Homemade sweets without artificial color	Flavored syrups Prepared dessert fillings Prepared icings Spreads with restricted ingredients Commercial candies Cake decorations and other confectionery Fruit Rollups® Fun Fruits® Fruit peel, citrus peel Glacé fruit
Other	Baking powder Baking soda Cream of Tartar Pure white cider or wine vinegar Baking chocolate Pure cocoa Plain gelatin Homemade pickles, ketchup, and relishes without added color Pure soy sauce without added color	Whipped toppings Topping mixes All vinegars with "flavorings" Chocolate candy Cake sprinkles Flavored gelatin Commercial pickles, relishes, and olives Some soy sauces Commercial ketchup Colored chewing gum Snacks such as Cheese Puffs®

Tartrazine and Other Food Color Restricted Diet

Type of Food	Foods Allowed	Foods Restricted
Beverages	Plain milk and buttermilk Pure juices of fruits and vegetables Plain and carbonated mineral water Plain coffee and tea Beer, wine, plain distilled alcoholic beverages	Flavored milks Fruit drinks, drinks, and cocktails All other carbonated drinks and soft drinks Liqueurs, coolers Drink mixes or pre-mixed drinks Fruit flavored drink powders and concentrates All drinks with "flavor", "spices", or "color" Diet drinks and shakes Meal replacement drinks

20

Sensitivity To Salicylates

The only form of salicylate proven to be allergenic is acetylsalicylic acid[1] or ASA (a drug known as "aspirin" in the USA, although this term is a registered trade name in Canada). Sensitivity to ASA is more common in persons with asthma than in other people. Up to 25% of persons sensitive to acetylsalicylic acid also react adversely to the azo dye tartrazine.[2] It is not known whether the mechanism of action of the two chemicals is similar. Sensitivity to acetylsalicylic acid has also been linked to sensitivities to benzoates and sulfites, but cross-reactivity to these substances has not yet been confirmed by research studies.

Salicylates (but not acetylsalicylic acid) occur naturally in many foods. Research studies have not proven that naturally occurring salicylates cause adverse reactions even in persons sensitive to acetylsalicylic acid. The level of salicylic acid may be the determining factor in salicylate sensitivity. Dietary consumption of salicylate is estimated to be 10 to 200 mg daily, whereas one dose of Aspirin® provides 600 to 650 mg of acetylsalicylic acid.[3]

Sensitivity to acetylsalicylic acid has been implicated in causing urticaria (hives), angioedema (tissue swelling), and in precipitating an asthmatic attack in persons with asthma. However, people with asthma who are sensitive to acetylsalicylic acid can usually ingest the salicylates in foods without difficulty.[2] No controlled research has been undertaken to study the effect of reduction of dietary salicylates on the course of asthma.

Mechanism of Action

Acetylsalicylic acid inhibits the cyclooxygenase pathway of arachidonic acid metabolism,[2] thus reducing the production of certain prostaglandins that mediate the sensation of pain. This reduction accounts for the analgesic properties of Aspirin®. Another result of this inhibition is enhanced production of leukotrienes that mediate the smooth muscle contraction that causes the bronchospasm of asthma. This effect explains why many persons sensitive to acetylsalicylic acid suffer from asthma.

Symptoms Associated with Salicylate Sensitivity

Wheezing, urticaria, and angioedema are reported symptoms of salicylate sensitivity.[2] Some investigators ascribe the hyperactivity experienced by some children to salicylate sensitivity; however, the role of salicylates in the attention deficit hyperactivity disorder has not been proven by controlled studies.[4] Investigations of the role of food components and additives in this disorder are currently in progress.[5] (Refer to Part V for further discussion of several of these disorders.)

Some practitioners in the field of food intolerance believe that, although avoiding foods high in salicylates is unlikely to diminish the symptoms of most persons sensitive to acetylsalicylic acid, a trial on a salicylate restricted diet may benefit those individuals who have a pronounced sensitivity and achieve no relief from other treatment modalities.[6]

Salicylates occur naturally in a large number of foods. The levels of salicylates may vary with the strain and species of the plant. The levels may also be altered by methods of farming, by type and length of storage. Food processing affects levels of salicylates in some foods and beverages.

The main sources of naturally occurring salicylates are fruits and vegetables, herbs, spices and condiments, nuts and seeds.

Pure cereals and grains contain practically no salicylates, with the exception of cornmeal. Other foods with very little or no salicylates are plain dairy products, plain meat, fish, poultry, and eggs.

Salicylates in Medications, Supplements, and Toiletries

Salicylates are in some medications, (both prescription and non-prescription). It is important to avoid:

Acetylsalicylic acid (ASA)
Aspirin ®
Menthol salicylate
Products flavored with mint, wintergreen, and menthol such as toothpaste, mouthwash, lozenges, cigarettes, medications

Read labels carefully on toiletries and cosmetics, such as sun screens and creams.

References

1.   Wright, R., and Robertson, D. Non-immune damage to the gut. In: Brostoff, J., and Challacombe, S.J. (Eds), *Food Allergy and Intolerance*. Baillière Tindall, London, 1987. 248-254.

2.   Nelson, J.K., Moxness, K.E, Jensen, M.D. and Gastineau, C.F. Food Allergy and Intolerance. In: *Mayo Clinic Diet Manual*, Seventh Edition. Mosby, 1994. 97-122.

3.   Virchow, C., Szczekik, A., and Bianco, S. Intolerance to tartrazine in aspirin-induced asthma: results of a multi-centre study. Respiration 1988 53:20-23.

4.   Wender, E.H. The food additive-free diet in the treatment of behaviour disorders: A review. Develop. Behav. Paediatr. 1986 7(1):35-42.

5.   Egger, J., Stolla, A., and McEwan, L.M. Controlled trial of hyposensitization in children with food-induced hyperkinetic syndrome. Lancet 1992 339:1150-1153.

6.   Brostoff, J., and Gamlin, L. *The Complete Guide to Food Allergy and Intolerance.* Crown Publishers, New York, 1991. 60-61.

Table 20-1: Level of Salicylates in Some Common Foods and Beverages

	Salicylates mg/100 g	Serving Size	Weight	Salicylates mg/serving
VEGETABLES, fresh and canned				
Asparagus, fresh	4	½ cup	83 g	3.32
Green pepper, fresh	1.2	1 large	100 g	1.2
Mushroom, canned	1.26	¼ cup	90 g	1.13
Endive, fresh leaves	1.9	10 leaves	50 g	0.95
Eggplant (with peel), fresh	0.88	½ cup	100 g	0.88
Zucchini, fresh	1.04	½ cup	76 g	0.79
Tomato, canned	0.53	½ cup	125 g	0.66
Broccoli, fresh	0.65	1 stalk	100 g	0.65
Squash, baby, fresh	0.63	½ cup	100 g	0.63
Radish, red, small, fresh	1.24	5 small	50 g	0.62
Okra, canned	0.59	8-9 pods	100 g	0.59
Spinach, fresh	0.58	3 ½ oz.	100 g	0.58
Chicory, fresh leaves	1.02	15-20 small	150 g	0.51
Potato, white, fresh, peeled	0.5	1 small	100 g	0.5
Corn, creamed, canned	0.39	½ cup	125 g	0.49
Sweet potato, fresh	0.45	½ cup	100 g	0.45
Parsnip, fresh	0.45	½ cup	100 g	0.45
Cucumber, no peel, fresh	0.78	½ medium	50 g	0.39
Asparagus, canned	0.32	½ cup	100 g	0.32
Mushroom, fresh	0.24	10 small	100 g	0.24
Carrot, fresh	0.23	1 large	100 g	0.23
Corn, niblets, canned	0.26	½ cup	83 g	0.22
Olives, green, canned	1.29	2 medium	13 g	0.17
Spinach, frozen	0.16	½ cup	100 g	0.16
Beans, green, French, fresh	0.11	½ cup	125 g	0.14
Tomato, fresh	0.13	1 small	100 g	0.13
Turnip, fresh	0.16	½ cup	76 g	0.12

Table 20-1: Level of Salicylates in Some Common Foods and Beverages

	Salicylates mg/100 g	Serving Size	Weight	Salicylates mg/serving
Pumpkin, fresh	0.12	2/5 cup	100 g	0.12
Corn, on the cob, fresh	0.12	½ cup	100 g	0.12
Watercress, fresh	0.84	10 sprigs	10 g	0.08
Cabbage, red, fresh	0.08	1 cup shredded	100 g	0.08
Leek, fresh	0.08	3-4 medium	100 g	0.08
Cauliflower, fresh	0.16	½ cup	50 g	0.08
Brussels sprouts, fresh	0.07	8 medium	100 g	0.07
Olives, black, canned	0.34	2 large	20 g	0.07
Peas, green, fresh	0.04	½ cup	67 g	0.03
Onion, fresh	0.16	1 tbsp	10 g	0.02
Shallots, fresh	0.03	1¾ oz	50 g	0.02
Squash, chayote, fresh	0.01	½ medium	100 g	0.01
Cabbage, green, fresh	0	1 cup shredded	100 g	0
Celery, fresh	0	1 stalk	50 g	0
Bamboo shoots, canned	0	1 cup	133 g	0
TOMATO, soup, juice, sauce, paste				
Heinz® tomato sauce	2.28	2/5 cup	100 g	2.48
Heinz® tomato paste	0.54	1 cup	240 g	1.29
Heinz® tomato juice	0.12	½ cup	122 g	0.15
Campbell® tomato soup	0.57	1 tbsp	15 g	0.09
LEGUMES, dried peas & beans				
Broad (fava) beans	0.73	½ cup	112 g	0.82
Yellow split peas	0.02	½ cup	125 g	0.03
Brown beans	0.002	½ cup	112 g	0.002
Soy beans	0	½ cup	112 g	0
Mung beans	0	½ cup	112 g	0
Lima beans	0	½ cup	112 g	0
Green split peas	0	½ cup	112 g	0

Table 20-1: Level of Salicylates in Some Common Foods and Beverages

	Salicylates mg/100 g	Serving Size	Weight	Salicylates mg/serving
Chickpeas (garbanzo beans)	0	½ cup	112 g	0
Brown lentils	0	½ cup	112 g	0
Red lentils	0	½ cup	112 g	0
Blackeye beans	0	½ cup	112 g	0
FRUIT, fresh, frozen, canned, dried, juice				
Raisins, sultana, dried	7.8	½ cup	76 g	5.93
Prunes, letona, canned	6.87	5 medium	86 g	5.91
Raisins, dried	6.62	½ cup	76 g	5.03
Currants, dried	5.8	½ cup	72 g	4.18
Dates, dried	4.5	10	83 g	3.74
Blueberries, canned	2.78	½ cup	128 g	3.53
Cherries, canned	2.78	½ cup	125 g	3.48
Orange, fresh	2.39	1 medium	140 g	3.35
Raspberries, fresh	5.14	½ cup	61 g	3.14
Currants, red, frozen	5.06	½ cup	56 g	2.83
Apricots, fresh	2.58	3 medium	106 g	2.74
Boysenberries, canned	2.04	½ cup	128 g	2.61
Blackberries, canned	1.86	½ cup	128 g	2.38
Raspberries, frozen	3.88	½ cup	61 g	2.37
Currants, black, frozen	3.06	½ cup	56 g	1.71
Pineapple, canned	1.36	½ cup	125 g	1.7
Strawberries, fresh	1.36	½ cup	125 g	1.7
Pineapple, fresh	2.1	½ cup	78 g	1.64
Apricots, canned, Ardmona®	1.42	4 halves	90 g	1.28
Tangelo, fresh	0.72	1 medium	170 g	1.22
Guava, canned	2.02	½ cup	60 g	1.21
Cantaloupe, fresh	1.5	½ cup	80 g	1.2
Figs, calamata, dried	0.64	10	187 g	1.2

Table 20-1: Level of Salicylates in Some Common Foods and Beverages

	Salicylates mg/100 g	Serving Size	Weight	Salicylates mg/serving
Grape, juice	0.88	½ cup	126 g	1.11
Plums, red, canned	1.16	3 medium	95 g	1.1
Cranberry sauce	1.44	¼ cup	69 g	0.99
Cherries (sweet), fresh	0.85	15	102 g	0.87
Grapes, fresh	1.88	½ cup	46 g	0.86
Peaches, canned	0.68	½ cup	124 g	0.84
Cranberries, canned	1.64	½ cup	50 g	0.82
Apple, Granny Smith, fresh	0.59	1 medium	138 g	0.81
Grapefruit, fresh	0.68	½ cup	118 g	0.8
Orange, mandarin, fresh	0.56	1	135 g	0.76
Nectarine, fresh	0.49	1 medium	136 g	0.67
Apple, canned, Ardmona®	0.55	½ cup	102 g	0.56
Apple, Jonathan, fresh	0.38	1 medium	138 g	0.52
Avocado, fresh	0.6	½ medium	87 g	0.52
Grapefruit, juice	0.42	½ cup	123 g	0.52
Pear, William (with skin), fresh	0.31	1 medium	166 g	0.52
Peach, fresh	0.58	1 medium	87 g	0.51
Kiwi fruit, fresh	0.32	2 medium	152 g	0.49
Pear, Packham (with skin), fresh	0.27	1 medium	166 g	0.45
Grapes, red Malaita, fresh	0.94	½ cup	46 g	0.43
Watermelon, fresh	0.48	½ cup	80 g	0.38
Cherries, sour, canned	0.3	½ cup	125 g	0.38
Lychee, canned	0.36	10 medium	100 g	0.36
Plums, red, fresh	0.21	2 medium	132 g	0.28
Apple, red Delicious, fresh	0.19	1 medium	38 g	0.26
Figs, kadota, canned	0.25	3	85 g	0.21
Grapes, light seedless, canned	0.16	½ cup	128 g	0.21
Pineapple juice	0.16	½ cup	125 g	0.2

Table 20-1: Level of Salicylates in Some Common Foods and Beverages

	Salicylates mg/100 g	Serving Size	Weight	Salicylates mg/serving
Figs, fresh	0.18	2	100 g	0.18
Persimmons, fresh	0.18	3 medium	75 g	0.14
Plums, green, fresh	0.095	2 medium	132 g	0.13
Mango, fresh	0.11	½ medium	103 g	0.11
Apple, Golden Delicious, fresh	0.08	1 medium	138 g	0.11
Pomegranate, fresh	0.07	1 medium	154 g	0.11
Lemon, fresh	0.18	1 medium	58 g	0.1
Rhubarb, fresh	0.13	½ cup	68 g	0.09
Papaya, (pawpaw), fresh	0.08	3 ½ oz	100 g	0.08
Passion fruit (granadilla), fresh	0.14	1 medium	18 g	0.03
Pear, Packham (no skin), fresh	0	1 medium	166 g	0
Pear, Bartlett, letona, canned	0	½ cup	125 g	0
Banana, fresh	0	1 medium	114 g	0
NUTS AND SEEDS				
Water chestnuts, canned	2.92	8 medium	50 g	1.46
Almonds, fresh	3	12-15	15 g	0.45
Peanuts, unshelled, fresh	1.12	1 oz.	28 g	0.31
Pistachio nuts, fresh	0.55	30 nuts	15 g	0.08
Macadamia nuts, fresh	0.52	6 nuts	15 g	0.08
Pine nuts, fresh	0.51	2 tbsp	15 g	0.08
Brazil nuts, fresh	0.46	4 medium	15 g	0.07
Walnuts, fresh	0.3	8-15 halves	15 g	0.05
Peanut butter	0.23	1 tbsp	15 g	0.04
Sunflower seeds, dry	0.12	3 tbsp	28 g	0.03
Coconut, desiccated, dry	0.26	2 tbsp	11 g	0.03
Hazelnuts, fresh	0.14	10-12	15 g	0.02
Sesame seed, dry	0.23	1 tbsp	8 g	0.02
Pecans, fresh	0.12	12 halves	15 g	0.02

Table 20-1: Level of Salicylates in Some Common Foods and Beverages

	Salicylates mg/100 g	Serving Size	Weight	Salicylates mg/serving
Cashews, fresh	0.07	6-8	15 g	0.01
Poppy seed, dry	0	1 tsp	3 g	0
SEASONINGS				
Curry spices, dry powder	218	1 tsp	2 g	4.36
Paprika, hot, dry powder	203	1 tsp	2 g	4.06
Worcestershire sauce	64.3	1 tsp	5 g	3.22
Dill, dry powder	94.4	1 tsp	2 g	1.89
Thyme, dry leaves	183	1 tsp	1 g	1.83
Turmeric, dry powder	76.4	1 tsp	2 g	1.53
Rosemary, dry powder	68	1 tsp	2 g	1.36
Garam masala, dry powder	66.8	1 tsp	2 g	1.34
Oregano, dry powder	66	1 tsp	2 g	1.32
Mixed herbs, dry leaves	55.6	1 tsp	2 g	1.11
Cumin, dry powder	45	1 tsp	2 g	0.9
Tarragon, dry powder	34.8	1 tsp	2 g	0.7
Mace, dry powder	32.2	1 tsp	2 g	0.64
Five spice, dry powder	30.8	1 tsp	2 g	0.62
Fenugreek, dry powder	12.2	1 tsp	4 g	0.49
Aniseed, dry powder	22.8	1 tsp	2 g	0.46
Mustard, dry powder	26	1 tsp	1.5 g	0.39
Cayenne, dry powder	17.6	1 tsp	2 g	0.35
Cinnamon, dry powder	15.2	1 tsp	2 g	0.3
Sage, dry leaves	21.7	1 tsp	1 g	0.22
Celery, dry powder	10.1	1 tsp	2 g	0.2
Vinegar, white, liquid	1.33	1 tbsp	14 g	0.19
Cardamom, dry powder	7.7	1 tsp	2 g	0.15
Pepper, black, dry powder	6.2	1 tsp	2 g	0.12
Cloves, whole, dry	5.74	1 tsp	2 g	0.12

Table 20-1: Level of Salicylates in Some Common Foods and Beverages

	Salicylates mg/100 g	Serving Size	Weight	Salicylates mg/serving
Paprika, sweet, dry powder	5.7	1 tsp	2 g	0.11
Allspice, dry powder	5.2	1 tsp	2 g	0.1
Mint, fresh	9.4	1 tsp	1 g	0.09
Ginger root, fresh	4.5	1 tsp	2 g	0.09
Caraway, dry powder	2.82	1 tsp	2 g	0.06
Nutmeg, dry powder	2.4	1 tsp	2 g	0.05
Chili peppers, red, fresh	1.2	1 tsp	3 g	0.04
Vegemite spread	0.81	1 tsp	5 g	0.04
Chili, dry powder	1.3	1 tsp	3 g	0.04
Marmite spread	0.71	1 tsp	5 g	0.04
Dill, fresh	6.9	1 tsp	0.5 g	0.04
Basil, dry powder	3.4	1 tsp	1 g	0.03
Chili, dry flakes	1.38	1 tsp	2 g	0.03
Bay leaf, dry leaf	2.52	1 tsp	1 g	0.03
Horseradish, canned	0.18	1 tbsp	18 g	0.03
Chili peppers, green, fresh	0.64	1 tsp	3 g	0.02
Chili peppers, yellow green, fresh	0.62	1 tsp	3 g	0.02
Tabasco® sauce	0.45	1 tsp	5 g	0.02
Pepper, white, dry powder	1.1	1 tsp	2 g	0.02
Fennel, dry powder	0.8	1 tsp	2 g	0.02
Vanilla essence, liquid	1.44	1 tsp	1 g	0.01
Coriander, fresh leaves	0.2	1 tsp	2 g	0.004
Chives, fresh	0.031	1 tbsp	10 g	0.003
Parsley, fresh leaves	0.08	1 tsp	3 g	0.002
Garlic, fresh bulbs	0.1	1 tsp	2 g	0.002
Vinegar, malt, liquid	0	1 tbsp	14 g	0
Soy sauce, liquid	0	1 tbsp	18 g	0
Saffron, dry powder	0	1 tsp	1 g	0

Table 20-1: Level of Salicylates in Some Common Foods and Beverages

	Salicylates mg/100 g	Serving Size	Weight	Salicylates mg/serving
Tandoori spice, dry powder	0	1 tsp	2 g	0
SUGARS				
Honey, liquid, assorted	2.2-11.24	1 tbsp	20 g	0.50-2.25
Molasses, liquid	0.22	1 tbsp	20 g	0.04
Golden syrup, liquid	0.1	1 tbsp	20 g	0.02
Maple syrup, liquid, Camp®	0	1 tbsp	20 g	0
Sugar, white, granulated	0	1 tbsp	12 g	0
CONFECTIONERY				
Licorice Nibs (1.2 cms x 6 cms)	7.96-9.78	15 pieces	20 g	1.59-1.96
Peppermints	0.77-7.58	3 pieces	12 g	0.09-0.91
LifeSavers®, peppermint	0.86	5 pieces	10 g	0.09
Pascall® Cream Caramel	0.12	3 pieces	28 g	0.03
BEVERAGES				
Coca-Cola®	0.25	½ cup	125 g	0.31
Tea, lemon scented, Twinings®	7.34	1 bag	1 g	0.07
Tea, orange pekoe, Tetley®	5.57	1 bag	1 g	0.06
Tea, Irish Breakfast, Twinings®	3.89	1 bag	1 g	0.04
Tea, Earl Grey, Twinings®	3	1 bag	1 g	0.03
Tea, English Breakfast, Twinings®	3	1 bag	1 g	0.03
Tea, green, Burmese, leaves	2.97	1 tsp	1 g	0.03
Tea, green, Indian, leaves	2.97	1 tsp	1 g	0.03
Tea, orange pekoe, Twinings®	2.75	1 bag	1 g	0.03
Tea, Lapsang Souchong, Twinings®	2.4	1 bag	1 g	0.02
Tea, Chinese, leaves	1.9	1 tsp	1 g	0.02
Tea, peony, jasmine, leaves	1.9	1 tsp	1 g	0.02
Coffee, instant, powder, Maxwell House®	1	2 tsp	2 g	0.02
Coffee, instant, granules, Nescafé®	0.59	2 tsp	2 g	0.01

Table 20-1: Level of Salicylates in Some Common Foods and Beverages

	Salicylates mg/100 g	Serving Size	Weight	Salicylates mg/serving
Tea, herbal, peppermint	1.1	1 bag	1 g	0.01
Tea, herbal, rosehip	0.4	1 bag	1 g	0.004
Tea, herbal, fruit	0.36	1 bag	1 g	0.004
Tea, herbal, chamomile	0.006	1 bag	1 g	0
Cocoa, dry powder	0	1 tbsp	21 g	0
Carob, dry powder	0	1 tbsp	21 g	0
Coffee, instant, powder, decaffeinated, Nescafé®	0	2 tsp	2 g	0
Ovaltine®, powder	0	3 tsp	19 g	0
ALCOHOLIC DRINKS				
Ale and beer	0.32-1.26	12 fl oz	360 g	1.15-4.54
Liqueur, Benedictine®	9.04	1 fl oz	28 g	2.53
Champagne/Sparkling Wine (1 sample)	1.02	4 fl oz	120 g	1.22
Port	1.4-4.2	1 fl oz	28 g	0.39-1.18
Wine	0.35-0.90	4 fl oz	120 g	0.42-1.08
Cider, sweet and dry	0.16-0.19	12 fl oz	360 g	0.58-0.68
Liqueur, Drambuie®	1.68	1 fl oz	28 g	0.47
Rum, Captain Morgan®	1.28	1 fl oz	28 g	0.36
Liqueur, Tia Maria®	0.83	1 fl oz	28 g	0.23
Liqueur, Cointreau®	0.66	1 fl oz	28 g	0.19
Sherry, sweet and dry	0.46-0.56	1 fl oz	28 g	0.13-0.16
Vermouth, dry	0.46	1 fl oz	28 g	0.13
Brandy, Hennessey®	0.4	1 fl oz	28 g	0.11
Vodka, Smirnoff®	0	1 fl oz	28 g	0
Whiskey, Scotch, Johnnie Walker®	0	1 fl oz	28 g	0
Gin, Gilbey's®	0	1 fl oz	28 g	0

References

1. Swain, A., Dutton, S., and Truswell, A.S. Salicylates in foods. J. Am. Diet. Assoc. 1985 85(8):950-960.

2. Pennington, J.A.T., and Church, H.N. *Food Values of Portions Commonly Used.* Fourteenth Edition. Harper and Row, New York, 1985.

3. Margen, S. *The Wellness Encyclopedia of Food and Nutrition.* University of California at Berkeley. Random House Press, New York, 1992.

Method: Salicylate Restricted Diet

Salicylate Restricted Diet

Type of Food	Foods Allowed	Foods Restricted

Milk and Dairy	Plain milk, buttermilk, cream, sour cream, and yogurt
	All plain uncolored cream cheese, cheddar, mozzarella, cottage cheese, Quark®, Parmesan
	Additive-free ice cream made with allowed ingredients
	Butter
		Chocolate flavored milk
		Milkshakes
		Flavored yogurt
		Prepared:
		  Cheese foods
		  Cheese slices
		  Dips
		  Spreads
		Other ice cream and frozen treats

Breads and Cereals	Any pure flour or grain except cornmeal Any prepared, plain bread, buns, biscuits, pizza dough with allowed ingredients	Products made with restricted items Cornmeal
	Homemade or purchased baked cookies, pies, etc., made with allowed ingredients	
	Prepared breakfast cereals with allowed ingredients Oats and oatmeal Red River Cereal® Plain oat bran All plain grains and their flakes, except cornmeal	

	Plain crackers such as:
	  Grissol Melba Toast®
	  RyVita®
	  Rye Krisp®
	  Wasa® Light or Golden Crackers
	  Homemade crackers
		Crackers with color, flavor, or restricted ingredients

	Plain pasta All homemade crackers, cereals, and pasta dishes with allowed ingredients Plain and wild rice General Foods Minute Rice®	Pasta or rice dinners

Salicylate Restricted Diet

Type of Food	Foods Allowed	Foods Restricted
Vegetables	Bamboo shoots, canned* Beans, fresh, green Brussels sprouts, fresh Carrots, fresh Cauliflower, fresh Celery, fresh* Cabbage, green, fresh* Cabbage, red, fresh Corn, niblets, canned Corn on the cob Leeks, fresh Lettuce Mushrooms, fresh Onion, fresh Peas, green, fresh Potato, white, peeled, fresh Pumpkin, fresh Shallots, fresh Spinach, frozen Tomato, fresh Turnip, fresh Watercress, fresh	All others

Fruit	Apple, Golden Delicious
	Banana, fresh*
	Figs, fresh*
	Figs, kadota, canned
	Lemon, fresh
	Mango, fresh
	Papaya (pawpaw), fresh
	Passion fruit (granadilla),
	  fresh
	Pear, Bartlett, canned*
	Pear, Packham, peeled,
	  fresh*
	Pineapple juice
	Pomegranate, fresh
	Rhubarb, fresh
		All others

Meat, Poultry, and Fish	All pure fresh, frozen, or
	  canned meat, poultry, or fish
	Processed meat made with
	  allowed ingredients
		Processed with restricted
		  ingredients, such as spices

Eggs	All	All prepared with restricted foods

Salicylate Restricted Diet

Type of Food	Foods Allowed	Foods Restricted
Legumes	Blackeye beans* Brown beans* Brown lentils* Chickpeas (garbanzos)* Green split peas* Lima beans* Mung beans* Red lentils* Soy beans* Yellow split peas Pure, natural peanut butter	All others
Nuts and Seeds	Brazil nuts, fresh Cashew nuts, fresh Coconut, dry, desiccated Hazelnuts, fresh Macadamia nuts, fresh Pecan nuts, fresh Pine nuts, fresh Pistachio nuts, fresh Poppy seed, dry* Sesame seeds, dry Sunflower seeds, dry Walnuts, fresh	All other nuts and seeds Any with spices or seasoning

Fats and Oils	Pure butter, cream,
	  shortening
	Pure vegetable oils including:
	  canola, olive, sunflower, soy,
	  peanut
	Homemade salad dressings
	  with allowed ingredients
	Lard and meat drippings
	Homemade gravy with
	  allowed ingredients
		Margarine
		Prepared salad dressings
		  with restricted foods
		Commercial gravies and
		  sauces

Fresh Herbs and Seasonings	Chili peppers, green, red and yellow, fresh Chives, fresh Coriander, fresh leaves Dill, fresh Garlic, fresh bulbs Ginger root, fresh Horseradish	All others

Salicylate Restricted Diet

Type of Food	Foods Allowed	Foods Restricted
Dry Spices and Herbs	Allspice, dry powder Basil, dry powder Bay leaf, dry leaf Caraway, dry Cardamom, dry powder Chili, powder and flakes Cloves, whole, dry Fennel, dry powder Nutmeg, dry powder Paprika, sweet, dry powder Pepper, black and white, dry powder Saffron	All others Seasoning salts Flavoring extracts Flavoring packets Any product labeled with "spices"
Sweets and Sweeteners	Sugar, molasses Maple syrup, corn syrup Icing sugar Pure jams, jellies, marmalades, and conserves made with allowed fruit and without added color or flavor Plain artificial sweeteners Homemade sweets with allowed ingredients	Honey Prepared dessert fillings Prepared icings and frostings Spreads with restricted foods Prepared candies Cake decorations Other confectionery Commercial candies Fruit Rollups® Fun Fruits® Fruit peel Glacé fruit Flavored syrups Licorice Peppermints
Other	Baking powder Baking soda Cream of Tartar Distilled white vinegar Malt vinegar Baking chocolate Pure cocoa Plain gelatin Pure vanilla extract Relishes with allowed ingredients Black and green olives Pure soy sauce made with allowed ingredients Vegemite® and Marmite®	Whipped toppings Topping mixes All other vinegars with "flavorings" Chocolate candy, sprinkles, and syrup Flavored gelatin Prepared pickles Other relishes Worcestershire Sauce® Mustard

Salicylate Restricted Diet

Type of Food	Foods Allowed	Foods Restricted

Beverages	Plain and carbonated mineral water
	Plain coffee
	Ovaltine® powder*
	Tetley® tea
	Twinings® teas:
	  Lemon scented
	  Irish Breakfast
	  English Breakfast
	  Orange Pekoe
	Indian/Burmese green tea
	Jasmine tea
	Rosehip herbal tea
	Chamomile herbal tea*
	Alcohol:
	  Sherry
	  Dry vermouth
	  Hennessey Brandy®
	  Smirnoff Vodka®
	  Johnnie Walker Whiskey®
	  Gilbey's Gin®
		All other carbonated drinks and soft drinks
		Flavored coffee and coffee mixes
		Other tea
		Fruit flavored powders, concentrates
		All drinks with color, flavor or spices
		Diet drinks, shakes
		Meal replacement drinks
		
		Liqueurs, coolers
		Drink mixes and pre-mixed drinks

* These fruits, vegetables, legumes, seeds, herbs, and beverages contain no salicylates.

21

Benzoate Sensitivity

Benzoic Acid and Sodium Benzoate

Use in Manufactured Foods

Both benzoic acid and sodium benzoate are used to prevent spoilage by micro organisms in a wide variety of processed foods, beverages, and pharmaceuticals, thus extending their shelf life.[1]

Benzoic acid is a common ingredient in flavorings (specifically: chocolate, lemon, orange, cherry, fruit, nut, and tobacco) that are used in carbonated and non-carbonated beverages, ice cream, ices, candies, baked goods, pie and pastry fillings, icings, and chewing gum. It may also be used in pickles and margarine.[2] In such processed foods, benzoic acid is used up to a level of 0.1%.[1]

Benzoic acid occurs naturally in foods at varying levels (see Table 21-1, *Level of Benzoates in Common Foods*, page 208).[3] High levels occur in:

- Most berries, especially strawberries and raspberries
- Prunes
- Tea
- Spices such as cinnamon, nutmeg, clove, and anise
- Cherry bark and cassia bark

Sodium benzoate may be used as a preservative in margarine, codfish, bottled soft drinks, maraschino cherries, mincemeat, fruit juices, pickles, fruit jelly preserves, and jams. In addition, it may be added to the ice used for cooling fish, and may be an ingredient in eye creams, vanishing creams, and toothpastes.[2]

Absorption and Excretion

Benzoic acid and sodium benzoate are rapidly absorbed; on reaching the liver they combine with the amino acid glycine and are excreted.[4] As long as liver function is healthy and adequate glycine is available, both chemicals are completely eliminated from the body.[4]

Benzoyl Peroxide

Use in Manufactured Foods

Benzoyl peroxide is used primarily as a bleaching agent in the manufacture of:

- White flour
- Some cheeses (especially blue cheeses such as Gorgonzola and bleached white Italian cheeses)
- Lecithin

Lecithin is an emulsifier used in manufactured foods containing fats and oils. Its action is improved when benzoyl peroxide, hydrogen peroxide, acetic or lactic acid, or sodium hydroxide is added to produce hydroxylated lecithin, which disperses more readily in water and acts as a better emulsifier than pure lecithin.[1] Certain vitamins can be destroyed by the addition of benzoyl peroxide to food. Where the loss could be significant, such as in the destruction of beta-carotene in milk, US government regulations require that the vitamin be replaced, such as in the addition of vitamin A to cheese made from bleached milk.[2]

Absorption and Excretion

Most benzoyl peroxide added to food has been converted to benzoic acid by the time the food is eaten. Only a small fraction of the bleach is ingested, most of which is converted in the intestine to benzoic acid or a similar product that is readily excreted in the urine.[4]

Adverse Reactions to Benzoates

Mechanism of Action

The mechanism of adverse reactions to foods containing benzoate is unknown, but evidence suggests that the cyclooxygenase pathway of arachidonic acid metabolism may be affected.[4] Persons sensitive to acetylsalicylic acid (ASA or Aspirin®) are particularly vulnerable to benzoate sensitivity.[4]

Symptoms

The following symptoms have been reported by persons sensitive to benzoates:[4]

- Asthma
- Urticaria (hives)
- Angioedema (tissue swelling)
- Headaches

Persons who have experienced Type I hypersensitivity reactions (atopic allergy) such as respiratory tract symptoms including asthma or skin reactions such as hives and eczema may be particularly vulnerable to benzoate sensitivity.[4]

Benzoic acid can act as a mild irritant to the skin, eyes, and mucous membranes. Its adverse effects often increase when combined with other additives.[4]

Role of Benzoates in Unusual Skin Rashes

One study[5] has indicated a possible causative role for benzoates in an acute inflammatory disorder known as *erythema multiforme*, which is characterized by lesions on the skin and mucous membranes of the mouth, eyes, and genitals. Patch testing with a variety of food additives showed that patients in the study reacted strongly to benzoic acid. Subsequent elimination and challenge testing confirmed a role for ingested benzoates in the exacerbation and possible etiology of the condition.

Recommendations for Managing Benzoate Sensitivity

People differ in their sensitivity to chemicals like benzoates. Consequently, it is impossible to define a limit of benzoate intake that applies to all persons intolerant of benzoate. The general recommendation is to reduce benzoate intake by avoiding foods known to contain added benzoates.

Benzoate sensitive persons should avoid:

- Natural sources of benzoic acid (see Table 21-1, page 208)
- Any processed foods containing benzoic acid or sodium benzoate
- Bleached flour
- Products containing hydrolyzed lecithin such as:
    margarine
    salad and cooking oils
    frozen desserts
    chocolate
    baked goods

Benzyl and Benzoyl Compounds

A large number of benzyl and benzoyl compounds are allowed in foods.[6] Examples are benzyl acetate, benzyl alcohol, benzyl ether, benzyl butyrate, benzyl cinnamate, benzyl formate, benzyl propionate, and benzyl salicylate. (For a complete list see Reference 2.) On food labels, this ingredient will include the word "benzyl" or "benzoyl." Most of these compounds are used as synthetic flavorings and perfumes in a wide variety of processed and manufactured foods, beverages, chewing gum, soaps, hair sprays, hair dyes, skin creams, sunscreens, perfumes, and cosmetics.

Some of these compounds are skin irritants and can cause hives and contact dermatitis. Others are digestive tract irritants and can cause intestinal upset, vomiting, and diarrhea, and in very high concentrations can have a narcotic effect. A few of these compounds irritate the eyes and cause respiratory symptoms when inhaled.

Parabens

Parabens, a class of derivatives of benzoic acid, are sometimes used as preservatives in foods. Persons who are sensitive to benzoates may also react to parabens because paraben metabolism mimics that of benzoates in the later stages.[4] There are no naturally occurring parabens. On food labels parabens will be indicated by the term "methyl p-hydroxybenzoate" or "propyl p-hydroxybenzoate".[4]

Parabens are used in processed fruits and vegetables, baked goods, fats, oils, and seasonings. They may be present in foods such as cakes, pies, pastries, icings, fillings, fruit products (e.g., sauces, and juices, fruit salads, syrups, preserves, jellies), syrups, olives, pickles, beers, ciders, and carbonated beverages.[2]

The following table contains only those foods that have been analyzed for benzoate content.[3,7,8,9] Other foods may contain benzoates. It is not necessary to avoid all food containing natural benzoates.

Table 21-1: Level of Benzoates in Common Foods

	Benzoates mg/kg	Serving Size	Weight	Benzoates mg/serving
FRUITS				
Navel orange	2.3	1 medium	140 g	0.322
Peach	2.7	1 medium	87 g	0.24
Papayas (Pawpaw)	1.5	½ medium	152 g	0.23
Nectarine	1.3	1 medium	136 g	0.18
Avocado	1.7	½ medium	86 g	0.15

Table 21-1: Level of Benzoates in Common Foods

	Benzoates mg/kg	Serving Size	Weight	Benzoates mg/serving
Grapefruit	0.7	½ medium	123 g	0.086
Cherry	1.1	10	68 g	0.075
Valencia orange	0.6	1 medium	121 g	0.073
Quince	0.7	1 medium	92 g	0.064
Mandarin orange	0.5	½ cup	126 g	0.063
Pomegranate	0.3	1 medium	154 g	0.046
Plum	0.4	1 medium	66 g	0.026
Watermelon	0.3	½ cup	80 g	0.024
Banana	0.2	1 medium	114 g	0.023
Lemon	0.7	½ medium	29 g	0.02
Fig	0.2	5	93 g	0.019
Lime	0.4	½ medium	33 g	0.013
Pineapple	0.1	½ cup	77 g	0.008
Kumquats	0.4	1 medium	19 g	0.008
Kiwi	0	1 medium	76 g	0
Grape	0	½ cup	46 g	0
Japanese pear	0	1 small	166 g	0
Persimmons	0	2 medium	50 g	0
Apple	0	1 medium	138 g	0
GRAINS/ BEANS				
Soy bean	1.9	½ cup	100 g	0.19
Red bean	1.8	½ cup	100 g	0.18
Rice	0.4	½ cup	115 g	0.046
Barley	0.3	½ cup	96 g	0.029

Table 21-1: Level of Benzoates in Common Foods

	Benzoates mg/kg	Serving Size	Weight	Benzoates mg/serving
Corn	0.2	½ cup	100 g	0.02
Wheat	0.3	½ cup	56 g	0.017
NUTS AND SEEDS				
Walnuts	1.2	8 -10 halves	15 g	0.018
Pistachios	0.5	30 nuts	15 g	0.008
Almonds	0.4	12 -15 nuts	15 g	0.006
Sesame seed	0.6	1 tbsp	8 g	0.005
Hazelnuts	0.3	10 -12 nuts	15 g	0.005
Cashews	0.3	6 - 8 nuts	15 g	0.005
SEASONINGS				
Cinnamon	336	1 tsp	2 g	0.672
Soy sauce	8.9	1 tbsp	18 g	0.16
Nutmeg	44.1	1 tsp	2 g	0.088
Worcestershire sauce	4.9	1 tbsp	15 g	0.074
Clove	28.1	1 tsp	2 g	0.056
Pimento	14.1	1 tsp	2 g	0.028
Light soy sauce	1.4	1 tbsp	18 g	0.025
Celery seed	8.9	1 tsp	2 g	0.018
Tomato ketchup	1.1	1 tbsp	15 g	0.017
Thyme	15.9	1 tsp	1 g	0.016
Cayenne pepper	7.0	1 tsp	2 g	0.014
Black pepper	4.7	1 tsp	2 g	0.009
Mustard seed	5.0	1 tsp	1.5 g	0.008
Coriander	3.2	1 tsp	2 g	0.006

Table 21-1: Level of Benzoates in Common Foods

	Benzoates mg/kg	Serving Size	Weight	Benzoates mg/serving
Cumin	3.2	1 tsp	2 g	0.006
White pepper	2.6	1 tsp	2 g	0.005
Paprika	2.3	1 tsp	2 g	0.0046
Bay leaf	4.3	1 tsp	1 g	0.004
Garlic	0.8	1 tsp	2 g	0.002
VEGETABLES				
Pumpkin	1.4	½ cup	100 g	0.14
Spinach	1.0	3½ oz	100 g	0.1
Chinese cabbage	0.7	1 cup	50 g	0.035
Carrots	0.3	1 large	100 g	0.03
Tomato	0.2	1 small	100 g	0.02
Parsley	0.6	1 tbsp	10 g	0.006
Radish	0.1	5 small	50 g	0.005
Broccoli	0	½ cup	50 g	0
Potato	0	1 medium	100 g	0
Cabbage	0	1 cup	100 g	0
Lettuce	0	3½ oz	100 g	0
Celery	0	½ cup or 1 stalk	50 g	0
Cauliflower	0	½ cup	50 g	0
Onion	0	1 tbsp	10 g	0

References

1. Freydberg, N., and Gortner, W.A. *The Food Additives Book.* Bantam Books, Toronto and New York, 1982.

2. Winter, R. *A Consumer's Dictionary of Food Additives.* Third Edition. Crown Publishers, New York, 1989.

3. Heimhuber, B., und Herrmann, K. Benzoe-, Phylessig-, 3-Phenylpropan- und Zimtsäure sowie Benzoylglucosen in einigen Obst- und Fruchtgemüsearten . Deutsche Lebensmittel-Rundschau 86 Jahrg. Heft 7 1990.

4. Jacobsen, D.W. Adverse reactions to benzoates and parabens. In: Metcalfe, D.D., Sampson, H.A., Simon, R.A. (Eds), *Food Allergy: Adverse Reactions to Foods and Food Additives.* Blackwell Scientific Publications, Oxford, London, 1991. 276-287.

5. Lewis, M.A.O. Erythema Multiforme: A possible role for foodstuffs. British Dental J. 1989 166(10):371-373.

6. Canadian Food & Drug Regulations, Part B, Div. 16. Health Protection Branch, Health and Welfare Canada, Ottawa, 1995.

7. Pennington, J.A.T. and Church, H.N. *Food Values of Portions Commonly Used,* Fourteenth Edition. Harper and Row, New York, 1985.

8. Margen, S. *The Wellness Encyclopaedia of Food and Nutrition,* University of California at Berkeley. Random House Press, New York, 1992.

9. *Mayo Clinic Diet Manual: A Handbook of Nutrition Practices.* Seventh Edition. Mosby, St. Louis, Baltimore, 1994. 112-113.

Method: Benzoate Restricted Diet

Sources of Benzoates

Benzoic acid occurs naturally in:

- Most berries, especially strawberries and raspberries
- Prunes
- Tea
- Spices such as cinnamon, nutmeg, cloves, anise
- Cherry bark and cassia bark

Notable levels of naturally occurring benzoates have also been found in:

- Naval orange
- Peach
- Papaya (pawpaw)
- Nectarine
- Avocado
- Soy beans
- Red beans
- Soy sauce
- Pumpkin
- Spinach

Benzoic acid and sodium benzoate are used in manufacturing to prevent spoiling by micro organisms in a wide variety of processed foods, beverages, and pharmaceuticals.

Benzoic acid is commonly used in flavoring:

- Chocolate, lemon, orange, cherry, fruit, nut, and tobacco
- Carbonated and non-carbonated beverages
- Ice cream and ices
- Candies
- Baked goods
- Pie and pastry fillings
- Icings
- Chewing gum
- Pickles
- Margarine

Sodium benzoate may be used as a preservative in:

- Margarine
- Codfish
- Bottled soft drinks
- Maraschino cherries
- Mincemeat
- Fruit juices
- Pickles
- Fruit jelly, preservatives, and jam
- May be used in the ice for cooling fish
- May be used in eye cream, vanishing cream, toothpaste

Para-aminobenzoic acid (PABA) is found in many sun screen creams and lotions.

Benzoyl peroxide is used in a variety of ways in manufactured foods:

- White flour as a bleaching agent
- Some cheeses (especially blue cheese such as Gorgonzola and some white Italian cheeses)
- Lecithin in manufactured fats and oils listed as "hydrolyzed lecithin"

Hydrolyzed lecithin is used in:

- Margarine
- Salad and cooking oils
- Frozen desserts
- Chocolate
- Baked goods

Benzyl and benzoyl compounds are used as synthetic flavorings and perfumes. On food labels, the ingredient will include the word "benzyl" or "benzoyl". These compounds are used in a wide variety of products including:

- Processed and manufactured foods
- Beverages
- Chewing gum
- Soaps, hair sprays, hair dyes, skin creams, sunscreens, perfumes, and cosmetics

Parabens are sometimes used as preservatives in food. On food labels they appear as "methyl p-hydroxybenzoate" or "propyl-p-hydroxybenzoate". Parabens may be used in:

- Cakes, pies, pastries, icings, fillings
- Fruit products (sauces, juices, salads, syrups, preserves, jellies)

- Syrups, olives, and pickles
- Beverages such as beers, ciders, and carbonated beverages

Note: Some of these compounds are skin irritants and can cause hives and contact dermatitis. Others are digestive tract irritants and can cause intestinal upset, bleeding, and at very high concentrations can have a narcotic effect. A few cause irritation of the eyes and respiratory symptoms when inhaled.

Benzoate Restricted Diet

Type of Food	Foods Allowed	Foods Restricted
Vegetables	All pure fresh and frozen vegetables, except those listed opposite	Avocado Pumpkin Red beans Soy beans Spinach All vegetables prepared with restricted ingredients
Milk and Dairy	Plain milk, buttermilk, cream, sour cream, and yogurt All plain cheese, cottage cheese, ricotta, Quark®, feta Ice cream made with allowed ingredients	All prepared milk products made with restricted ingredients Blue cheese Gorgonzola cheese
Breads and Cereals	Any pure unbleached flour or grain Any plain fresh bread, buns, biscuits, pizza dough with allowed ingredients Homemade or purchased baked cookies, pies, etc. made with allowed ingredients Baking chocolate and pure cocoa	Products made with: Bleached flour Restricted fruit Cinnamon Cloves Anise Artificial flavors Margarine Maraschino cherries Some fruit juices Some jams & jellies Some cheeses Other chocolate Oils with hydrolyzed lecithin Some commercial pie and pastry fillings

Benzoate Restricted Diet

Type of Food	Foods Allowed	Foods Restricted
	Breakfast cereals with allowed foods, including: 　All plain grains 　Corn flakes 　Oats and oatmeal 　Plain Cream of Wheat® 　Puffed rice and wheat 　Shredded Wheat® 　Shreddies® Plain crackers without benzoates	All others
	Plain pasta All homemade crackers, cereals and pasta dishes with allowed ingredients	**Read labels carefully** on all packaged pasta meals
Fruit	All pure fresh or frozen fruit except those listed opposite Pure frozen and canned allowed fruit juices Fruit dishes made with allowed ingredients	Berries, especially strawberries and raspberries Prunes Peaches Papaya (pawpaw) Nectarines Fruit dishes, jams, juices with benzoates or "flavoring"
Meat, Poultry, and Fish	All pure fresh, frozen or canned meat, poultry or fish Processed meat made with allowed ingredients	Meat, poultry, or fish processed with restricted ingredients Cod Pickled products
Eggs	All	All prepared with restricted foods
Legumes	All plain legumes except those on restricted list Pure peanut butter	Red beans Soy beans
Nuts and Seeds	All plain nuts and seeds	All with restricted ingredients

Benzoate Restricted Diet

Type of Food	Foods Allowed	Foods Restricted
Fats and Oils	Pure butter and cream Shortening Pure vegetable oils Homemade salad dressings with allowed ingredients Lard and meat drippings Homemade gravy	All fats and oils with hydrolyzed lecithin Margarine Prepared salad dressings with restricted ingredients
Spices and Herbs	All fresh, frozen or dried herbs and spices except those listed opposite	Anise Cinnamon Cloves Seasoning packets with restricted foods Foods labeled with "spices"
Sweets and Sweeteners	Sugar, honey, molasses Maple syrup, corn syrup Icing sugar Pure jams, jellies, marmalade, and conserves made with allowed ingredients and without added benzoates Plain artificial sweeteners Homemade sweets with allowed ingredients	Flavored syrups Prepared dessert fillings Prepared icings and frostings Spreads with restricted ingredients Prepared candies Cake decorations and other confectionery Commercial candies
Other	Baking powder Baking soda Cream of Tartar Distilled white cider or wine vinegars Baking chocolate Pure cocoa Plain gelatin Homemade pickles and relishes with allowed ingredients Homemade ketchup with allowed ingredients	All other vinegars with "flavorings" Chocolate candy, sprinkles, and syrup Flavored gelatin Mincemeat Prepared pickles, relishes, and olives Soy sauce Commercial ketchup Chewing gum Most commercial salad dressings

Benzoate Restricted Diet

Type of Food	Foods Allowed	Foods Restricted
Beverages	Plain milk, buttermilk Pure juices of allowed fruits and vegetables Plain and carbonated mineral water Coffee	Flavored milks Fruit drinks and cocktails with restricted ingredients All other carbonated drinks Flavored coffee All tea All drinks with "flavor" or "spices" Some cider and beer

Cosmetics

The following may contain benzoates, and labels should be carefully checked:

Eye cream
Hair sprays
Hair dyes
Other cosmetics
Other skin creams

Perfumes
Soaps
Sun screen
Vanishing cream

22

Butylated Hydroxyanisole and Butylated Hydroxytoluene

The antioxidants butylated hydroxyanisole (BHA) and butylated hydroxytoluene (BHT) are used to prevent fat from becoming rancid and developing objectionable tastes and odors.[1] These two preservatives are often used together and/or with other antioxidants.

Sensitivity to BHA and BHT

Extremely high doses of BHA and BHT in experimental animals have consistently resulted in enlargement of the liver. Both kidney and liver functions have been affected. In addition, adverse effects on the brain have resulted in abnormal behaviour patterns in experimental animals.[2]

Clinical trials have indicated that these chemicals may induce urticaria (hives)[3] and may be implicated in hyperactivity in children.[4]

In 1978 the United Nations Joint FAO/WHO Expert Committee on Food Additives suggested that daily ingestion of these chemicals should not exceed 0.5 mg per kg body weight (e.g., 34 mg for a 68 kg adult).[2] However, intake should be much lower for individuals who are sensitive to these chemicals. The goal should be to eliminate BHA and BHT by careful reading of food labels and avoiding all possible sources of these preservatives.

References

1.   Winter, R. *A Consumer's Dictionary of Food Additives.* Third Edition. Crown Publishers, New York, 1989. 72-74.

2.   Freydberg, N., and Gortner, W.A. *The Food Additives Book.* Bantam Books, Toronto and New York, 1982.

3.   Bosso, J.V., Simon, R.A. Urticaria, angioedema, and anaphylaxis provoked by food additives. In: Metcalfe, D.D., Sampson, H.A., Simon, R.A. (Eds), *Food Allergy: Adverse Reactions to Foods and Food Additives.* Blackwell Scientific Publications, Oxford, London, 1991. 288-300.

4.   Egger, J., Stolla, A., and McEwan, L.M. Controlled trial of hyposensitization in children with food-induced hyperkinetic syndrome. Lancet, May 9, 1992 339:1150-1153.

Method: Butylated Hydroxyanisole (BHA) and Butylated Hydroxytoluene (BHT) Restricted Diet

Sources of BHA and BHT

BHA and BHT are antioxidants that are used as preservatives to prevent or delay fats, oils, and fat-containing foods from becoming rancid and developing objectionable tastes and odors.

They are often used together with other antioxidants.

In Food Products:

BHA and BHT are commonly found in food products such as:

- Dehydrated potatoes
- Dried fruits
- Dry yeast
- Vegetable oils
- Foods cooked in or containing vegetable oils such as :
    Baked goods
    Breakfast cereals
    Doughnuts
    Nut meats
    Pastries and pie crusts
    Potato chips

Additional foods that sometimes contain BHA and BHT include:

Animal fats	Gelatin desserts
Beverages	Glacé fruits
Cake mixes	Ice cream
Candies	Lard and shortening
Chewing gum	Potato and sweet potato flakes
Dry yeast	Soup bases
Dry dessert mixes	Unsmoked dry sausage
Enriched rice	

In Food Packaging:

BHA and/or BHT may be added to the packaging of cereals, crackers etc. to help maintain the freshness of the food. Foods packaged in such materials should be avoided. BHA and BHT will appear on the label if the food contains the preservatives, or if they are present in the packaging materials.

Avoid any commercial packaged and prepared food with BHA and/or BHT on the label.

BHA and BHT Restricted Diet

Type of Food	Foods Allowed	Foods Restricted

Milk and Dairy	Plain milk, buttermilk, cream, sour cream, and yogurt
	All plain cheese, cottage cheese, ricotta, Quark®
	Ice cream made with allowed ingredients
	Butter
		All prepared dairy products made with unknown fats or oils, such as:
		  cheese foods
		  cheese spreads
		  cream sauces
		  drink mixes
		  dry dessert mixes
		  ice cream

Breads and Cereals	Any pure flour or grain Any plain fresh bread, buns, biscuits, pizza which is labeled "preservative-free" Check with baker or manufacturer whether oil or packaging used contains BHA and/or BHT Most fat-free baked goods should be safe, but check Homemade breads, buns, baked cookies, pies, etc., made with allowed ingredients	All other grains and baked goods, including those fried in fat, such as doughnuts Pie crusts Pastries Cake and other baking mixes Dry dessert mixes

	Breakfast cereals with allowed ingredients and packaging, including:
	  Puffed rice and wheat
	  Post Bran Flakes®
	  All plain grains and their flakes
	  Original Cream of Wheat®
	  Red River Cereal®
	  Pure oat bran
	Read all cereal labels
		All others

	Crackers Homemade Melba toast Grissol Melba Toast® RyVita Rye Krisp® RyVita Snackbread® Wasa Light or Golden Crackers® Almost all rice cakes Read all cracker labels	All others

BHA and BHT Restricted Diet

Type of Food	Foods Allowed	Foods Restricted
	Plain pasta Plain and wild rice General Foods Minute Rice® All homemade cereals, crackers, and pasta dishes with allowed ingredients	Enriched rice Read labels on all packaged pasta meals and rice meals
Vegetables	All pure fresh, frozen and canned vegetables and their juices V-8 Vegetable Cocktail® Homemade French fries	Prepared vegetable dishes with unknown fats or oils Salads with commercial salad dressings Some commercial French fries Potato and sweet potato flakes Dehydrated potatoes
Fruit	All pure fresh, frozen, or canned fruit and juices Pure fruit ices, sorbets and ice pops	Prepared fruit dishes with unknown fats or oils Glacé fruits Dried fruits
Meat, Poultry, and Fish	All pure fresh or frozen meat, poultry, or fish Fish canned in broth or water, not in oil Processed meat made with allowed ingredients Read all meat labels	Processed with unknown oils or fats Unsmoked dry sausage Processed meats with restricted ingredients
Eggs	All	All prepared with restricted foods
Legumes	All plain legumes except those listed opposite Pure, natural peanut butter	Prepared legume dishes with unknown fats or oils Some regular peanut butter
Nuts and Seeds	All plain nuts and seeds Pure almond butter and sesame seed butter (tahini)	All with restricted ingredients, especially snack nuts and seeds
Fats and Oils	Pure butter and cream Vegetable oils Homemade salad dressings with allowed ingredients Lard and meat drippings Homemade gravy	All fats with BHA and/or BHT Margarine Shortening Lard Most commercial salad dressings Prepared gravy

BHA and BHT Restricted Diet

Type of Food	Foods Allowed	Foods Restricted
Spices and Herbs	All fresh, frozen, or dried herbs and spices	Seasoning packets with BHA and/or BHT
Sweets and Sweeteners	Sugar, honey, maple syrup Maple syrup, corn syrup Icing sugar Pure jams, jellies, marmalades, and conserves made with allowed ingredients Plain artificial sweeteners Homemade sweets with allowed ingredients Pure baking chocolate and cocoa	Syrups and sauces with restricted ingredients Commercial candies Commercial icings and frostings Commercial chocolates
Other	Baking powder Baking soda Cream of Tartar Fleischmann's Quick-Rise Yeast® Distilled vinegar Baking chocolate Pure cocoa Plain gelatin	Dry dessert mixes Cake and baking mixes Most dry yeast Glacé and dried fruit Chocolate candy, sprinkles, and syrup Flavored gelatin Soup bases Chewing gum

23

Sulfite Sensitivity

Sensitivity to sulfites is most common in people with asthma.[1] Of these people, individuals who are steroid dependent are considered most at risk for sulfite sensitivity.[2] Although the incidence of adverse reactions to sulfites is estimated to be as high as 1% of the US population, sulfite sensitivity in people without asthma is considered rare.[3] Reported symptoms have occurred in most organ systems, including the lungs, gastrointestinal tract, and skin and mucous membranes. Incidences of life threatening anaphylactic reactions in persons with sulfite sensitivity and asthma have been reported, but are very rare.

Symptoms of Sulfite Sensitivity

Symptoms reported to result from sulfite sensitivity are:[3]

- Severe respiratory reactions, including bronchospasm, wheezing, and a feeling of tightness in the chest; asthma in asthmatics
- Flushing, feeling of temperature change
- Onset of hypotension (low blood pressure)
- Gastrointestinal symptoms (abdominal pain, diarrhea, nausea, vomiting)
- Swallowing difficulty
- Dizziness, loss of consciousness.
- Urticaria (hives), angioedema (swelling, especially of the mouth and face)
- Contact dermatitis

- Anaphylaxis (in persons with asthma), anaphylactoid reaction (in persons without asthma).

There is no evidence that avoiding all dietary sources of sulfites improves asthma.

For people who are not sensitive to sulfites, exposure to sulfiting agents poses very little risk. Toxicity studies in volunteers showed that ingestion of 400 mg of sulfites daily for 25 days produced no adverse effects.[4]

Mechanism of Action of Sulfites

Respiratory symptoms caused by sulfites are thought to be caused by sulphur dioxide, which acts as a direct irritant on hypersensitive airways. Sulphur dioxide is released from sulphurous acid, which forms when sulfites dissolve in water.[1] Persons with asthma can experience significant bronchospasm after inhaling as little as one part per million of sulphur dioxide.[5] Wheezing, flushing, and other symptoms of asthma have been induced by the inhalation of the vapors from a bag of dried apricots.[5]

An IgE-mediated reaction has been suggested, in which sulfite acts as a hapten, combining with protein to form a neoantigen that elicits antigen specific IgE.[1] However, because the levels of IgE, eosinophils, and histamine are normal in most persons demonstrating sulfite sensitivity and because sulfite specific IgE has not been demonstrated, IgE-mediated reactions are considered to be unlikely or very rare.[6]

A deficiency in the enzyme sulfite oxidase, which converts sulfite to the inert sulphate, has been suggested as a possible cause of abnormally high levels of sulfites, which may provoke an adverse reaction.[1] This hypothesis has not yet been substantiated.

Use of Sulfites in Foods and Medications

Sulfites are used as preservatives in beverages, fruits, vegetables, prepared and pre-sliced foods, and packaged snack foods.[5] They are also used to control browning in foods such as potatoes, apples, coconut, dehydrated vegetables, dried fruits, white wines, white grape juice, and some vinegars; in the modification of dough texture, especially in frozen pizza dough and pie shells; for bleaching, particularly in the production of maraschino cherries, glacé fruits, and citron peel; and for their antimicrobial effects.[7] In addition, sulfites occur naturally in some foods, including wines.[5]

Sulfites are also used as preservatives in some medications, including inhalable and injectable drugs. Some forms of epinephrine (adrenalin) contain sulfite as a preservative. However, the action of epinephrine appears to overcome any adverse effects of sulfite, and administration of epinephrine in anaphylactic emergencies is the recommended treatment.[5]

Cooking foods does not cause sulfites to lose their effect.[8] In addition, because sulfites bind to several substances in foods, such as protein, starch and sugars, washing foods may not remove sulfites.[9]

Sulfates in foods do not cause the same adverse reactions as sulfites, and need not be avoided by persons who are sensitive to sulfites.

Detection of Sulfites in Foods

Chemically treated strips have been developed to test foods for the presence of sulfites. Because of a high number of false positive and false negative results obtained with these test strips, their use is not recommended.[10]

References

1.   Simon, R.A. Sulfite sensitivity. Ann. Allergy 1987 57:100-105.

2.   Bush, R.K., Taylor, S.L., Holden, K., Nordlee, J.A., and Busse, W.W. Prevalence of sensitivity to sulfiting agents in asthmatic patients. Am. J. Med. 1986 81:816-820.

3.   Bush, R.K., Taylor, S.L., and Busse, W.W. A critical evaluation of clinical trials in reactions to sulfites. J. Allergy Clin. Immunol. 1986 78(1):191-202.

4.   Stevenson, D.D., Simon, R.A. Sensitivity to ingested metabisulfites in asthmatic subjects. J. Allergy Clin. Immunol. 1981 68:26-32.

5.   Taylor, S.L., Bush, R.K., and Nordlee, J.A. Sulfites. In: Metcalfe, D.D., Sampson, H.A., and Simon, R.A. (Eds), *Food Allergy: Adverse Reactions to Foots and Food Additives.* Blackwell Scientific Publications, Oxford, London, 1991. 239-260.

6.   Settipane, G.A. Adverse reactions to sulfites in drugs and foods. J. Am. Acad. Dermatol. 1984 10(6):1077-1080.

7.   Perkin, J.E. In: Perkin, J.E. (Ed), *Food Allergies and Adverse Reactions.* Aspen Publishers, Gaithersburg, MD, 134-140.

8.   Bahna, S.L. Food sensitivity - handling reactions to foods and food additives. Postgrad. Med. J. 1987 82(5):195-205.

9.   Taylor, S.L., Bush, R.K., Selner, J.C. Sensitivity to sulfited foods among sulfite-sensitive subjects with asthma. J. Allergy Clin. Immunol. 1988 81(6):1159-1167.

10.   Nordlee, J.A., Naidu, S.G. and Taylor, S.L. False positive and false negative reactions encountered in the use of sulfite test strips for the detection of sulfite-treated foods. J. Allergy Clin. Immunol. 1988 81:537-541.

Method: Sulfite Restricted Diet

Sulfites in Foods

Sulfites are used as a preservative and to prevent foods and beverages from discoloring. The use of sulfites on fresh fruits and vegetables, except for sliced potatoes and raw grapes, has been banned in the USA by FDA regulation since 1986, and in Canada since 1987.

Sulfites are permitted for use in the form of:

Sodium metabisulfite
Potassium metabisulfite
Sodium bisulfite
Potassium bisulfite

Sodium sulfite
Sodium dithionite
Sulphurous acid
Sulphur dioxide

A specified level of sulfites (calculated in parts per million) may be added to the following foods and beverages because no suitable alternatives are currently available:

Fruits and Vegetables

Dried fruits and vegetables
Fruit juices except frozen concentrated
    orange juice
Frozen sliced apples
Frozen sliced mushrooms
Grapes
Sliced potatoes

Beverages

Alcoholic
Non-alcoholic wines and beers
Cider
Sulfites occur naturally in some
    wines

Sweeteners

Glucose solids and syrup
Dextrose (used in making sweets)
Molasses including: fancy, refiner's,
    and table

Fish

Canned flaked tuna
Processed crustaceans (crab, crayfish, lobster,
    prawn, shrimp, squid)

Others

Jams, jellies, marmalades (sulfite is in the
    pectin)
Mincemeat
Some vinegars
Pickles and relishes
Tomato paste, pulp, ketchup, purée
Gelatin
Pectin
Snack foods
Candies and confectioneries
Maraschino cherries, glacé fruits, and citron
Coconut
Frozen pizza dough
Frozen pastry shells
Biscuit dough

Not all manufacturers of these foods use sulfites.

Labeling of Sulfite-containing Foods and Beverages

Canadian Government regulations require that if sulfites are used, they must be listed on the label, except in the case of alcoholic beverages.

USA Government regulations state that if any food contains 10 parts per million or more, the sulfite must be identified on the ingredient label.

In Canada, ingredients including sulfites in alcoholic beverages, need not be listed on the label. In the USA, if sulfite levels are 10 parts per million or more in wine, distilled spirits, and malt beverages, sulfites must be listed on the labels.

Preparations of meat, fish, and poultry (other than tuna and crustaceans listed above), as well as foods listed as a good source of thiamine, are not allowed to contain sulfites.

Sometimes the sulfite is contained in a prepared ingredient whose contents do not appear on the food label. For example, if one of the ingredients in a prepared cake is jam that contains sulfites, the jam must be listed, but not the sulfite contained in it. This is because the final level of sulfite in the finished product is below the amount required by law to be disclosed.

Some bulk foods do not require ingredient labels. Deli foods do not require ingredient labels. Individually sold candies do not require ingredient labels.

Food processing equipment and food packaging materials such as plastic bags, may be sanitized with sulfites. These sources of sulfites will not be listed on any labels.

Sulfites in Medications

Sulfites are used in a wide range of medications and pharmaceuticals. The Compendium of Pharmaceuticals and Specialties (CPS) provides a list of sulfite-containing products. Consult your pharmacist about the sulfite content of any medications required.

Sulfite Restricted Diet

Type of Food	Foods Allowed	Foods Restricted
Milk and Dairy	Plain milk, buttermilk, cream, sour cream, and yogurt All plain cheese, cottage cheese, ricotta, Quark® Ice cream made with allowed ingredients Butter	All prepared dairy products made with restricted ingredients
Breads and Cereals	Any pure flour or grain Any plain fresh bread, buns, biscuits, pizza dough with allowed ingredients Homemade or purchased baked cookies, pies, etc., made with allowed ingredients	Biscuit dough Frozen pizza dough Frozen pastry shells Any baked goods with dried or glacé fruit, molasses, coconut, dehydrated vegetables, or commercial frozen apple slices, or confectionary icing

Sulfite Restricted Diet

Type of Food	Foods Allowed	Foods Restricted

	Breakfast cereals without dried fruit or coconut, including:
	  Puffed rice and wheat
	  Shreddies®
	  Shredded Wheat®
	  Corn flakes
	  Oats and oatmeal
	  Plain Cream of Wheat®
		All others, including granola and muesli with dried fruit and/or coconut
		
		Instant oatmeal and Cream of Wheat® with dried fruit

	All plain grains Plain crackers without sulfites Plain pasta All homemade crackers, cereals, and pasta dishes with allowed ingredients	All others All packaged pasta meals All canned, frozen and dried commercial pasta dishes
Vegetables	All pure fresh and frozen vegetables and their juices, except those listed opposite	Dried vegetables Frozen sliced mushrooms Processed sliced potatoes Pickled vegetables Tomato paste, pulp, purée All prepared vegetables with restricted ingredients
Fruit	All pure fresh or frozen fruit except those listed opposite Frozen orange juice All canned and bottle juices, except those listed opposite **Check labels**	Grapes Frozen apple slices Dried and glacé fruit Maraschino cherries All other frozen juices Grape juice Cider Most bottled lime and lemon juice
Meat, Poultry, and Fish	All unprocessed, pure, fresh or frozen meat, poultry, or fish Fish canned with water, or water and salt only Freshly caught crab, crayfish, lobster, prawns, shrimp, squid which has not had a sulfite wash Processed meat made with allowed ingredients	Processed with restricted ingredients Canned tuna with sulfites All processed crustaceans Processed meats with restricted ingredients Gelatin
Eggs	All	Any prepared with restricted ingredients

Sulfite Restricted Diet

Type of Food	Foods Allowed	Foods Restricted
Legumes	All plain legumes Pure peanut butter	All others
Nuts and Seeds	All plain nuts and seeds	Any with restricted ingredients
Fats and Oils	Pure butter and cream Shortening, margarine Pure vegetable oils Homemade salad dressings with allowed ingredients Lard and meat drippings Homemade gravy	All others

Spices and Herbs	All fresh, frozen, or dried
	  herbs and spices
		All herb or spice mixes and
		  seasoning packets with
		  restricted ingredients, such as
		  dehydrated vegetables

Sweets and Sweeteners	White sugar, honey
	Maple syrup, corn syrup
	Icing sugar
	Pure jams, jellies, marmalade,
	  and conserves made without
	  added pectin or gelatin, and
	  with allowed ingredients
	Plain artificial sweeteners
	Homemade sweets with
	  allowed ingredients
		Brown sugar, molasses
		Glucose solids and syrup
		Dextrose (used in sweets)
		Spreads with restricted
		  ingredients
		Commercial icing and
		  frosting
		Cake decorations and other
		  confectionary
		Commercial candies

Other	Baking powder, baking soda,
	  Cream of Tartar
	Distilled white vinegar
	Baking chocolate
	Pure cocoa
	Homemade pickles and
	  relishes
	Homemade ketchup with
	  allowed ingredients
		Gelatin and pectin
		All other vinegars
		Chocolate candy, sprinkles
		  and syrup
		Mincemeat
		Prepared pickles and relishes
		Commercial ketchup

Alcohol	None	All
Medications	All without sulfites and dextrose **Check with pharmacist**	All others

24

Monosodium Glutamate (MSG) Sensitivity

Monosodium glutamate (MSG), a flavor enhancer common in Chinese cooking, is used increasingly to flavor Western foods. In addition, some foods such as tomatoes, mushrooms, and cheese contain MSG naturally.[1]

Persons sensitive to MSG report a variety of symptoms known as the "Chinese Restaurant Syndrome" or "Kwok's Syndrome". Symptoms may include facial flushing, pain in the face and the back of the neck, headache, tingling and burning sensations, blurred vision, nausea and vomiting, increased heartbeat, and chills and shaking.[2] Several incidents of severe asthma have been attributed to the ingestion of MSG,[3] depression, irritability, and other mood changes have also been reported.

Experts are widely divided on the subject of MSG sensitivity. A recent review[4] stated that results of a number of research studies "led to the conclusion that 'Chinese Restaurant Syndrome' is an anecdote applied to a variety of postprandial illnesses: rigorous and realistic scientific evidence linking the syndrome to MSG could not be found". On the other hand, some clinicians have estimated that the prevalence of "Chinese Restaurant Syndrome" may be as high as 1.8% of the adult population.[5]

A recent double blind placebo controlled study of people with a history of "Chinese Restaurant Syndrome" indicated that the majority of individuals did not react to MSG.[6] In the cases where a reaction occurred, the response was reported as mild. The threshold dose that led to the development of symptoms was measured at 2.5 grams. A report on MSG by the U.S. Food and Drug Administration issued in 1995 indicated that healthy individuals may respond to an oral intake of 3 grams of MSG within an hour in the absence of food.[7]

Mechanism of Action of MSG

MSG is the sodium salt of glutamic acid, an amino acid. Glutamate is the active ingredient in the compound.[8]

One theory to explain sensitivity to MSG links its action to abnormally high levels of acetylcholine,[9] a neurotransmitter that acts on the brain and central nervous system. Because glutamate acts as a precursor in the synthesis of acetylcholine, as well as other physiological chemicals, the symptoms ascribed to MSG sensitivity may be caused by excessive levels of neurotransmitters that develop in a short period of time. Toxic levels of acetylcholine may explain the symptoms of the "Chinese Restaurant Syndrome".[10]

The usual source of exogenous glutamate is food proteins, where it is combined with other amino acids. Before glutamate is free to be absorbed, the peptide bonds in these proteins must be broken by enzymes. Because this process is gradual, it controls the level of free glutamate in the body. According to the theory of "neurotransmitter toxicity," when MSG is eaten, glutamate enters the blood stream rapidly because no peptide linkages need to be broken. Clinical studies have shown that an MSG dose of 0.1 g/kg body weight can induce plasma glutamate levels to peak to 15 times the basal concentration in approximately one hour.[6] However, a correlation between plasma glutamate levels and symptoms has not been demonstrated.[4]

Some practitioners have noticed a deficiency of Vitamin B_6 (pyridoxine) in a number of MSG sensitive persons.[8] This factor could retard hepatic catabolism of glutamate, thus prolonging high plasma glutamate levels and exacerbating symptoms.

Symptoms Possibly Caused by MSG

The following symptoms are reported to be caused by MSG:[2,3]

- Flushing
- Tightness around face, jaw and chest; numbness of face
- Tingling, burning of face and chest
- Rapid heartbeat
- Nausea, diarrhea, stomach cramps
- Headache, especially at back of head and neck
- Weakness, dizziness, balance problems, staggering
- Confusion, slurred speech
- Blurring of vision, difficulty focusing, seeing shining lights
- Chills and shaking, excessive perspiration
- Difficulty in breathing
- Symptoms of asthma (in persons with asthma)
- Water retention, thirst
- Insomnia, sleepiness
- Stiffness, heaviness of arms and legs
- Mood changes, irritability
- Depression, paranoia

Symptoms of the "Chinese Restaurant Syndrome" are reported to usually occur within 30 minutes of eating a meal high in MSG. Symptoms of asthma, however, have been reported to occur 1 to 2 hours after MSG ingestion, and even as long as 12 hours later.[3]

Management of MSG Sensitivity

A safe level of MSG in foods cannot be set because a number of different factors contribute to plasma levels of glutamate, only one of which is the MSG added to food. Glutamate is a natural constituent of the body, where it plays an essential role in metabolism. Transaminases in the liver allow glutamate to interact in a variety of reactions, and free glutamate is also found in muscle, brain, kidneys, and other organs. The average person weighing 70 kg has the equivalent of about 12 g of MSG in their body.[6] Whether or not any particular plasma level can be considered safe is not known.

Milk contains natural free glutamate. The daily glutamate intake of a 3 kg infant obtained from 480g of mother's milk is 3.75 g (1.25 g/kg body weight).[6]

The Joint FAO/WHO Expert Committee on Food Additives has evaluated MSG and has deemed that no numerical limitation is necessary for the use of MSG in food.[11]

MSG sensitive persons should be advised to restrict their intake of MSG as much as possible. Because alcohol seems to increase the rate of absorption of many foods as well as MSG, drinking alcoholic beverages while eating MSG containing foods probably increases both the severity and rate of onset of symptoms. In addition, eating foods containing MSG on an empty stomach seems to increase the adverse effects of MSG.

Sources of MSG

The following flavorings containing MSG:

Accent®	Hydrolyzed vegetable protein (HVP)
Ajinomoto	Hydrolyzed plant protein (HPP)
Zest	Natural flavorings (may be HVP)
Vetsin	Flavorings
Gourmet powder	Kombu extract
Subu	Mei-jing
All Chinese seasonings	Wei-jing
Glutavene	RL-50
Glutacyl	

Many prepared foods contain MSG or one of the above flavorings. Foods containing these additives include:[12]

Canned meats	Freeze-dried foods
Prepared dinners and side dishes	Frozen foods
Canned soups	Potato chips
Dry soup mixes	Prepared snacks
Gravy and seasoning mixes	Prepared salads, salad dressings and
Cookies and crackers	mayonnaise
Cured meats	Croutons
Smoked meats and sausages	Bottled and canned sauces
Diet foods	Spices and seasonings

Glutamate is also present in monopotassium glutamate, monoammonium glutamate, calcium glutamate and other salts of glutamic acid. Some MSG sensitive persons may react to these salts also.[13]

Restaurants, Cafeterias, and Fast Food Restaurants

The majority of eating places in North America include MSG in some form in most of their dishes, unless they specifically state otherwise. Most reputable establishments can supply a list of the ingredients in their menu items.

Table 24-1: MSG Levels in Representative Foods[10]

Food Group	Mean % MSG (g/100 g)
Meat and Meat Products	
Cured ox tongue with brine	0.81
Cured pork leg with brine	0.06
Bacon and ham, uncooked	0.23
Canned ham	0.83
Other canned meats	0.41
Sausages, pork, uncooked	0.02
Sausages, beef, uncooked	0.54
Meat pie, ready to eat	0.10
Sausage roll, ready to eat	0.11
Frozen meat burgers	0.56
Frozen meat pies	0.32
Delicatessen type sausages (salami, etc.)	0.26
Meat pastes and spreads	0.49
Lasagne, ready to eat	0.10
Meat loaf	0.53

Table 24-1: MSG Levels in Representative Foods[10]

Food Group	Mean % MSG (g/100 g)
Fish	
Frozen, ready-to-eat, fish products (fish sticks, fish cakes)	0.39
Vegetables	
Canned beans with sausage	0.14
Canned mushrooms	0.24
Potato chips	0.91
Nuts	
Nuts and nut products	0.48
Grains and Flours	
Crackers	0.20
Frozen pizza	0.29
Canned pasta	0.18
Fresh pizza	0.17
Packaged rice or noodles with sauce mixes	2.06
Cereals	0.92
Miscellaneous	
Soups, canned	0.33
Soups, dehydrated and powdered (reconstituted)	3.78
Meat and yeast extracts (e.g. Bovril®, Marmite®, Vegemite®)	8.70
Pickles and sauces (e.g., ketchup)	0.62

References

1. McBride, R.L. MSG and the bliss point factor. ILSI MSG Symposium Food Australia, July 1991 43(7):S16-S19.

2. Schwartz, G.R. *In Bad Taste: The MSG Syndrome.* New American Library, Signet Books, Scarborough, Ont., 1988.

3. Allen, D.H., and Baker, G. J. Chinese restaurant asthma. New Eng. J. Med. 1981 305(19):1154-1155.

4. Tarasoff, L., and Kelly, M.F. Monosodium L-glutamate: A double-blind study and review. Food Chemistry and Toxicology 1993 31(12):1019-1035.

5. Kerr, G., Wu-Lee, M, and El-Lozy, M. Prevalence of the "Chinese restaurant syndrome". J. Am. Diet. Assoc. 1979 75:29-33.

6. Yang, W.H., Drouin, M.A., Herbert, M., Mao, Y,. Double-blind, placebo-controlled, randomized study (DBPCRS) to evaluate reactions allegedly due to the consumption of monosodium glutamate (MSG) - the Canadian study. J. Allergy Clin. Immunol. (Abst.) 1995 95 (1 pt 2) 304.

7. Zardakas,M., Scott, F., Salimen, J., and Ham Pong, A. Project 19. Development of a list of foods known to cause severe adverse reactions in Canadians. Agriculture and Agri-Food Canada and Health Canada, March 1996.

8.   Rand, M.J. The international status of MSG. ILSI MSG Symposium. Food Australia, July 1991 <u>43</u>(7).

9.   Moneret-Vautrin, D.A. Food intolerance masquerading as food allergy: False food allergy. In: Brostoff, J., and Challacombe, S.J. (Eds) *Food Allergy and Intolerance.* Baillière-Tindall, London and Philadelphia, 1989.

10.   Ghadimi, J., Kumar, S, et al. Studies on monosodium glutamate ingestion: biochemical explanations of Chinese Restaurant Syndrome. Biochem. Med. 1971 <u>5</u>:447-456.

11.   Rhodes, J. Titherley, A.C., Norman, J.A., Wood, R., and Lord, D.W. A survey of the monosodium glutamate content of foods and an estimation of the dietary intake of monosodium glutamate. In: *Food Additives and Contaminants.* 1991 <u>8</u>(3):265-274.

12.   Scopp, A.L. MSG and hydrolyzed vegetable protein induced headache: Review and case studies. Headache, February 1991. 107-110.

13.   JECFA-L-glutamic acid and its ammonium, calcium, monosodium and potassium salts. In: *Toxicological Evaluation of Certain Food Additives.* Joint FAO/WHO Expert Committee on Food Additives. WHO Food Additives Services, 1987 <u>22</u>:97-161. Cambridge University Press, Cambridge.

Method: Monosodium Glutamate (MSG) Restricted Diet

Monosodium Glutamate (MSG) Restricted Diet

Type of Food	Foods Allowed	Foods Restricted
Milk and Dairy	Plain milk, buttermilk, cream, sour cream, and yogurt All plain cheese, cottage cheese, ricotta, Quark® Pure vanilla ice cream Plain salted or unsalted butter	Flavored milk Commercial dips Flavored yogurt All flavored and smoked cheese, cheese slices, and cheese foods All other ice cream All seasoned butter
Breads and Cereals	Any pure flour or grain Any bread, bun, pita or pizza dough without flavoring, except plain sourdough	Bread, baking mixes or grain mixes with flavoring or seasoning packets Sourdough bread and buns All others, such as croutons, stuffing, meat coating mixes
	Breakfast cereals without flavorings, including: Puffed rice and wheat Shreddies® Shredded Wheat® Corn flakes Cereals with malt or malt syrup Oats and oatmeal Plain Cream of Wheat® All plain grains	All others, especially the colored and flavored cereals made to appeal to children Flavored oatmeal and Cream of Wheat®
	Plain crackers without flavoring (read labels) Plain pasta All homemade baked goods, cereals and pasta dishes with allowed ingredients	All flavored crackers All flavored pasta All canned, frozen and dried commercial pasta dishes
Vegetables	All pure fresh and frozen vegetables and their juices	Canned vegetables and juices Read labels on plain frozen vegetables Commercially prepared vegetables with sauces and flavorings

Monosodium Glutamate (MSG) Restricted Diet

Type of Food	Foods Allowed	Foods Restricted
Fruit	All pure fresh or frozen fruits and their juices Homemade fruit dishes and drinks with allowed ingredients	Fruit dishes with flavoring Fruit drinks and cocktails

Meat, Poultry, and Fish	All unprocessed, pure, fresh or frozen meat, poultry, or fish
	Fish canned with water, or water and salt, only
	Processed meat such as ham, with "MSG-free" on the label
	Homemade sausages, etc.
		Processed or with restricted ingredients, e.g.:
		  stuffing
		  butter basted
		  in broth
		  with spices or seasoning
		  cured or smoked sausages, patties, etc.
		Canned, except as listed opposite

Eggs	All	All prepared with restricted foods
Legumes	All plain legumes Pure peanut butter	All others
Nuts and Seeds	All plain nuts and seeds	All others
Fats and Oils	Pure butter and cream Shortening Pure vegetable oils Homemade salad dressing Lard and meat drippings Gravy	All others
Spices and Herbs	All fresh, frozen, or dried herbs and single spices	All herb or spice mixes and seasoning packets See listing of flavorings containing MSG
Sweets and Sweeteners	Sugar, honey, molasses Pure jams and jellies Pure corn and maple syrup Plain artificial sweeteners Homemade sweets and fruit drinks with allowed ingredients	Artificially flavored and colored sweeteners, jams, jellies, icings, cake decorations, candies, and drink mixes

25

Nitrate and Nitrite Sensitivity

Nitrates and nitrites are used in foods as preservatives, particularly as protection against the deadly bacterium *Clostridium botulinum*. They are also used to impart flavor and color to manufactured foods, especially processed meats.[1]

Symptoms of Sensitivity

Some reports indicate that nitrates and nitrites can provoke headache in persons sensitive to these compounds.[2]

Nitrates and Nitrites in Foods

The presence of nitrates or nitrites in manufactured foods will be indicated on the label as sodium nitrate, potassium nitrate, sodium nitrite, or potassium nitrite.[3] High levels are found in processed meats such as pepperoni, frankfurters, wieners, sausages, salami, bologna, other luncheon meats, bacon, and ham, as well as in smoked fish and some imported cheeses.[4]

Plants can contain naturally occurring nitrates derived mainly from nitrate containing fertilizers. The following plant species tend to accumulate nitrates more than others:[2]

- Beets
- Celery
- Collards

- Eggplant (aubergine)
- Lettuce
- Radishes
- Spinach
- Turnip greens

Nitrates may be converted to nitrites in the mouth and intestine. Thus, the level of the chemical in food does not always reflect the level in the body after digestion.

References

1. Simon, R.A. Adverse reactions to food additives. New Eng. Regional Allergy Proc. 1986 7(6):533-542.

2. Raskin, N.H. Chemical headaches. Ann. Rev. Med. 1981 32:63-71.

3. Winter, R. *A Consumer's Dictionary of Food Additives*. Crown Publishers, New York, 1989. 227-230.

4. Vaughan, T.R., and Mansfield, L.E. Neurologic reactions to foods and food additives. In: Metcalfe, D.D., Sampson, H.A., and Simon, R.A. (Eds), *Food Allergy: Adverse Reactions to Foods and Food Additives*. Blackwell Scientific Publications, Oxford, London, 1991. 355-369.

Method: Nitrate and Nitrite Restricted Diet

The levels of nitrates and nitrites vary according to:

- The quantity added to processed meat
- The level found in the soil in which a plant is grown

It is not possible to provide an accurate measure of the chemicals in each food.

People vary in their tolerance of nitrates and nitrites. It is difficult to give directives concerning the quantity of food that can be eaten without eliciting symptoms.

If a person is intolerant to nitrites and nitrates it is important to avoid foods containing the highest levels of these chemicals as indicated in Table 25-1.

Table 25-1: Level of Nitrates and Nitrites in Some Meats and Vegetables

Food	Mean Level (mg/100 g)
Nitrites	
Meats	
Bacon	1.3
Bacon, smoked	3.1
Luncheon meat	0.3
Ham, smoked	3.0
Salami	0.3
Salami, kosher	38.0
Vegetables	
Asparagus, raw	2.1
Beet, raw	276.0
Beans, dry	1.3
Broccoli, raw	78.3
Cabbage, raw	63.5
Carrot, raw	11.9
Cauliflower, raw	84.7
Corn, raw	4.5
Cucumber, raw	2.4
Green beans, raw	25.3
Eggplant (aubergine), raw	30.2
Lettuce, raw	85.0
Lima beans, raw	5.4
Melon, raw	43.3
Onion, raw	13.4
Peas, raw	2.8
Pepper, sweet raw	12.5

Table 25-1: Level of Nitrates and Nitrites in Some Meats and Vegetables

Food	Mean Level (mg/100 g)
Nitrites	
Vegetables	
Pickles	5.9
Potato, raw	11.9
Pumpkin, raw	41.3
Sauerkraut	19.1
Spinach, raw	186.0
Sweet potato, raw	5.0
Tomato, raw	6.2

Part IV

Pediatric Allergy

26

Pediatric Allergy

Early infancy is considered to be the time when infants are at maximum risk of being sensitized to allergens. Many experts believe that, when factors predictive of early sensitization to allergens are present, preventive measures can be taken to reduce or avoid the possibility of allergy developing.[1]

Critical Periods for Sensitization to Allergens

The last trimester of pregnancy, the neonatal period, and the first months of life are cited as critical periods for allergic sensitization.[1] If exposure to highly allergenic foods is avoided during these periods, the likelihood of the infant becoming allergic to these foods can be reduced or eliminated.[2]

Incidence of Allergy in Children

A 1994 report[3] suggests that the prevalence of food allergy in childhood is less than 4 to 5%, and that a conservative estimate of the incidence of cow's milk allergy in infants is 2 to 3%. In contrast, other reports suggest that the incidence of food allergy in childhood is up to 8%, and that "food related complaints" afflict as many as 28% of children.[4]

Early Allergy Predictors

The first requirement in prevention of allergy of any sort is to identify the potentially allergic infant so preventive measures can be initiated at the earliest appropriate time.

Family History of Allergy

The most important factor in predicting the likelihood that allergy will develop is a history of allergy in first degree relatives (parents and siblings). A number of studies have attempted to quantify the incidence of allergy. The findings are limited by the lack of definitive, objective tests for allergy, especially to foods. The numbers most frequently quoted from a 1977 study of 1327 children[5] indicate that the incidence of allergy of any type is as follows:

Total incidence of atopic disease	15%
Both parents with identical allergy symptoms	72%
Both parents with non-identical allergy symptoms	43%
One parent with allergy symptoms	20%
One sibling with allergy symptoms	32%
Neither parent allergic	12%

Elevated Total IgE in Cord Blood

Several research studies have attempted to establish a level of IgE in cord blood that can be used to identify the potentially allergic infant at birth. At present there is no consensus on the usefulness of IgE levels in cord blood as a predictive indicator.

Values of IgE in cord blood of greater than 0.7 kU/L[6] to greater than 0.9 kU/L[7] have been cited as indicative of the development of allergy in children before the age of 18 months. Other studies[8] have suggested that free IgE (i.e., that produced by the fetus in utero) is an inadequate predictor of potential atopy. These investigators recommend that a more accurate measure of fetal IgE is the sum of free IgE in cord blood plus IgE complexed with anti-IgE IgG that was produced by the mother and crossed the placenta.

To add further to the confusion regarding the predictive value of cord blood IgE, a report published in 1994[9] indicates that many variables can influence the level of cord blood IgE and therefore diminish its value as a predictor of potential atopy. These factors include:

- Single and bi-parental atopic heritage
- Maternal eczema and perennial rhinitis
- Month of birth (levels peak in infants born in late autumn)
- Gender (boys have significantly higher levels than girls)
- Alcohol and caffeine consumption by mother during pregnancy
- Mother's pre-pregnancy weight

The authors of this report concluded that "the fact that many factors presumably not related to infant allergy seem to influence the regulation of fetal IgE production could explain the questionable value of cord blood IgE in predicting allergy in childhood."[9] Thus, despite interest in cord blood analysis as a possible predictor of childhood allergy, the strongest predictive factor at present is a positive family history of allergy in one or both parents and/or one or more siblings.

Additional Factors Contributing to Childhood Food Allergy Sensitization of the Fetus to Allergens in Utero

Reports of acute adverse reactions to foods on the first prenatal contact provide circumstantial evidence that sensitization to food allergens is likely to have occurred in utero.[10] The fetus is capable of producing its own IgE as early as 17 weeks after conception.[11] Theoretically, levels of IgE in the fetus are adequate during the last trimester of pregnancy for an antigen-specific response to food allergens that might cross the placenta from the maternal diet. No study has conclusively demonstrated the presence of antigen-specific IgE in cord blood, in particular to wheat[12] and cow's milk.[13]

A 1988 study[14] indicated that dietary manipulation from week 28 to the end of pregnancy did not affect the atopic status of the infant. The placenta seems to protect the fetus against the effects of maternal food, even in pregnancies considered as high risk for atopy.[14] Based on available evidence, the view now held is that sensitization to food allergens in utero does occur occasionally but is uncommon, appearing in less than 0.4% of pregnancies.[1]

As there is no definitive evidence of food allergen sensitization in utero and because unnecessarily restricting the maternal diet risks nutritional deficiency, rigorous exclusion of food allergens during pregnancy is rarely considered necessary. The rare occasion occurs when a previous offspring is severely allergic and the mother is strongly motivated to prevent sensitizing the unborn infant. Otherwise, the recommendations for a pregnant mother with a familial history of allergy are:

- To avoid the foods to which the mother is allergic
- To reduce the mother's intake of the most highly allergenic foods, particularly during the last trimester of pregnancy.

The most highly allergenic foods need not be eliminated entirely, only reduced. These foods are:

- Peanut
- Nuts
- Eggs
- Shellfish
- Fish
- Cow's milk and dairy products

Developmental Immaturity of the Digestive Tract

During the first three years of life, and in particular during the first year, the intestine is highly permeable to the absorption of large molecules. It is during this time that sensitization to food allergens occurs and food allergy is most likely to develop.[15]

Protective Antibodies

In addition to having a hyperpermeable intestinal tract, the newborn lacks secretory IgA (sIgA), the antibody that provides the first line of defense against microorganisms entering the body through a mucous membrane. Saliva and secretions of the mature digestive tract contain protective substances, including sIgA. Human colostrum and milk contain sufficient sIgA to supply the infant with adequate protection until it can produce amounts sufficient to protect itself. This level of production is not achieved until about 6 months of age in the normal infant.[11] Research studies have indicated that sIgA may also act as a barrier to food allergens.[16] Inadequate sIgA may contribute further to sensitization to foods in the potentially allergic infant. It is especially important that the atopic infant have the early protection afforded by breast-feeding.

Food Allergy in the Breast-fed Infant

The majority of breast-fed infants are free from allergies. For the few who exhibit allergy signs, the initial reactions are mainly in the skin and digestive tract.[17] These reactions are responses to food allergens ingested by the mother and transferred to her breast milk.[18]

Sometimes a sensitizing dose of cow's milk allergen is introduced through one or two feedings of infant formula in the newborn nursery. For potentially atopic infants, avoiding these early formula feedings is particularly important.[19]

Prevention of Early Food Allergen Sensitization

As long as the lactating mother continues to eat the major allergenic foods, the potentially allergic infant is vulnerable to developing allergy to food allergens in the maternal diet.[1] To achieve optimum protection from food allergy, the lactating mother should be advised to avoid all sources of the most highly allergenic foods. Peanut, egg, and cow's milk are the allergens most often detected in breast milk and are the ones most likely to cause infant sensitization.[1,17,18,20]

If a history of severe allergy in the mother or a first degree relative indicates that problems might be caused by one or more other foods, especially major allergenic foods such as tree nuts, shellfish, and fish, these foods should be excluded from the mother's diet.

When an infant exhibits signs of food allergy while being exclusively breast-fed, the mother should keep an exposure diary to determine the foods that might be implicated as possible allergens, (see the method for *Exposure Diary*, page 40). Foods that appear to be implicated should then be tested by elimination and challenge. When the culprit foods have been identified they should be excluded from the maternal diet for as long as breast-feeding continues.

Maternal Diet During Breast-feeding

It is extremely important that lactating mothers obtain equivalent nutrients from alternative sources when excluding a major food group from the diet, especially milk and dairy products. Appropriate substitution of foods and nutrient supplements should be implemented during any dietary restriction.

Exclusive breast-feeding of the potentially atopic infant to the age of six months, with the mother avoiding the most highly allergenic foods (i.e., peanut, egg, and cow's milk) and other allergens as implicated, is the ideal.[1,20] This approach should ensure that the infant obtains the optimum amount of protective secretory IgA antibodies until adequate amounts are produced by the infant. In addition, the infant is not exposed to the most highly allergenic food antigens during the most vulnerable period of life.

Association of Food Allergy and Infant Colic

Colic may be the earliest sign of allergy in the atopic infant. Several research studies have implicated cow's milk proteins in infant formulas as a cause of colic in the first four months of life.[21] Proteins such as bovine alpha-lactalbumin, beta-lactoglobulin, and IgG have been cited as possible etiological factors.

In the infant who is exclusively breast-fed, cow's milk proteins in the mother's diet appear to be a frequent cause of colic.[22] Treating the formula-fed infant by changing to a product without cow's milk and treating the breast-fed infant by excluding all milk and dairy products from the maternal diet have led to resolution of colic in a significant number of cases.[22]

Symptoms Indicating Food Allergy in the Infant

A number of symptoms can indicate possible food allergy in the young infant, especially if they occur within a short period (about two hours) of ingesting the food.[23] As in all allergy treatment, other pathology should be ruled out before food allergy is considered. In the exclusively breast-fed infant, symptoms usually occur about 6 to 8 hours after the mother has ingested the culprit food.

In all cases, a detailed food record of the infant's food and formula intake or, in the case of a breast-fed infant, of the mother's diet, should indicate the food allergens that most likely are responsible for the reaction.

Symptoms most commonly associated with food allergy in the young infant are:

Gastrointestinal Tract

- Persistent colic
- Frequent "spitting up"
- Vomiting
- Diarrhea

Skin

- Urticaria (hives)
- Swelling and reddening around the mouth
- Eczema or a rash
- Dry itchy skin
- Persistent diaper rash
- Redness around anus
- Redness on cheeks
- Scratching and rubbing
- Reddened ears

Respiratory Tract

- Nasal stuffiness
- Sneezing
- Nose rubbing
- Noisy breathing
- Persistent cough
- Wheezing
- Asthma
- Itchy, runny, reddened eyes
- Frequent earaches

Other

- "Feeding problems" (the infant may forcibly reject food)
- Failure to thrive

Formulas for the Food Allergic or Food Intolerant Infant

Although exclusive breast-feeding without supplemental infant formula is the ideal for the potentially allergic infant, this regimen is sometimes impossible and feeding of infant formula is unavoidable. The chosen formula should achieve the best possible outcome for the allergic infant.

Many authorities suggest that, because cow's milk is the most likely source of allergens, formulas based on cow's milk should be avoided until after the first year.[1] Initially soy-based formulas were considered to be hypoallergenic alternatives. However, it has been demonstrated that these formulas also induce allergy in the highly susceptible infant.[1,24]

Several formulas based on hydrolyzed milk casein (Alimentum®, Nutramigen®, Pregestimil®) have proved useful in feeding infants who are allergic to cow's milk and soy. In a few instances, infants have also developed allergies to the hydrolyzed milk casein formulas.[1,25]

A formula based on hydrolyzed whey proteins (Good Start®) may be used as a prophylactic formula to reduce the possibility of sensitizing the potentially allergic infant to cow's milk proteins.[26] This formula is not suitable for the infant in whom milk allergy is already established because molecules of incompletely hydrolyzed whey in the formula can induce an allergic reaction.[1]

Selecting the most appropriate infant formula is based on the infant's reactivity according to the following guidelines:

- If the infant shows no signs of allergy, has no evidence of lactose intolerance, and is free from colic, a conventional formula based on cow's milk and containing lactose should be suitable.

- If the infant has no evidence of cow's milk allergy but shows digestive upset with diarrhea indicating possible lactose intolerance (which might occur following infection in the gastrointestinal tract), a lactose-free formula based on cow's milk (such as Alactamil®) should be tried.

- If the infant is allergic (or suspected to be allergic) to cow's milk, a soy-based formula with sucrose should be tried. If gastrointestinal upsets persist and are the only symptoms, a disaccharide-free formula (such as Prosobee®) should be tried.

- If the infant is allergic (or suspected to be allergic) to both cow's milk and soy, a casein hydrolysate formula should be tried. Alimentum® is often tried first because the sucrose in this formula makes the taste more acceptable. However, if gastrointestinal symptoms persist with Alimentum®, then Nutramigen® or Pregestimil® (neither of which contain disaccharides) should be tried. The disadvantage in using any formula containing a casein hydrolysate is its high cost.

Introducing Solid Foods

Introduction of the multiple allergens in solid foods to the allergic infant should be delayed until after six months of age. Up to this age the immaturity of the infant's digestive tract and immune system increases the risk of sensitization and development of allergy.

Most pediatric allergists recommend that the most highly allergenic foods should not be introduced until one year of age or later. These foods are milk (of any species except human), egg, peanut, soy, corn, wheat, and citrus fruits.[1] Some authorities also recommend the delayed introduction of beef, shellfish, and fish.[27]

Sequence for Introducing Solid Foods

The safest method of introducing solid foods to the allergic infant is to follow an incremental dose protocol.

- Start with a very small quantity of the least allergenic food in each category and increase the amount gradually.

- Use Table 5-1, the Joneja Food Allergen Scale (page 28) as a guide for foods that are least likely to cause allergy. Start at the bottom of the scale in each category (grains, fruits, vegetables, meat and alternates) and use the infant friendly foods. Gradually move up the scale, reserving the foods at the top for one year of age or older.

- For the introduction of solid foods follow Table 26-1, *Sequence of Adding Solid Foods for the Allergic Infant*, page 263. This table is based on Table 5-1: Joneja Food Allergen Scale.

- Before introducing foods to the infant who demonstrates a strong allergic reaction, apply the new food to the cheek and wait 20 minutes to see if a reddened area appears at the site of application.[27] This early warning sign indicates the release of histamine, which presages any allergic response to the food.

- If a reddened area does not appear, apply a little of the food to the infant's outer lower lip. If no reactions occur, give 1 to 2 mL (½ teaspoonful or less) and observe the infant's reactions for up to 4 hours.

- If no adverse reactions occur, give about 5 mL (1 teaspoon) of the food.

- If no adverse reactions occur after a further 4 hours, give 10 mL (2 teaspoons) of the food.

- Observe the infant for the next 24 hours, looking for delayed reactions, which may develop in several ways, including disturbed sleep patterns, irritability, and overt allergic symptoms.

- If no adverse reactions are observed, give more of the food on the third day.

- Use the fourth day as a second monitoring day, looking for delayed reactions.

- If the infant is free from signs of allergy after the fourth day, the food is assumed safe and is included in the infant's diet.

References

1.   Zeiger, R.S. Prevention of food allergy in infancy. Review article. Ann. Allergy December 1990 65:430-441.

2.   Johnstone, D.E. The natural history of allergic disease in children and its intervention. Pediatric Asthma Allergy Immunol. 1989 3:161-189.

3.   Hide, D.W. Food allergy in children. Clin. Exper. Allergy 1994 24:1-2.

4.   Bock, S.A. Prospective appraisal of complaints of adverse reactions to foods in children during the first three years of life. Pediatrics 1987 79:683.

5.   Kjellman, N.I.M. Atopic disease in seven-year-old children. Incidence in relation to family history. Acta Paediatr. Scand. 1977 66:465-471.

6.   Chandra, R.K., Puri, S., Cheema, P.S. Predictive cord blood IgE in development of atopic disease and role of breast-feeding in its prevention. Clin. Allergy 1985 15:517-522.

7.   Kjellman, N.I.M., and Croner, S. Cord blood IgE determination for allergy prediction: a follow-up to seven years of age in 1,651 children. Ann. Allergy 1984 53:167-171.

8.   Vassell, C.C., deWeck, A.L., and Stadler, B.M. Natural anti-IgE auto-antibodies interfere with diagnostic IgE determination. Clin. Exper. Allergy 1990 20:295-303.

9.   Bjerke, T., Hedegaard, M., Henriksen, T.B., Nielsen, B.W., and Schiotz, P.O. Several genetic and environmental factors influence cord blood IgE concentration. Pediatr. Allergy Immunol. 1994 5:88-94.

10.   Collins-Williams, C. Prevention of allergy in the "at-risk" infant. Documents Scientifiques Guigoz, March 1993.

11.   Miller, D.L., Hirvonen, T., and Gitlin, D. Synthesis of IgE by the human conceptus. J. Allergy Clin. Immunol. 1973 52:182-188.

12.   Kaufman, H.S. Allergy in the newborn: skin test reactions confirmed by the Prausnitz-Kustner test at birth. Clin. Allergy 1971 1:363.

13.   Businco, L., Marchetti, F., Pellegrini, G., and Perlini, R. Predictive value of cord blood IgE levels in "at-risk" newborn babies and influence of type of feeding. Clin. Allergy 1983 13:503-508.

14.   Kjellman., N.I.M. Allergy prevention: Does maternal food intake during pregnancy or lactation influence the development of atopic disease during infancy? In: Hanson, L.A. (Ed), *Biology of Human Milk*. Nestlé Nutrition Workshop Series 15, Vevey/Raven Press, New York, 1988. 197-203.

15.   Eastham, E.J., Lichauco, T., Grady, M.I., and Walker, W.A. Antigenicity of infant formulas: Role of immature intestine in protein permeability. J. Pediatr. 1978 93:561-564.

16.   Goldman, A.S., and Goldblum, R.M. Human milk: Immunologic-nutritional relationships. Ann. N.Y. Acad. Sci. 1990 587:236-245.

17.   Gerrard, J.W. Allergy in breast-fed babies to ingredients in breast milk. Ann. Allergy 1979 42(2):69-72.

18.   Jakobsson, I. Food antigens in human milk. Europ. J. Clin. Nutr. 1991 45(Suppl.1):29-33.

19.   Kjellman. N.I.M. Natural history and prevention of food hypersensitivity. In: Metcalfe, D.D., Sampson, H.A., and Simon, R.A. (Eds) *Food Allergy: Adverse Reactions to Foods and Food Additives*. Blackwell Scientific Publishers, Boston, 1991. 319-331.

20.   Hamburger, R.N., Heller, S., Mellon, R., O'Connor, R., and Zieger, R.S. Current status of the clinical and immunological consequences of a prototype allergic disease prevention program. Ann. Allergy 1983 51:281-290.

21.   Lothe, L., and Lindberg, T. Cow's milk whey protein elicits symptoms of infantile colic in colicky formula-fed infants: a double-blind cross-over study. Pediatrics 1989 83:262-266.

22.   Clyne, P., and Kulczycki, A. Human breast milk contains bovine IgG. Relationship to infant colic? Pediatrics 1991 87:439-444.

23.   Ham Pong, A.J. Pinpointing and treating food allergy in children. Allergy: A Canadian Perspective, September 1990. 7-14.

24.   Kjellman, N.I.M., and Johansson, S.G.O. Soy versus cow's milk in infants with a biparental history of atopic disease: development of atopic disease and immunoglobulins from birth to four years of age. Clin. Allergy 1979 9:347-358.

25.   Dean, T.P., Adler, B.R., Ruge, F., and Warner, J.O. *In vitro* allergenicity of cow's milk substitutes. Clin. Exper. Allergy 1993 23:205-210.

26.   Chandra, R.K., Singh, G., and Shridhara, B. Effect of feeding whey hydrosylate, soy and conventional cow milk formulas on incidence of atopic disease in high risk infants. Ann. Allergy 1989 63:102-106.

27.   Chandra, R.K., Puri, S., Suraiya, C., and Cheema, P.S. Influence of maternal food antigen avoidance during pregnancy and lactation on incidence of atopic eczema in infants. Clin. Allergy 1986 16:563-571.

Method: Preventive Measures to Reduce Food Allergy in Infants

The following guidelines will ensure the best possible outcome by avoiding allergens during the most vulnerable period of the infant's life. In certain medical conditions, these guidelines may need to be altered. It is important to follow the physician's advice.

Phase One: Preventive Measures During Pregnancy (Especially in the Third Trimester)

All foods to which the mother is allergic or intolerant should be avoided.

The importance of a well balanced, healthy diet, including the greatest variety of foods possible, is essential. Nutritionally equivalent foods should be eaten as substitutes for foods which are avoided, and supplementation of calcium and Vitamin D must be used if milk and dairy products are eliminated. If entire food groups are eliminated, a complete vitamin and mineral supplement should be taken.

Moderate amounts of a variety of foods should be eaten. Binging produces an unbalanced diet as well as the possibility of allergic sensitization to the food.

Tobacco smoke, caffeine, alcohol, prescription and non-prescription drugs (such as painkillers and laxatives) are to be avoided.

There should be no smoking pre- or post-natally in the home.

Food and beverages containing caffeine should be used in moderation and should not replace healthier beverages like fruit and vegetable juices. Caffeine is found in chocolate, cocoa, tea, coffee, and cola.

Medications containing caffeine should be used only on the advice of a physician. Caffeine is found in cold, allergy, stay-awake, and headache medications.

Alcoholic beverages are not advised for pregnant women. For the allergic mother, there is the possibility of intolerance of some of the ingredients in the beverages.

Prescription and non-prescription drugs should be taken only on the advice of a physician.

Phase Two: Preventive Measures Early Postnatally

Breast-feeding should commence as soon as possible after delivery. Ideally, the infant should be breast-fed within the first half hour of life. The early breast milk provides the infant with protective colostrum.

Measures should be taken to ensure that the infant be given no supplemental feedings. This includes both glucose water and infant formula. Sterile distilled water is safe if the infant requires extra fluid. If the infant spends time in the nursery, a visible sign with this information should be attached to the bassinet.

Phase Three: Preventive Measures in Infancy

Because allergenic components of foods from the mother's diet can pass into the breast milk, the nursing mother should avoid the foods most likely to cause allergy in the infant.

The foods to be avoided include:

Egg

Small amounts of egg in baking should be tolerated. All products containing egg as the main ingredient should be avoided, including:

Hen's eggs: boiled, scrambled, fried, poached, etc.
Eggs from other poultry: ducks, quail, goose, turkey, etc.

Other sources of egg: eggnog, omelette, custard, soufflé, quiche, egg noodles, angel food cake, Caesar salad, some salad dressings, sauces such as Hollandaise, Bearnaise, and Newburg, egg swirl and Wonton soup, some ice cream, meringues (pavlova), some packaged dessert mixes.

All Milk and Dairy Products

All products containing milk, components of milk, or dairy products should be avoided including:

Milk	Ricotta
Condensed milk	Quark®
Evaporated milk	Sherbet
Milk solids	Ice cream
Milk powder	Cream
Yogurt	Sour cream
Butter	Casein
Buttermilk	Sodium caseinate
Curd	Potassium caseinate
Cheese	Calcium caseinate
Cottage cheese	Whey
Cream cheese	Lactoglobulin
Feta	Lactose

All Peanut and Peanut Containing Foods

All products containing peanut or components of peanuts must be avoided including:

Peanut	Satay sauces
Peanut protein	Goober peas
Hydrolyzed peanut protein	Goober nuts
Peanut oil*	Prepared soups (especially dried packaged
Peanut butter	soup mixes)
Peanut flour	Baked goods
Mixed nuts	Cookies
Mandalona nuts**	Candies
Artificial nuts	Chocolate bars
Marzipan (almond paste)	Prepared and frozen desserts
Chili	Vegetable oil
Egg rolls	Hydrogenated vegetable oil
Chinese dishes	Vegetable oil shortening
Thai dishes	

* Pure peanut oil is non-allergenic and will not cause an allergic reaction. However, there is a good chance that the oil is contaminated with peanut protein in its manufacture, so persons allergic to peanut, especially those who have experienced an anaphylactic reaction, are advised to avoid peanut oil.

** "Mandalona" nut is one of the names given to a manufactured product made from de-flavored, de-colored peanut meal that is pressed into molds, re-flavored and colored and sold as a cheaper substitute for tree nuts such as almonds, pecans, and walnuts. Persons with peanut allergy must avoid such products. One manufacturer of such peanut products is Nu-nuts Flavored Nuts Co., Division of Seabrook Blanching Corp., Tyrone, Pennsylvania, USA.

Foods to Which the Infant Appears to React

Reactions in the breast-fed infant typically appear about 6 to 8 hours after the food is eaten by the mother. When trying to identify problem foods, the mother should keep a careful diary of her diet and time of onset of the infant's adverse reaction. This should provide a good idea of which foods mother should avoid, on a trial basis at first. Reintroduction of the food and careful observation of the infant's reactions should identify the culprit foods. The mother should avoid these foods and find a nutritionally equivalent food as a substitute.

The mother's diet should include the greatest variety of foods tolerated by both mother and infant.

Supplementation with 1500 mg of elemental calcium is necessary when all milk and dairy products are eliminated.

If many foods need to be eliminated, an additive-free multivitamin and mineral supplement should be taken by the mother, and the diet made nutritionally complete with the substitution of alternative foods for those restricted.

Avoiding Food Allergens in the Infant's Diet

The infant should be breast-fed exclusively for 6 months. If it is unavoidable, a casein hydrolysate formula can be used. These include Nutramigen® (Mead Johnson), Pregestimil® (Mead Johnson) or Alimentum® (Ross).

If the infant tolerates soy, a soy-based formula can be given. These include Isomil® (Ross), Nursoy® (Wyeth), Prosobee® (Mead Johnson).

The introduction of solids should be delayed until 6 months. Introduce the least allergenic foods first, (see *Table 26-1: Sequence of Adding Solid Foods for the Allergic Infant* page 263). Continue breast-feeding while introducing solids.

After one year, at two week or one month intervals, add one of the following more highly allergenic foods:

- Milk and dairy products
- Wheat
- Soy (if not used earlier as formula)
- Corn
- Citrus (including orange, grapefruit, lemon, lime etc.)
- Egg (delay longer in obviously food allergic infants.)
- Fish (delay longer in obviously food allergic infants.)

Breast-feeding should be continued as long as possible.

Do not feed the infant peanuts, nuts, or chocolate until after two years of age.

Important Environmental Factors

Inhalant allergens to be avoided include house dust mites, tobacco smoke, animal dander, feathers, pollens and other air pollutants. Frequent dusting will reduce house dust mites. Smoking in the house before or after the infant is born should not be allowed. Electronic air filters may be useful in reducing air-borne allergens.

The infant's exposure to infections should be minimized.

Egg, Milk, Dairy, and Peanut Restricted Diet for Pregnant and Breast-feeding Women

Type of Food	Foods Allowed	Foods Restricted
Milk and Dairy	Substitutes: Soy milk Soy infant formula Casein hydrosylate formula Rice Dream® Coconut milk Whey-free margarine Tofu without milk solids	All milk and dairy products Dairy substitutes containing egg or peanut
Breads and Cereals	Breads and baked goods without milk, egg or peanut French or Italian bread Some whole wheat bread Some rye bread Soda crackers Egg-free pasta Plain or wild rice General Foods Minute Rice® Plain cooked or ready-to-eat cereals Homemade granola or muesli without peanut All plain grains, flours, and starches All homemade baked goods with allowed ingredients	Baked products with milk or milk products, peanut, or with egg as a major ingredient Packaged, canned or frozen prepared pasta or rice dishes Cereals processed with milk or milk solids, or peanut All commercial baking mixes All grain products with "peanut" or "nuts" on the label
Fruit	All pure fruit and pure fruit juices	Fruit dishes prepared with restricted foods
Eggs	To be used only in moderation in baking	See list of egg restrictions, page 255

Vegetables	All vegetables and their juices except those listed opposite	Prepared as:
		  Creamed
		  Scalloped
		  Mashed with milk
		  Breaded or battered
		  Butter or margarine added
		  Instant potatoes
		All vegetable dishes made with peanut or with unknown ingredients
		Salads with dressings containing unknown ingredients

Egg, Milk, Dairy, and Peanut Restricted Diet for Pregnant and Breast-feeding Women

Type of Food	Foods Allowed	Foods Restricted
Meat, Poultry, and Fish	All plain, fresh, or frozen meat, poultry, or fish Fish canned in water, broth or disclosed oil other than peanut Pure deli meats such as ham, sliced beef, smoked chicken, smoked turkey	Meat, poultry, or fish that is breaded, battered, or creamed Dishes made with peanut or undisclosed oils Chinese and Thai dishes Egg rolls Commercial chili Vegetarian burgers, unless known to be peanut-free
Legumes	All plain legumes except peanuts Soy milk Milk-free tofu	Products containing milk or dairy products or peanut, or egg, as a major ingredient Peanut butter
Nuts and Seeds	All packaged, plain, pure nuts and seeds All pure nut and seed oils and their butters, such as tahini, or almond butter	Prepared with milk or milk products Mixed nuts Mandalona nuts Artificial nuts Any oils or nuts of undisclosed origin
Fats and Oils	Pure vegetable oils except peanut Milk-free margarine, e.g.: Fleischmann's Low Sodium® Parkay Diet Spread® Lard Meat drippings Homemade gravy	Butter Peanut oil Margarine containing whey, milk, or peanut Salad dressings with restricted ingredients Shortening
Spices and Herbs	All pure herbs and spices Blends of herbs and spices without added oil	Seasoning packets with undisclosed ingredients Vegetables such as sun-dried tomato or garlic in oil, unless source of oil is disclosed
Sweets and Sweeteners	Plain sugar, honey, molasses, maple syrup, corn syrup Pure chocolate and cocoa Pure jams and jellies Homemade cookies, candies, and sweets with allowed ingredients Sugar Twin®	The following, unless sources are revealed and ingredients are allowed: Other chocolate Chocolate bars Marzipan (almond paste) Most commercial sweets Sugar substitutes containing lactose

Method: Feeding the Allergic Infant Solid Foods After Six Months of Age

General Information

When adding solid food to the allergic infant's diet, there are two goals:

- To increase the chances of the development of tolerance
- To avoid sensitization and the development of allergic reactions.

Mechanism of Intolerance

The precise immunological mechanisms that will lead to tolerance or sensitization are not fully known.   The following method of introducing new foods has proved to be the best so far devised for achieving these objectives.

Guidelines for Testing Foods

The least allergic foods should be introduced first, (see *Sequence of Adding Solid Foods for the Allergic Infant*, page 263).

For the exclusively breast-fed infant, no foods should be introduced prior to six months of age. New foods may be added every week, every second week, or for exceptionally allergic infants, once a month. This will depend on the infant's reactions.

Introduction of the most highly allergenic foods should be delayed until after twelve months. Chocolate, peanuts, and nuts should not be introduced until after two years of age.

Breast-feeding should be continued while adding new foods, as human milk provides protection.

Table 26-1: Sequence of Adding Solid Foods for the Allergic Infant, page 263, includes foods which are:

- Usually acceptable to infants
- Easily digested at the times of introduction suggested
- Most commonly introduced to North American infants.

The foods should be introduced first in their pure form. Cook in plain water. Sieve or purée.

Some Heinz® Beginner Foods (carrots, green beans, squash, sweet potatoes, peaches, pears, plums) and Gerber® First Foods (carrots, green and yellow beans, squash, sweet potatoes, peaches, pears) are suitable.

Gerber® and Heinz Infant® chicken, beef, and veal are suitable, but the lamb has lemon added.

Pure grains should be cooked in water and pureed for initial introduction.

Infant cereals (Pablum) contain other ingredients including malt and soy which might cause an adverse reaction. Tolerance for soy should be tested prior to introducing the infant cereals, once tolerance to the cereal grain is established.

Foods on the Infant Food Allergen Scale are least allergenic at the top of the list and increase in allergenic potential from the top to the bottom of the list.

If the infant has an adverse reaction to the food at any time, discontinue the food immediately and do not test the same food again for about 2 months.

Wait at least 48 hours after the symptoms have *subsided* before testing a new food.

Day 1

Apply a small amount of a new food to the cheek. Wait for 20 minutes to see if a reddened area appears at the site of application. If redness does appear, this "early warning sign" indicates a probable allergic response to the food.

If a reddened area does not appear, a little may be applied to the outer lower lip. If no response to this is observed, the following feeding can be given.

Morning:	Feed ½ teaspoon of the new food. Monitor the infant's reaction. Wait four hours. If no adverse reaction is apparent, continue as follows:
Afternoon:	Feed 1 teaspoon of the same food. Monitor the infant's reaction. Wait four hours. If no adverse reaction is apparent, continue as follows:
Evening:	Feed 2 teaspoons of the same food. Monitor the infant's reaction. Be alert for any changes in sleeping patterns (restlessness, crying, difficulty settling down to sleep) which might indicate a reaction to the new food.

Day 2

Do not feed any of the new food. Monitor the infant's reactions during the day. Look for delayed reactions to the food eaten on Day 1.

Day 3

If no adverse reactions have appeared, test the same food as on Day 1 (eliminating the cheek and lip test), but use larger quantities at each feeding.

Morning:	Feed 2 tablespoons of the food. Monitor the infant's reaction, as on Day 1. If no adverse reaction is apparent, continue as follows:
Afternoon:	Feed ¼ cup of the same food. Monitor the infant's reactions. If no adverse reaction is apparent, continue as follows:
Evening:	Feed as much of the food as the infant wants. Monitor the infant's reactions.

Day 4

Monitor the infant's reactions as described for Day 2. If no adverse reactions occur, the food may be considered safe and can be included in the infant's diet.

If the food is tolerated, include it in the infant's diet. Some authorities believe that by including the food in the infant's diet at least once every 4 days, tolerance to the food will be maintained. Including large doses frequently every day, on the other hand, is thought to risk sensitizing the infant to develop an allergic reaction to the food. Moderation is the best strategy.

Wait two days or up to one week depending on the infant's potential to develop allergic-type reactions, then test a different food in the same way.

Adverse Reactions

Discontinue the food immediately if:

- The infant obviously rejects the food by grimacing or spitting it out forcibly; she/he may be responding to an unpleasant sensation due to an allergic reaction inside the mouth

- The infant takes the food, but a visible reaction appears around the mouth (reddening, red patches, hives), or hives (itchy, flat, red patches) appear anywhere on the body

- The infant shows obvious signs of abdominal discomfort (increased crying, drawing up of the legs, abdominal bloating), itching, or irritability; these are clear signs of an adverse reaction

- the infant spits up, vomits, or has diarrhea. These are all strong adverse reactions.

Delayed reactions (occurring 6-8 hours or longer after eating the food) often include respiratory symptoms (stuffy nose, frequent sneezing, persistent coughing, wheezing), or skin reactions (exacerbation of eczema, hives).

Table 26-1: Sequence of Adding Solid Foods for the Allergic Infant

Time of Introduction	Grains and Cereals	Vegetables	Fruits	Meat and Alternates	Milk and Dairy	Nuts, Seeds, Other

Six to nine months	Rice
	Millet
		All cooked
		Yam
		Sweet
		  potato
		Squash (all
		  types)
		Carrot
		Beets
		Broccoli
		Potato
		Green
		  beans
		Cabbage
			All cooked
			Pear
			Peach
			Banana
			Apricot
			Nectarine
			Blueberry
				Lamb
				Turkey
					Breast milk
					
					If absolutely
					  necessary,
					  casein
					  hydrolysate
					  formula.
						None

Nine to twelve months	Barley
	Rye
	Oats
		Asparagus
		Avocado
		Cauliflower
		Brussels
		  sprouts
			Plum
			Prune
			Pineapple
			Grape
			Apple,
			  cooked
			Cranberry
			Raisins
				Chicken
				Veal
				Beef
					Breast milk
					  or casein
					  hydrolysate
					  formula
						None
						except
						vegetable
						oils
						in formula

Twelve to twenty-four months	Corn
	Wheat
	Other grains
		Green pea
		Spinach
		Tomato
		Celery
		Cucumber
		Lettuce
		Onion
		Garlic
		Lima beans
		Broad beans
		Other
		  legumes
		  including
		  soy
		Any raw
		vegetables
			Citrus
			fruits
			(orange,
			  grapefruit
			  lemon,
			  lime)
			Berries:
			
			Strawberry
			Raspberry
			Other
			Melons
			Mango
			Fig
			Date
			Cherry
			Any raw
			fruits
				Ham
				Pork
				Fish
				Egg
					Yogurt (plain)
					Homogenized
					  milk
					White cheese
					Cottage cheese
						Seed oils:
						Canola
						Safflower
						Sunflower

After two years	All	All	All	Shellfish	All others
					  including ice
					  cream
						Peanut
						Nuts
						Chocolate
						Seeds

Composition of Infant Formulae*

Appropriate Choices in the Management of Food Allergy and Disaccharide Intolerance. Numbers refer to products listed in the table below.

<u>Formulation</u>

1. Cow's milk base with lactose
2. Cow's milk base without lactose
3. Whey hydrolysate with lactose (Prophylactic)
4. Soy base with sucrose
5. Soy base without sucrose
6. Casein hydrolysate with sucrose
7. Casein hydrolysate without sucrose
8. Soy hydrolysate without sucrose

<u>Suitable for:</u>

CMA -; Lactose intolerance -
CMA -; Lactose intolerance +
CMA -; Lactose intolerance -
CMA +; Disaccharide intolerance -
CMA +; Disaccharide intolerance +
CMA+; Soy allergy+; Disaccharide intolerance
CMA +; Soy allergy +; Disaccharide intolerance +
CMA +; Soy allergy +; Disaccharide intolerance +
CMA = cow's milk protein allergy
+ and - indicate presence or absence of the indicated condition

Table 26-2: Composition of Infant Formulae*

Protein Source	Carbohydrate	Name	Manu-facturer	Fat
1. Cow's Milk Base With Lactose				
Demineralized whey Skim milk powder	**Lactose**	Enfalac	Mead Johnson	Palm oil Soy oil Coconut oil Sunflower oil
Skim milk	**Lactose** Corn starch Glucose solids	Milumil	Milupa	Coconut oil Soy oil
Skim milk powder	**Lactose**	Similac	Ross	Coconut oil 40% Soy oil 60%
Lactalbumin 60% Casein 40%	**Lactose**	SMA	Wyeth	Coconut oil Soy oil Safflower oil Beef fat
Demineralized skim milk Whey	**Lactose**	Aptamil	Milupa	Coconut oil Soy oil
Skim milk powder	**Lactose** Corn syrup solids	Enfalac Next Step	Mead Johnson	Coconut oil Sunflower oil Palm olein Soy oil Soy lecithin

Table 26-2: Composition of Infant Formulae*

Protein Source	Carbohydrate	Name	Manu-facturer	Fat
Skim milk powder	**Lactose** Maltodextrin	Follow Up	Carnation	Palm oil Safflower oil Corn oil Soy oil Coconut oil
2. Cow's Milk Base Without Lactose				
Milk protein	<u>Lactose-free</u> **Glucose** Corn syrup solids	Enfalac Lactose-free (formerly Alactamil)	Mead Johnson	Coconut oil Sunflower oil Palm olein Soy oil
3. Cow's Milk Base: Modified Whey				
Whey hydrolysate Promoted as a <u>prophylactic</u> formula for infants <u>at risk</u> for cow's milk allergy (<u>Not</u> suitable for infants with cow's milk allergy)	**Lactose** Maltodextrin	Good Start	Carnation	Palm oil Safflower oil Coconut oil
4. Soy Base With Sucrose				
Soy protein isolate	**Sucrose** Corn syrup solids	Isomil	Ross	Coconut oil Soy oil
	Sucrose Corn syrup solids	Nursoy	Wyeth	Oleo Coconut oil Safflower oil Soy oil
	Sucrose Corn syrup solids	Soyalac	Loma Linda	Soy oil
	Sucrose Dextrin Tapioca	I-Soyalac	Loma Linda	Soy oil
5. Soy Base Without Sucrose				
	Corn syrup solids	Prosobee	Mead Johnson	Coconut oil Soy oil

Table 26-2: Composition of Infant Formulae*

Protein Source	Carbohydrate	Name	Manu-facturer	Fat
6. Hydrolyzed Cow's Milk Protein With Sucrose				
Casein hydrolysate free amino acids 60% small peptides 40%	**Sucrose 71%** Modified tapioca starch 29%	Alimentum	Ross	MCT 50% Safflower oil 40% Soy oil 10%
7. Hydrolyzed Cow's Milk Protein Without Sucrose				
Casein hydrolysate (amino acids)	Corn syrup solids Modified corn starch	Enfalac Nutramigen	Mead Johnson	Corn oil Soy oil
Casein hydrolysate (amino acids)	Corn syrup solids Modified tapioca starch	Pregestimil	Mead Johnson	MCT Corn oil Soy oil
8. Hydrolyzed Soy Without Sucrose				
Hydrolysate of: Bovine collagen Soy (low molecular weight peptides and amino acids)	Maltodextrins Predigested gluten free starch (Free from lactose, sucrose, galactose, fructose)	Prejomin (Not presently available in Canada)	Milupa	"Vegetable oils"

Note: Because of frequent changes in formulation, the ingredients indicated do not represent a complete list of nutrient sources for each formula. Apply to the manufacturer for a comprehensive list of ingredients.

* Source of data: Manufacturer

Part V

Therapeutic Diets for Specific Conditions

Note On the Therapeutic Diets

The therapeutic diets described in this book have been compiled from a variety of sources. References to the relevant literature are found in each chapter.

The management protocols have been used successfully in the Allergy Nutrition Program at the Vancouver Hospital and Health Sciences Centre for a number of years, and at other centers on an experimental basis. Controlled studies are underway in the management of several conditions, but the results are not yet available.

Users are cautioned that these therapeutic diets are still experimental at the present time and should be undertaken with this in mind. No diet should take the place of currently recognized medical treatment for any condition, but may have value as an adjunct to standard medical protocols.

All dietary protocols should be followed only with the approval of the attending physician. For maximum benefit and safety, these diets should be supervised by a registered dietitian/nutritionist.

The author and publisher disclaim any responsibility for any adverse consequences resulting from the use of drugs, diet, supplements, or procedures mentioned in this book.

27

Disaccharide Intolerance

Carbohydrate malabsorption may occur in a variety of conditions, such as lactase deficiency, sucrase-isomaltase-deficiency, cow's milk and soy protein sensitive enteropathy, gluten sensitive enteropathy, infections with micro organisms such as *Giardia lamblia* and viruses such as the rotavirus group.[1] In the infant, additional causes may include immaturity, or congenital absence of enzymes or components of the transport systems needed to assimilate sugars.

Normal Digestion of Dietary Carbohydrates

Carbohydrates cross the intestinal mucosa as monosaccharides (glucose, galactose, fructose). All dietary carbohydrates must be broken down to the hexose form to be absorbed. Several enzymes are produced by cells in the brush border at the surface of the small intestine.[2] These enzymes hydrolyze specific disaccharides and break them down into their constituent monosaccharides.

The carbohydrate composition of the normal diet is about 60% starch, 30% sucrose, and 10% lactose. Each carbohydrate is treated slightly differently in the process of digestion.[3]

Starch

Starches are long polymers of glucose. They are initially cleaved into shorter glucose chains by amylase from saliva and pancreatic secretions in the intestinal lumen. These resulting sugars pass into the intestinal lumen as maltose, maltotriose, and α-dextrins. They are further split into the free monosaccharide by sucrose-α-dextrinase and glucoamylase in the brush border.[4] Alpha-glucosidases are sometimes referred to as maltases.

Maltase and α-dextrinase (isomaltase) break the disaccharides down to glucose. Glucose is carried into circulation through the epithelial cells of the small intestine by a process of active transport.

The normal range of maltase is 128-461 units per gram of protein. The normal range of α-dextrinase is 50-160 units per gram of protein.[3] These levels ensure that adequate amounts of enzymes are available for the breakdown of starches, even when the brush border cells are damaged and the enzymes are produced at only a fraction of their normal levels.

The step that determines the speed of starch digestion is he transport of glucose across the epithelium, not the amount of enzyme available to break down the disaccharide to glucose.

Sucrose

Sucrose is broken down to its constituent monosaccharides glucose and fructose by the enzyme sucrase produced by the brush border cells of the small intestine.

In the normal diet, the 30% sucrose content results in 15% glucose and 15% fructose. Both glucose and fructose are carried into circulation by an active transport system across the epithelium of the intestine.

The normal range of sucrase is 40-165 units per gram of protein.[3] The amount of enzyme in most cases is adequate to process the sucrose in the diet, leading to a rapid production of glucose and fructose. These monosaccharides may quickly saturate the transport system, and, like dietary starch, the rate-limiting step in sucrose digestion and absorption is the transport of the monosaccharides across the epithelium.

Lactose

Lactose is present in all animal milk, including human milk and is the major source of sugar and energy for the newborn infant. Lactose is broken down to glucose and galactose by a β-galactosidase enzyme commonly called lactase. The 10% lactose of the normal diet produces 5% glucose and 5% galactose which are carried into circulation by an active transport system across the epithelium.

Lactase is produced in small amounts compared to the other disaccharidases, averaging 45 units per gram of protein (the normal range is 15-95 units per gram protein).[3]

The hydrolysis of lactose proceeds at half the rate of sucrose, and the glucose and galactose released are not sufficient to produce maximal rates of transport. Therefore, the rate-limiting step in lactose digestion is the amount of enzyme and its action on lactose, and not the transport of the monosaccharides across the epithelium.

In Summary

In the digestion of starch and sucrose, the transport of the monosaccharides glucose and fructose into circulation determines the rate of utilization and uptake of the carbohydrate. In lactose digestion, the amount of available enzyme limits the rate of digestion.

In addition, in non-specific intestinal injury such as inflammation, lactase is depressed earlier than the other disaccharidases and is the last of these enzymes to return to normal after the disease process has resolved. It is not uncommon to find secondary lactase deficiency with normal intestinal sucrase, maltase, and α-dextrinase.[3]

This difference explains why lactase deficiency occurs more frequently than sucrase and maltase-isomaltase deficiency after damage to the mucosal cells.[2]

Deficiencies of Disaccharidases

Persons with carbohydrate malabsorption complain of abdominal fullness, bloating, and cramping pain within 5 to 30 minutes after eating the offending carbohydrate. The undigested disaccharide moves down into the colon where the excess osmotic pressure draws fluid into the intestinal lumen, resulting in watery diarrhea containing carbohydrate, which may start within a few minutes and persist for several hours.[1] Bacteria in the lower ileum and colon metabolize the carbohydrate to fatty acids, which causes a low pH (<6.0) in children, but not consistently in adults. The increased fluid in the intestinal lumen and the acid environment stimulate intestinal mobility and accelerate the rate of intestinal transit.[5]

Lactose Intolerance

Persons with symptoms of abdominal fullness, nausea, and diarrhea after ingestion of one to three glasses of milk should be investigated for lactase deficiency.

Most children have full capacity to digest lactose at birth, even if they are members of population groups with a high prevalence of adult lactase deficiency. Congenital lactase deficiency is extremely rare. It becomes evident soon after birth as a watery diarrhea when the infant is first given milk in any form. Human milk contains about 6 percent lactose, in contrast to cow's milk, which contains about 4 percent. Elimination of milk and dairy products from the mother's diet will not affect the lactose content of her milk, which will remain at 6 percent.

Adult onset primary lactase deficiency is much more common and is due to the gradual loss of lactase after weaning.[6]

Sucrase-Isomaltase Deficiencies

Congenital sucrase-isomaltase deficiency is reported to be more common than congenital lactase deficiency. It is especially prevalent in Greenland and Northern Canadian Inuit, in whom the incidence has been reported to be as high as 10% of the population.[7] When sucrose is first fed to the infant, (usually in the form of fruit), watery diarrhea, abdominal bloating, and gas result.

Secondary Disaccharidase Deficiencies

Secondary disaccharidase deficiencies can result from mucosal damage due to infection, inflammation caused by food allergy, especially to milk proteins, and a variety of enteropathies.[8,9] Secondary disaccharidase deficiency is much more common in infants and children than in adults. Management involves restriction of dietary disaccharides. In the case of a transient disaccharidase deficiency, restrictions can be phased out gradually as the mucosal damage is repaired.[10]

References

1.   Perman, J.A. Carbohydrate malabsorption. In: Lifshitz, F. (Ed), *Nutrition for Special Needs in Infancy.* Marcel Dekker, New York, 1985. 145-157.

2.   Gray, G. Intestinal disaccharidase deficiencies and glucose-galactose malabsorption. In: Stanbury, J.B., Wybgaarden, J.B., Fredrickson, D.S., Goldstein, J.S., and Brown, M.S. (Eds), *The Metabolic Basis of Inherited Disease*, 5th Edition. McGraw-Hill, New York, 1983. 1729-1742.

3.   Gray, G.M. Intestinal disaccharidase deficiencies and glucose-galactose malabsorption. In: Stanbury, J.B., Wybgaarden, J.B., Fredrickson, D.S., Goldstein, J.S., and Brown, M.S. (Eds), *The Metabolic Basis of Inherited Disease.* McGraw-Hill, New York, 1972. 1453-1464.

4.   Gray, G.M., Lally, B.C., and Conkin, K.A. Action of intestinal sucrase-isomaltase and its free monomers on an alpha-limit dextrin. J. Biol. Chem. 1979 254:6038-6043.

5.   Lifshitz, F. Carbohydrate problems in paediatric gastroenterology. Clinics Gastroenterol. 1977 6:415-429.

6.   Littman, A., and Hammond, J.B. Diarrhoea in adults caused by deficiency in intestinal disaccharides. Gastroenterology 1965 48:237-249.

7.   McNair, A., Gudmand-Hoyer, E., Jarnum, S., and Orrild, L. Sucrose malabsorption in Greenland. Br. Med. J. 1972 2:19-21.

8.   Lee, P.C. Transient carbohydrate malabsorption and intolerance in diarrhea disease of infancy. In: Lebenthal, E. (Ed), *Chronic Diarrhea in Children.* Nestle Vevey, Raven Press, New York, 1984.

9.   Freier, S. Paediatric gastrointestinal allergy. J. Hum. Nutr. 1976 30:187-192.

10. Brunser, O., and Araya, M. Damage and repair of small intestinal mucosa in acute and chronic diarrhea. In: Lebenthal, E. (Ed), *Chronic Diarrhea in Children.* Nestle Vevey, Raven Press, New York, 1984.

Method: Disaccharide Restricted Diet

General Description

This eating plan is designed to restrict dietary carbohydrates for people who have disaccharide intolerances.

The Problem Disaccharides

Lactose

Lactose is the sugar in milk. It occurs mostly in the whey (liquid) fraction of milk, although foods made mainly of casein (such as cheeses) may still contain a small amount of lactose. The enzyme that breaks down lactose is called lactase. It splits lactose into two monosaccharides: glucose and galactose.

A person whose intestinal cells are producing very little lactase will not be able to break down much lactose.

Lactose intolerance is different from milk allergy, in which a person's immune system fights the protein in milk.

Sucrose

Sucrose is table sugar. It is usually derived from sugar beet or sugar cane, but is also present in many plants, especially fruits, grains, and vegetables.

The enzyme that breaks down sucrose is called sucrase. It splits sucrose into the two monosaccharides: glucose and fructose.

Maltose

Maltose is derived mostly from grains and starchy vegetables. The enzymes that break down maltose include maltase and isomaltase. They split maltose and starches into molecules of glucose.

Starches

Starches are made up of long chains of glucose molecules. The linkages between the glucose molecules have to be split to release the free glucose before it can be absorbed. If there is a deficiency in the enzymes that split these linkages, free glucose molecules will not be released. The remaining undigested starch or sugar will be passed into the large bowel, where bacteria will ferment it.

Identifying the Disaccharidase that is Deficient

Except in the case of a lactase deficiency, which improves dramatically when lactose is removed from the diet, it is often difficult to separate specific disaccharide intolerances from each other.

If the deficiency is due to damaged intestinal cells, loss or reduction in activity of all the disaccharidases often results. In such a case, it is usually advisable to follow a diet restricting all disaccharides at first. Since this is usually a temporary situation, avoidance will lead to healing, and the foods may be tolerated in increasingly larger dosages the longer the diet is followed.

If the deficiency is permanent, it is often due to loss, or lack, of the ability to produce one specific disaccharidase. In this case, efforts should be made to identify the specific deficiency. In the majority of cases, it will be a lactase deficiency as this is usually an inherited tendency, often associated with certain racial groups (such as the Oriental, most African and Mediterranean races, and North American First Nations peoples). Eighty percent of these people tend to lose the ability to produce lactase on aging, and culturally, these groups tend not to drink milk after infancy. Northern Europeans tend to retain the ability to produce lactase throughout life.

Nutritional Supplements Required on this Diet

In general, if a wide range of allowed foods are eaten and the condition is a secondary (temporary) deficiency, a supplement is not needed.

The amount of supplement that may be required will depend on individual tolerances to the disaccharide-containing food. Some people will be able to tolerate a small amount of the food and any nutritional deficiencies will be minimal.

For people with primary (permanent) deficiencies, or those who need to follow the diet for an extended period of time, the following supplements may be necessary:

- Lactose restricted: calcium, and possibly Vitamin D
- Sucrose restricted: Vitamin C
- Maltose restricted: Vitamin B complex

Feeding the Disaccharide Intolerant Infant

Infant formulas that are lactose-free and sucrose-free can be given to a disaccharidase deficient infant.

If the infant is not allergic to milk, the milk based formula Alactamil® (Mead Johnson), which is free from lactose and sucrose, is suitable.

If the infant is allergic to cow's milk proteins but tolerates soy, the soy based, sucrose-free formula Prosobee® (Mead Johnson), is suitable.

If the infant is allergic to both cow's milk and soy proteins, a casein hydrolysate formula such as Nutramigen® (Mead Johnson) or Pregestimil® (Mead Johnson) may be tolerated. These formulas are free from lactose and sucrose.

A breast-fed infant will ingest significant quantities of lactose in mother's milk. The lactose composition of the mother's milk will remain constant, regardless of whether or not mother consumes milk and dairy products. If the lactose intolerance is secondary to a gastrointestinal tract infection or other condition that is expected to be transient, some authorities advise continuing breast-feeding and expect the diarrhea to gradually diminish as the underlying inflammation disappears.

Alternatively, the mother can pump her breast milk and treat it with Lactaid® drops (4 drops per 250 mL milk), and allow the enzyme to act for 24 hours in the fridge. The infant can be fed the lactose-free milk the next day. This procedure is continued until the diarrhea subsides and the infant may then be gradually put back to the breast.

Disaccharide Restricted Diet

Restriction of all disaccharides will be required initially.

Phase I   To determine if disaccharidase deficiency is the cause of the gastrointestinal symptoms, specifically diarrhea, the Phase I diet should be followed for a minimum of four weeks. When the diarrhea improves, liberalization of these restrictions will determine each individual's limit of tolerance for each disaccharide.

Phase II   This phase involves the introduction of one food from the "restricted" lists every other day until diarrhea recurs. Maltose tolerance is determined by introducing grains, especially white grains and flours. Sucrose tolerance is determined by introducing vegetables, fruits, nuts and seeds, and finally sugars. Lactose tolerance is determined by introducing dairy products and milk. Specific details of lactose intolerance are provided in the method for *Lactose Restricted Diet*, page 92.

Phase I: Restriction of All Types of Disaccharides

Disaccharide Restricted Diet

Type of Food	Foods Allowed	Foods Restricted
Milk and Dairy	Cheeses (**not** processed): 　Brie 　Camembert 　Cheddar 　Cream 　Gruyere 　Limburger 　Monterey Jack 　Mozzarella 　Port au Salut Non-dairy creamers: 　Coffee Rich®	All except those listed 　opposite
Meat, Poultry, and Fish	All fresh or frozen: 　Lamb　　　Duck 　Beef　　　Turkey 　Pork　　　Game birds 　Wild game　Fin fish 　Chicken　　Shellfish	Processed Breaded Smoked Cured Canned Corned Beef

Disaccharide Restricted Diet

Type of Food	Foods Allowed	Foods Restricted
Grains, Breads and Cereals	None	All; they contain starches. Flours made from grains. Amaranth Quinoa Barley Rice Buckwheat Rye Bulgur Spelt Corn Triticale Millet Wheat Oats
Vegetables	Fresh, frozen, canned, without added sugar or starch: Celery Chives Cucumber Endive Garlic Green onion Kale Lettuce Mushrooms Parsley Parsnips Radishes Spinach Swiss chard Tomatoes Tomato juice Turnip Watercress Avocado Peppers, green and red Potatoes, French fried or hash browns	Canned with additives Added sauces Added butter or margarine Asparagus Artichokes Broccoli Carrots Cauliflower Corn Kohlrabi Leeks Okra Pumpkin Yams Sweet potatoes Onion (mature, cooking) Potatoes (boiled) Squash, all types Cabbage, green and red V-8 Vegetable Juice®

Fruit	Fresh, frozen, canned in own juice.
	Berries:
	  Blackberry
	  Blueberry
	  Cranberry
	  Gooseberry
	  Loganberry
	Cherry
	Currants, red and black
	Damson plums
	Figs, raw
	Guava
	Grapes
	Grape juice
	Kiwi fruit
	Lemon
	Lime
	Passion fruit (Granadilla)
		Added sugar or syrup
		Apple
		Apricot
		Banana
		Date
		Grapefruit
		Mango
		Melon, all types
		Nectarine
		Orange
		Papaya (Pawpaw)
		Peach
		Pear
		Pineapple, raw
		Plum, prune type
		Raspberry
		Strawberry
		Tangerine
		Watermelon

Eggs	Cooked, plain (e.g., fried, boiled, scrambled)	With added milk, flour or sugar

Disaccharide Restricted Diet

Type of Food	Foods Allowed	Foods Restricted
Legumes	Tofu	Bean sprouts Black eyed peas Broad beans (fava beans) Chickpeas (garbanzos) Green and wax beans Kidney beans Lentils Navy beans Peanut Peas Soy beans Split peas
Fats and Oils	Pure vegetable oil: 　Canola 　Corn 　Flaxseed 　Olive 　Safflower 　Soy 　Sunflower Margarine without milk 　solids, e.g.: Fleischmann's low sodium, 　no salt margarine® Parkay Diet Spread® Some other diet spreads Lard and meat drippings	Butter Margarine containing whey 　or milk solids.
Nuts and Seeds	None	All, including: 　Almond　　Beechnut 　Brazil nut　Butternut 　Cashew　　Walnut 　Hickory　　Macadamia 　Peanut　　Pecan 　Pistachio　Pumpkin seed 　Sesame seed 　Soybean (roasted) 　Sunflower seed 　Hazelnut (Filbert

Disaccharide Restricted Diet

Type of Food	Foods Allowed	Foods Restricted
Spices and Herbs	Allspice Anise seed Basil Bay leaf Caraway Cayenne Celery Chervil Chili powder Cinnamon Cloves Fennel seed Cumin seed Ginger Garlic Mace Marjoram Mustard Nutmeg Onion powder Oregano Paprika Parsley Poppy seed Rosemary Savory Sage Tarragon Thyme Turmeric Coriander, leaf or seed Pepper, black and white Dill, seed or weed Fenugreek seed Poultry seasoning	Herb or spice mixes or seasoning packets Curry Ginger

Sugars and Sweeteners	Glucose
	Dextrose
	Fructose (fruit sugar)
	Levulose
	Honey
	Sugar substitutes *(lactose-
	free, and in moderation)*
	   Aspartame
	   Cyclamate
	   Saccharine
	   Sugar Twin®
	   Equal®
	   Sweet 'n' Low®
		Sucrose (table sugar)
		Lactose (milk sugar)
		Maltose (grain sugar)
		Foods containing sugars
		Syrups

28

Crohn's Disease

Crohn's Disease is characterized by chronic granulomatous inflammation that may affect any part of the gut from mouth to anus, but predominantly affects the terminal ileum and the colon. Medical treatment involves corticosteroids, immunosuppressive drugs, and antibiotics, but is sometimes ineffective.[1] Many persons suffering from Crohn's disease undergo extensive surgery, which carries significant risk of morbidity and mortality.[2]

Crohn's disease may affect any age group but is most common in young adults.[1] Its onset often occurs shortly after puberty, and it lasts throughout life. The disease is most common in North America and Northern Europe, especially in Scandinavia, where it has the highest prevalence[2] and is an increasing public health concern. The cause of the disease is unknown.[3]

The Role of Diet in Crohn's Disease

Reports of links between gastrointestinal disease and diet have appeared from time to time in medical literature since the 1920's[4] and between Crohn's disease and diet since the 1970's. However, diet has not been considered a method for managing Crohn's disease in conventional therapy. Although remission of symptoms has occurred using periods of TPN (total parenteral nutrition), its effect has usually been explained on the basis of bowel rest rather than the avoidance of antagonistic foods.[5]

Use of Elemental Diets

The work of Alun Jones and colleagues during the last 10 years indicates that diet does indeed play a role in inflammatory bowel disease,[6] and that remission of symptoms in Crohn's disease can be achieved by dietary intervention.[7] In most reports of dietary management of Crohn's disease, initial remission of symptoms has been obtained by enteral nutrition using an elemental formula; these formulas contain nutrients in their simplest forms: proteins as amino acids; carbohydrates as glucose; fats as triglycerides containing short chain fatty acids. In controlled trials in recent-onset Crohn's disease, an elemental diet was demonstrated to be as, or more, effective than prednisone, the usual anti-inflammatory therapy.[8,9] Long term remission has been reported in affected children treated with an elemental diet for a prolonged period.[10]

The present view of dietary management of Crohn's disease was summarized by Ginsberg in 1992 as follows:[11]

"The conclusion that clinical remission of Crohn's disease can be induced in some patients with the use of fixed formula diets as the sole source of calories is inescapable."

Ginsberg points out that,

"Fixed formula diets, especially elemental diets, are expensive and unpalatable, and may have to be administered via a nasogastric tube. For these reasons, they are an acceptable therapeutic modality for only the most desperate patients who are highly motivated to avoid or eliminate corticosteroid therapy."

Selective Dietary Exclusion as a Management Strategy

An alternative to unpalatable elemental formulas may be available. A number of studies have indicated that remission of symptoms in Crohn's disease can been maintained by a diet excluding the foods to which the person is intolerant.[1,12,13] Using selective dietary exclusion as a management strategy, the approach is to achieve initial remission with an elemental formula and then to introduce each food separately. If the person tolerates the food, it is included in the diet; if an adverse reaction occurs, it is excluded.

This method can be criticized as being time consuming, socially inhibiting, and often expensive. It requires dedication on the part of the patient, together with skill on the part of the dietitian supervising the reintroduction of foods and designing the diet.[14] Despite these drawbacks, this approach offers an attractive alternative to surgery and to the debilitating side-effects of long term drug therapy.

A complicating factor in weaning a person from an elemental diet to regular food is the reported occurrence of gastrointestinal symptoms of "explosive diarrhea, gas, cramps, sweating, and feeling light headed".[15] These symptoms were reported by a group of healthy volunteers who had been on an elemental formula without regular foods for two weeks. Because the volunteers in this study had no history of food intolerance or gastrointestinal dysfunction, the symptoms may have been due more to motility disturbances resulting from adaptation to an elemental formula rather than to food intolerance.[14]

Such a response would certainly create a confounding problem in trying to identify the foods not tolerated by a person with Crohn's disease.

Immunology and Crohn's Disease

Recent research has attempted to identify specific food antigens that may induce an immunological response in susceptible individuals. The most likely response is an inflammatory reaction that could cause or exacerbate the symptoms of Crohn's disease. Foods most frequently responsible for intolerance in Crohn's disease appear to be various cereal grains, dairy products, and yeast.[13]

Antibodies to components of these foods have been detected in the sera of persons with Crohn's disease in a number of studies. Elevated serum IgG and IgA titres against the major cow's milk proteins (i.e., casein, bovine serum albumin, alpha-lactalbumin, beta-lactoglobulin A, and beta-lactoglobulin B) correlated well with disease activity in Crohn's disease but not in ulcerative colitis.[16] Antibodies to baker's and brewer's yeast (*Saccharomyces cerevisiae*) were detected in sera from persons with Crohn's disease, but not from those with ulcerative colitis or other bowel disease.[17,18,19,20]

More particularly, elevated levels of IgA anti-*Saccharomyces* antibodies appear to be a specific serological marker. The presence of these antibodies is consistent with an active immune response in gut-associated lymphoid tissue (GALT) in Crohn's disease, either as a primary or secondary effect.[21] The antigen most likely responsible for this response has been identified as a glycoprotein 200 kilodaltons in size.[22]

In another study, isolated peripheral blood lymphocytes from persons with Crohn's disease proliferated in response to baker's yeast, although similar blood lymphocytes from healthy controls showed no response.[23] A study of the effect of baker's yeast demonstrated that while subjects with Crohn's disease were taking capsules containing baker's yeast, their index of disease activity was significantly greater than during the test period when yeast was excluded.[24]

It is clear from these studies that diet has both a primary and adjunctive role in Crohn's disease.[25] The result of such studies is an increasing interest in the use of diet to promote remission of symptoms.

Overview of the Experimental Diet

The diet presented in this book is based on the research data linking Crohn's disease and diet. At present it is experimental, as controlled trials have not been completed. The diet should be used only on medical advice and under medical supervision.

Elimination

The following foods are eliminated:

- Wheat, rye, oats, barley, and corn
- Milk and dairy products
- *Saccharomyces* species in foods
- All foods inducing intolerance in the person being treated

Supplementation to Avoid Nutritional Deficiency

The equivalent nutrients needed to replace the nutrients in excluded foods are:

- Calcium to achieve the recommended daily allowance, (see *Non-dairy Sources of Calcium*, page 102)
- A multivitamin/mineral supplement, free from wheat, yeast, artificial color, flavor and preservatives

References

1.   Alun Jones, V., and Hunter, J.O. Irritable bowel syndrome and Crohn's disease. In: Brostoff, J., and Challacombe, S.J. (Eds), *Food Allergy and Intolerance*. Baillière Tindall, London and Philadelphia, 1987.

2.   Mayberry, J.F., and Rhodes, J. Epidemiological aspects of Crohn's disease: a review of the literature. Gut 1984 25:886-899.

3.   Sachar, D.B., Auslander, M.O., Walfish, J.S. Aetiological theories of inflammatory bowel disease. Clin. Gastroenterol. 1980 9:231-257.

4.   Duke, W.D. Food allergy as a cause of abdominal pain. Arch. Int. Med. 1921 28:151-165.

5.   Ostro, M.J., Greenberg, G.R., Jeejeebhoy, K.N. TPN and complete bowel rest in the management of Crohn's disease. Gastroenterol. 1984 86:1203.

6.   Alun Jones, V., Shorthouse, M., *et al.* Food intolerance: a major factor in the pathogenesis of irritable bowel syndrome. Lancet 1982 ii:1115-1117.

7.   Alun Jones, V., Workman, E., Freeman, A.H., Dickinson, R.J., Wilson, A.J., and Hunter, J.O. Crohn's disease: maintenance of remission by diet. Lancet 1985 ii:177-180.

8.   O'Morain, C., Segal, A.W., Levi, A.J. Elemental diet as primary treatment of acute Crohn's disease: a controlled trial. Br. Med. J. 1984 288:1859-1862.

9.   Seidman, E.G., Bouthillier, L., Weber, A.M., Roy, C.C., and Morin, C.L. Elemental diet versus prednisone as primary treatment of Crohn's disease (abstract). Gastroenterol. 1986 90:1625.

10.   Navarro, J., Vargas, J., Cezard, J.P., Charritat, J.L., Polonoviski, C. Prolonged constant rate elemental enteral nutrition in Crohn's disease. J. Pediatr. Gastroenterol. Nutr. 1982 1:541-546.

11.   Ginsberg, A.L. Diet therapy for Crohn's disease. Mayo Clinic Proceedings 1992 67:394-395.

12.   Workman, E.M., Alun Jones, V., Wilson, A.J., and Hunter, J.O. Diet in the management of Crohn's disease. Human Nutrition: Applied Nutrition 1984 38A:469-473.

13.   Riordan, A.M., Hunter, J.O., Cowan, R.E., Crampton, J.R., Davidson, A.R., *et al.* Treatment of active Crohn's disease by exclusion diet: East Anglian multi-center controlled trial. Lancet 1993 342:1131-1134.

14.   Pearson, M., Teahon, K., Levi, A.J., and Bjarnson, I. Food intolerance and Crohn's disease. Gut 1993 34:783-787.

15.   McCammon, S., Beyer, P.L., Rhodes, J.B. A comparison of three defined formula diets in volunteers. Am. J. Clin. Nutr. 1977 30:1655 1660.

16.   Knoflach, P., Park, B.H., Cunningham, R., Weiser, M.M. and Albini, B. Serum antibodies to cow's milk protein in ulcerative colitis and Crohn's disease. Gastroenterol. 1986 92:479-485.

17.   Main, J., McKenzie, J., Yeaman, G.R., Kerr, M.A., Robson, D., Pennington, C.R., Parratt, D. Antibody to *Saccharomyces cerevisiae* (baker's yeast) in Crohn's disease. Brit. Med. J. 1988 297:1105-1106.

18.   Lindberg, E., Magnusson, K-E., Tysk, C., Jarnerot, G. Antibody (IgG, IgA, and IgM) to baker's yeast (*Saccharomyces cerevisiae*), yeast mannan, gliadin, ovalbumin and betalactoglobulin in monozygotic twins with inflammatory bowel disease. Gut 1992 33:909-913.

19.   McKenzie, J., Main, J., Pennington, C.R., and Parratt, D. Antibody to selected strains of *Saccharomyces cerevisiae* (baker's and brewer's yeast) and *Candida albicans* in Crohn's disease. Gut 1990 31:536-538.

20.   Giaffer, M.H., Clark, A., Holdsworth, C.D. Antibodies to *Saccharomyces cerevisiae* in patients with Crohn's disease and their possible pathogenic importance. Gut 1992 33:1071-1075.

21.   Barnes, R.M.R., Allan, S., Taylor-Robinson, C.H., Finn, R., Johnson, P.M. Serum antibodies reactive with *Saccharomyces cerevisiae* in inflammatory bowel disease: Is IgA antibody a marker for Crohn's disease? Int. Arch. Allergy Appl. Immunol. 1990 92:9-15.

22.   Heelan, B.T., Allan, S., and Barnes, R.M.R. Identification of a 200-kDa glycoprotein antigen of *Saccharomyces cerevisiae*. Immunology Letters 1991 28:181-186.

23.   Young, C.A., Sonnenberg, A., Burns, E. Lymphocyte proliferation response to baker's yeast in Crohn's disease. Digestion 1994 55:40-43.

24.   Barclay, G.R., McKenzie, H., Pennington, J., Parratt, D., Pennington, C.R. The effect of dietary yeast on the activity of stable chronic Crohn's disease. Scand. J. Gastroenterol. 1992 27:196-200.

25.   O'Morain, C.A. Does nutritional therapy in inflammatory bowel disease have a primary or an adjunctive role? Scand. J. Gastroenterol. 1990 25(Suppl.172):29-34.

Method: Diet For Crohn's Disease

This diet is experimental at the present time; results of controlled trials are not currently available.

This diet should be used only under medical advice and supervision.

General Description

This eating plan is designed to achieve and maintain remission of symptoms in Crohn's disease.

The diet has been developed to eliminate the foods which may not be tolerated, and change the intake of other possible contributing factors (Phase 1). The Phase 1 diet is initially followed for a period of four weeks.

If symptoms have not improved in this time, diet is unlikely to be a contributing factor, and there will be no benefit in following the dietary restrictions any longer.

If significant improvement is experienced, the diet should be followed until all symptoms are in remission and a weight gain is experienced. At this time, certain modifications can be made to the diet (Phase 2).

Phase One Diet

Eliminate all milk and dairy products.

Eliminate grains: wheat, rye, oats, barley, corn.

Eliminate brewer's and baker's yeast (*Saccharomyces* species).

Eliminate spices (seed, root, bark of spice plant). Herbs (flowers, leaves) are allowed.

Eliminate coffee, tea, and chocolate. Herbal teas without spices should be tolerated.

Note: Caffeine intake is to be reduced gradually to avoid unpleasant side effects.

Avoid raw foods. Cook all vegetables and fruits (or use canned in their own juice or vegetable juice); no raw vegetables, including salads, are allowed.

Nuts and seeds should be ground to a flour or paste (nut "butters").

Avoid all alcoholic beverages.

Reduce fat: Select lean meats and reduce fats and oils in cooking.

Supplements

A multivitamin and mineral tablet or capsule should be taken once a day. These must be wheat-free, yeast-free, sugar and salt-free and free from additives such as artificial color, flavor, and preservatives. Suggested brands: Quest®, Jamieson®, Nulife®.

Additive-free calcium gluconate or calcium citrate malate are the better absorbed and utilized forms of calcium.

Phase Two Diet

Restricted foods can be gradually reintroduced **except**:

- Milk and dairy products
- Cereal grains
- Yeast.

According to individual tolerance (see the method for *Challenge Phase*, page 42):

- Gradually increase intake of raw fruits and vegetables, including raw salads.
- Small quantities of whole nuts and seeds can be introduced and increased gradually.
- If desired, small quantities of spices can be added to foods, and gradually increased.
- Small quantities of tea and coffee can be taken, and increased as tolerated.
- Fat can be increased as tolerated.
- Distilled alcohol can be taken in moderate quantities. Vodka made from potatoes is preferred. All fermented alcoholic beverages such as wines and beers should be avoided.

Foods and Products Allowed on the Diet

Each of the foods restricted on this diet can be found in many products and derivatives. Listing them all would require extensive lists of foods and their products.

This is a test diet, and the Phase Two testing should isolate specific intolerances. Only foods listed as allowed are used during this diet trial.

Phase I Diet For Crohn's Disease

Type of Food	Foods Allowed
Milk and Dairy	Rice Dream® (made from brown rice and safflower oil) Soy milk and plain tofu Non-dairy creamers such as Coffee Rich® Clarified light whipped butter Whey-free margarine In recipes: substitute fruit or vegetable juice or homemade soup stock
Vegetables	All cooked, plain fresh, frozen, and canned vegetables and their juices If juice is extracted from raw vegetables, heat (and chill if desired) before drinking
Fruit	All cooked, plain fresh, frozen, and canned fruits and their juices If juice is extracted from raw fruits, heat (and chill if desired) before drinking
Breads and Cereals	**Grains and Flours** Amaranth and amaranth flour Arrowroot starch and flour Buckwheat and buckwheat flour Chickpea or garbanzo flour (Besan) Lentil or pea flour Millet and millet flour (Bajri) Potato starch and flour Quinoa and quinoa flour Rice and rice flour Sago flour Soy flour Tapioca, tapioca starch, and flour Wild rice and wild rice flour
	Yeast-Free Breads and Baked Goods Baked goods and specialty baking mixes containing allowed foods Homemade baked goods made with allowed foods
	Crackers and Snacks Pure rice crackers/cakes without nuts, seeds, or restricted grains or yeast Nut and seed butters can be added as a spread
	Cereals Cream of Rice®, rice bran Any of the allowed grains, cooked Puffed rice Puffed millet Puffed amaranth

Phase I Diet For Crohn's Disease

Type of Food	Foods Allowed
	Pasta Rice noodles and pasta Brown rice pasta Wild rice pasta Mung bean pasta Pasta made from any allowed grain
Meat, Poultry and Fish	All plain, cooked, lean and well trimmed fresh or frozen meat and poultry Plain fish such as tuna canned in water **Note:** Avoid all high fat and spiced deli meats, as well as meats which are breaded, creamed, or otherwise prepared with restricted foods
Eggs	All plain eggs in moderation Egg whites are low in fat and not restricted
Legumes	All plain legumes and legume dishes cooked and prepared with allowed ingredients Pure peanut butter Plain tofu Cooked soy beans and their products
Nuts and Seeds	These foods are high in fat and may be tolerated only in small amounts at first Nut and seed butters, such as: Almond butter Cashew butter Sesame tahini Sunflower seed butter Butters can be made from any nuts or seeds in a blender
Fats and Oils	These foods are very high in fat and may be tolerated only in small amounts at first All pure vegetable oils except corn oil Pure vegetable shortening Margarine without milk solids Fleischmann's low sodium, no salt margarine® Parkay diet margarine® Meat drippings and poultry fat Homemade gravy made with allowed foods Lard

Phase I Diet For Crohn's Disease

Type of Food	Foods Allowed
Herbs	All dried herbs, including Basil · Bay leaf Chervil · Coriander leaf Dill weed · Garlic powder Marjoram · Mint Onion powder · Oregano Parsley · Poultry seasoning Rosemary · Sage Savory · Tarragon Thyme
Sweeteners	All, including white and brown sugar, maple sugar or syrup, pure jams, jellies, conserves
Beverages	Plain water Mineral water, plain or carbonated Herbal teas without spices, e.g., mint, peppermint, chamomile, rosehip, hibiscus Fruit juices and drinks made with fruits and sweeteners Vegetable juice cocktail made with allowed ingredients Commercial varieties contain spices
Other	Baking soda Allergen free baking powder Cream of Tartar Salt Guar gum Plain gelatin

References

Workman, E.M., Alun Jones, V., Wilson, A.J., and Hunter, J.O. Diet in the management of Crohn's disease. Human Nutrition: Applied Nutrition 1984 38A:469-473.

Alun Jones, V., Workman, E., Freeman, A.H., Dickinson, R.J., Wilson, A.J., and Hunter, J.O. Crohn's disease: maintenance of remission by diet. Lancet 1985 ii:177-180.

Teahon, K., Bjarnson, L., Pearson, M., Levi, A.J. Ten years experience with an elemental diet in the management of Crohn's disease. Gut 1990 31:1133-1137.

Riordan, A.M., Hunter, J.O., Cowan, R.E., Crampton, J.R., Davidson, A.R., et al. Treatment of active Crohn's disease by exclusion diet: East Anglian multi center controlled trial. Lancet 1993 342:1131-11

29

Irritable Bowel Syndrome

The term "irritable bowel syndrome" (IBS) refers to a variety of minor bowel disturbances of unknown origin. Terms with a similar meaning are "irritable colon" or "spastic colon".

Symptoms of IBS

The usual symptoms of IBS are constipation, diarrhea, and alternation of the two, with no sign of infection or other physical cause and no sign of structural damage to the intestinal wall (which is usually indicated by blood in the stool). There is no weight loss or night time diarrhea, symptoms usually suggestive of more serious conditions such as Crohn's disease or ulcerative colitis.[1]

Further symptoms include abdominal pain, excessive gas, flatulence and bloating, and indigestion.[2] Sometimes symptoms appear after a meal and are relieved by defecation. Occasionally nausea and fatigue are reported.

Diagnosis of IBS

A diagnosis of irritable bowel syndrome is made when all organic disease has been ruled out by appropriate medical tests.[2]

IBS is a chronic disorder that is more prevalent in women than in men and has been estimated to affect as many as 22 million people.[3] Although the causes of IBS are unknown, a variety of determinants have been suggested, including dietary factors (such as inadequate fibre, high fat intakes, and consumption of gas-producing foods and carbonated beverages), food intolerance, gut motility disorders, hormonal fluctuations, psychiatric disorder, side effects of medications, smoking, swallowing of air during eating, and stress.[2]

Management of IBS

One of the most favored approaches to treating IBS has been to increase the amount of dietary fibre by adding wheat bran and bulking agents such as psyllium, ispaghula, and methylcellulose.[2] However, controlled studies of added dietary fibre showed no difference between the effect of wheat bran and that of a placebo.[4] Furthermore, adding wheat bran to the diet can worsen symptoms if the IBS is caused by an undetected wheat allergy.[1] Some studies have shown that as many as 70% of persons with IBS are food intolerant.[5] One of the foods most frequently reported to cause food intolerance is wheat. Fortunately, adding bran and bulking agents to the diet in the treatment of IBS has now been largely discredited, especially if the predominant symptom is diarrhea.[1]

Abdominal gas and bloating is usually a result of microbial fermentation of unabsorbed carbohydrate in the bowel.[6]

Microbial Fermentation of Undigested Food in the Colon

Normal Digestion of Food

Digestion of food by enzymes produced in the body starts in the mouth and continues until the food has passed through the length of the small intestine. Most of the nutrients resulting from enzymatic digestion are absorbed into the body through the epithelium of the small intestine. The remaining food matter passes into the colon, where microorganisms continue the process. Further breakdown of the food components is thereafter carried out by enzymes produced by the colon microflora. The products of microbial metabolism are absorbed into the body through the colonic epithelium and provide an additional source of nutrients.[7]

All carbohydrate that is not digested and absorbed from the small intestine is a potential substrate for fermentation by the colonic microflora. An abnormal degree of fermentation of undigested food in the colon by microorganisms would certainly explain the abdominal bloating, gas, and constipation cycling with diarrhea which are the predominant symptoms in IBS.

Carbohydrate Digestion and Fermentation

Plant foods contain two broad classes of carbohydrates:[8]

- Free sugars (glucose, fructose, sucrose)
- Polysaccharides

Free sugars are found mainly in fruit and vegetables and are rapidly absorbed from the small intestine in healthy humans.

Plant polysaccharides can be separated into two broad categories:

- Starch: a storage polysaccharide
     It is an alpha linked glucan and is the major carbohydrate of cereal grains and potatoes
- Non-starch polysaccharides:
     These Non-alpha linked glucans are structural components of the plant cell wall and include a mixture of polymers such as cellulose, pectin, and hemicellulose which are considered the dietary fibre of foods.

Starch is susceptible to hydrolysis by pancreatic amylase. The alpha glucosidic linkages are broken by the enzyme in the human small intestine. Non-starch polysaccharides resist pancreatic amylase because they do not have the alpha glucosidic linkages, thereby escaping digestion in the small intestine of humans.

Digestion of Non-starch Polysaccharides (dietary fibre)

Using ileostomy patients (where the effluent collected in the ileostomy bag is the same as the digesta that in normal subjects would pass into the colon and would act as the substrate for microbial fermentation) researchers find that *non-starch polysaccharides* in the diet pass completely undigested through the small intestine and into the colon.[9]

After the fibre enters the colon it will either be fermented by microorganisms or pass unchanged out of the body in the feces. Non-starch polysaccharide is not affected by food processing or cooking.[9]

Digestion of Starches

Starch is found in many of the world's staple foods such as cereals, legumes, potatoes, and bananas. Most cereal and legume starches are readily hydrolyzed by alpha amylase in the small intestine and are absorbed from there into the body. Normally, very little starch passes into the colon. The digestive process can be sped up by cooking which gelatinizes the starch.[8]

However, some starches may pass undigested into the colon.[9] All starch entering the large intestine is a substrate for bacterial fermentation. Starch from cereal products and freshly cooked potato is usually well digested and absorbed in the small intestine.[8] In contrast, up to 89% of the starch from raw banana escapes digestion in the small intestine[10] and is consequently available for microbial fermentation in the colon. The starch that resists digestion by human enzymes has been designated resistant starch.[10]

Another dietary source of "resistant starch" results from food processing that leads to a retrogradation, rendering some starches partly resistant to enzymatic digestion.[9] Such resistant starch may be introduced into a food as a result of heating, cooling, freezing, or drying.[10] For example, cooled cooked potato was found to be less well digested than freshly cooked potato;[11] therefore, more of the cooled potato would be fermented in the colon than if the potato were eaten hot and freshly cooked. The decrease in digestibility of starch as a result of cooking, cooling, and processing also occurs with spaghetti[12] and undercooked rice.[13]

Table 29-1: A Comparison of Dietary Starch Fed and Recovered After Digestion in the Small Intestine of Humans

Type of Food	Starch Fed (Grams)	Starch Recovered (Grams)	Percentage Starch Recovered (%)
White bread	62	1.6	3
Oats	58	1.2	2
Cornflakes	74	3.7	5
Banana (raw)	19	17.2	89

Potato
  Freshly cooked
  Cooled
  Reheated
	
	45
	47
	47
		
		1.5
		5.8
		3.6
			
			3
			12
			8

Adapted from Englyst and Kingman 1990 (with permission from the authors).[10]

Physical Accessibility of Starch to Human Enzymes

There are other factors that can affect the amount of starch passing into the colon and becoming available for microbial fermentation. One of the most important is how physically accessible the starch is to the digestive enzymes in the small intestine.

Whole Grains, Nuts, and Seeds

When starch is contained within undisrupted plant structures, such as whole grains, nuts, and seeds, the cell wall entraps the starch and prevents its swelling and dispersion. This entrapment delays or prevents the hydrolysis of starch by pancreatic amylase in the small intestine.[9]

Incompletely Milled Grains and Vegetable Skins

Partly milled grains and seeds, vegetables with skins (such as sweet corn, peas, beans) and parboiled white rice[13] and spaghetti[12] are examples of foods with physical structures which retard or resist amylase digestion.

Digestion of Cooked Starches

Cooking disrupts the starch containing granules in the plant and facilitates the hydrolysis (digestion) of the starch. When foods containing high levels of resistant starch granules are eaten raw (e.g. banana), more undigested starch passes into the colon.

Other Dietary Factors Which May Contribute to IBS

The chronic diarrhea experienced with IBS may be the result of a deficiency of lactase and possibly other disaccharidases which are produced in the brush border of the small intestine. Undigested disaccharides remain unabsorbed and pass into the lower bowel where they act as a substrate for microbial fermentation.

Despite the strong association of food intolerance and IBS, it is not known whether wheat intolerance or disaccharidase deficiency is responsible for the symptoms of IBS. It is likely that a variety of factors contribute to IBS symptoms in an individual sufferer. For example, certain raw fruits and vegetables, spices, coffee, and/or alcohol may exacerbate existing symptoms.

A practical approach to the dietary management of IBS takes into account as many of these factors as possible and eliminates all foods that may be implicated. The prescribed diet is followed for a limited time period (usually four weeks). If significant improvement is achieved, a sequential incremental dose challenge usually identifies any foods that are causing intolerance. The intake of other restricted foods can be liberalized gradually as the condition dissipates.

References

1.   Brostoff, J., and Gamlin, L. *The Complete Guide to Food Allergy and Intolerance.* Crown Publishers, New York, 1989. 101-103; 127.

2.   Nelson, J.K., Moxness, K.E., Jensen, M.D., and Gastineau, C.E. Gastrointestinal diseases and disorders. In: *Mayo Clinic Diet Manual*, Seventh Edition. Mosby, St. Louis, Baltimore, 1994. 213-274.

3.   Drossman, D.A. Irritable bowel syndrome. Amer. Fam. Phys. 1989 36(6):159-164.

4.   Thompson, W.G. A strategy for management of the irritable bowel. Am. J. Gastroenterol. 1986 81(2):95- 100.

5.   Alun Jones, V., and Hunter, J.O. Irritable bowel syndrome and Crohn's disease. In: Brostoff, J., and Challacombe, S.J. (Eds), *Food Allergy and Intolerance*. Baillière Tindall, London, Philadelphia, 1987. 555- 569.

6.   Kellow, J.F., and Langluddecke, P.M. Advances in the understanding and management of the irritable bowel syndrome. Med. J. Austr. 1989 151(2):92-99.

7.   Asp,N G. Classification and methodology of food carbohydrates as related to nutritional effects. Amer.J.Clin.Nutr. 1995 61(Suppl):930S-937S

8.   Englyst,H.N. and Cummings,J.H. Digestion of the carbohydrates of banana (*Musa paradisiaca sapientum*) in the human small intestine. Amer.J.Clin.Nutr. 1986 44:42- 50

9.   Englyst,H.N. and Cummings,J.H. Digestion of the polysaccharides of some cereal foods in the human small intestine. Am.J.Clin.Nutr. 1985 42:778-787

10.   Englyst,H.N. and Kingman,S.M. Dietary fibre and resistant starch: A nutritional classification of plant polysaccharides. In: Kritchevski,D., Bonfield,C. and Anderson,J.W. (eds) *Dietary Fibre*, Plenum Publishing Co., New York. 1990 49-65

11.   Englyst,H.N. and Cummings,J.H. Digestion of the polysaccharides of potato in the small intestine of man. Amer.J.Clin.Nutr. 1987 45:423-431

12.   Hermansen,K., Rasmussen,O., Arnfred,J., Winther,E., and Schmitz,O. Differential glycemic effects of potato, rice and spaghetti in Type 1 (insulin dependent) diabetic patients at constant insulinaemia. Diabetologia 1986 29:358-361

13.   Wolever,T.M.S., Jenkins,D.J.A., Kalmusky,J., Jenkins,A., Giordano,C., Giudici,C., Josse,R.G., and Wong,G.S. Comparison of regular and parboiled rice: Explanation of discrepancies between reported glycemic responses to rice. Nutr.Res. 1986 6:349-357

Method: Diet For Irritable Bowel Syndrome (IBS)

General Description

This eating plan is designed to remove the foods and food additives which most frequently trigger the symptoms associated with irritable bowel syndrome. If there is significant improvement during the four week diet trial, foods will be systematically reintroduced in order to isolate specific dietary irritants.

Mechanism of Sensitivity in IBS

IBS tends to be an umbrella term for a variety of minor bowel disturbances. It is sometimes called "irritable colon" or "spastic colon". It is a chronic disorder, and a variety of causes have been suggested including dietary factors such as inadequate fibre, high fat intake, consumption of gas producing foods and carbonated beverages. Other suggested causes include: food intolerance, a disturbance of involuntary muscle movement in the large intestine, hormonal fluctuations, side effects of medications, smoking, swallowing of air while eating, and stress. A diagnosis of IBS is made when all organic disease has been ruled out by appropriate medical tests.

At the present time it is not known which mechanisms in the body are responsible for the symptoms of IBS.

Symptoms of IBS

Symptoms of IBS include: abdominal pain, excessive gas, flatulence and bloating, indigestion, constipation and diarrhea, and occasionally nausea and fatigue.

Dietary Management

Avoid: All milk and milk products (see *Milk-free Diet* page 89).
Add calcium and Vitamin D supplements as appropriate (*Non-dairy Sources of Calcium* page 102).

Avoid: Specific cereal grains and flours (wheat, rye, oats, barley) and corn (see *Restricted Grain Diet* page 116).
Use alternative grains to provide equivalent nutrients.

Cook: All vegetables, fruits, and fruit and vegetable juices, or use fruits canned in fruit juice.
Raw vegetables, salads, and fruits and juices are not allowed.

Avoid: Deli meats such as fermented sausages (salami, bologna, pepperoni, etc.).
Cook all meats and fish from fresh or frozen sources and do not use breaded, battered, sweet cured meats or smoked fish or meat. Do not add cream sauces.

Avoid: Legumes with non-starch polysaccharide outer skins such as navy beans, pinto beans, kidney beans, and green beans. Legumes without outer skins (lentils, split peas) are allowed.

Avoid: Whole nuts and seeds. Eat as spreads (paste) only. Try peanut butter (without any added sweeteners), almond butter, cashew butter, sesame tahini, sunflower seed butter, pumpkin seed butter, etc.

Avoid: Spices (root, seed, bark of plant): Herbs (leaves and flowers) are allowed as seasoning.
Cooked garlic and ginger are allowed, if tolerated.

Avoid: Caramel as a flavor or coloring in foods.

Avoid: All alcoholic beverages.

Avoid: Caffeine. Avoid coffee and black tea. Herbal teas (without spices) are allowed. Some decaffeinated coffees contain chemicals to which sensitive individuals react adversely.

Note: Caffeine intake is to be reduced gradually to avoid unpleasant side effects.

Avoid: Vinegars and all foods containing vinegar such as pickles, relish, and ketchup.

Reduce: Disaccharide sugars including lactose, sucrose, and maltose, (see *Disaccharide Restricted Diet* page 273). The degree to which this restriction will be advised depends on the severity of diarrhea being experienced. Use monosaccharides (honey, certain selected fruits, vegetables, and grains).

If diarrhea is a predominant symptom, a low fat diet is recommended until the stool becomes formed and the frequency of the bowel movements has decreased to one or two per day. If chronic diarrhea is a problem, a limited time trial on a disaccharide diet is worthwhile.

To ensure adequate intake of micronutrients, a multivitamin/mineral supplement is recommended. Select one that is wheat free, yeast free, lactose free, corn free, and free from additives such as artificial colors, flavors, and preservatives. Such products are made by Quest®, Jamieson®, Nulife®, Nutricology®, Natural Factors®.

Foods Allowed on this Diet

Each of the foods restricted on this diet can be found in many products and has many derivatives. It is important that only the foods listed as allowed are used during the trial period.

Testing to isolate specific foods causing the symptoms should be carried out after an initial trial period on the diet. Four weeks allows adequate time for the effects of the diet to be experienced.

Lists of restricted foods can be provided when specific dietary sensitivities have been isolated.

Diet For Irritable Bowel Syndrome

Type of Food	Foods Allowed
Milk and Dairy	Soy beverages free from milk ingredients Soy infant formulae Casein hydrolysate formulae Rice Dream® Coconut milk Nut milk Milk-free margarine Milk-free soy bean cake Non-dairy creamers such as Coffee Rich®
Vegetables	All cooked vegetables and their cooked juices are allowed if diarrhea is not a problem.

Breads and Cereals	Grains and Flours
	All allowed grains and legume flours such as:
	  Amaranth and amaranth flour
	  Arrowroot starch and flour
	  Buckwheat and buckwheat flour
	  Chickpea or garbanzo flour (Besan)
	  Lentil or pea flour
	  Millet and millet flour (Bajri)
	  Pea or bean flour
	  Potato starch and flour
	  Quinoa and quinoa flour
	  Rice and rice flour
	  Sago flour
	  Soy flour
	  Tapioca, tapioca starch, and flour
	  Wild rice and wild rice flour
	  T'ef flour

	Breads and Baked Goods
	Baked goods and specialty baking mixes containing allowed foods
	Specialty breads:
	    Ener G Rice®
	    Good 'n' Easy® bread and pastry mixes
	    Kingsmill® breads, cookies and muffin mixes
	  Homemade baked goods made with allowed flours

Diet For Irritable Bowel Syndrome

Type of Food	Foods Allowed

	Crackers and Snacks
	    Pure rice crackers
	    Cakes without nuts, seeds, or restricted grains.
	    Potato chips with allowed oil such as Nalley 100% Golden
	    Light Chips® *if a low fat diet is not being followed*

	Cereals
	    Cream of Rice®, rice bran
	    Any of the allowed grains, cooked
	    Puffed rice
	    Puffed millet
	    Puffed amaranth

	Pasta
	    Rice noodles and pasta
	    Brown rice pasta
	    Wild rice pasta
	    Mung bean pasta
	    Pasta made from any allowed grain

Legumes	Cooked peas and beans *without* the outer digestion resistant
	    skins such as:
	    Lentils (red, yellow, white)
	    Split peas (yellow, green)
	Pure "smooth" peanut butter without sweeteners
	Plain tofu
	Chickpea flour
	Red bean flour
	Soy bean flour
	Black bean flour

Fruit	All cooked fruits, fruits canned in fruit juice, cooked and cooled fruit
	    juices, and pasteurized fruit juices are allowed if diarrhea is not a
	    problem

Meat, Poultry, and Fish	All plain, cooked, lean and well trimmed fresh or frozen meat,
	    poultry, and fish
	Marinate in oil, herbs, lemon (cooked)
	Fish canned in water
	Note: Avoid all deli meats, smoked or pickled meats, as well as
	    meats which are breaded, creamed or otherwise prepared
	    with restricted foods

Eggs	All plain eggs.

Diet For Irritable Bowel Syndrome

Type of Food	Foods Allowed

Nuts and Seeds	Nut and seed butters only, such as:
	  Almond butter
	  Cashew butter
	  Sesame tahini
	  Sunflower seed butter
	  Peanut butter
	Butters can be made in a blender from any nuts or seeds.
	  (see recipes)

Fats and Oils	Pure oils, including canola, olive, sunflower, safflower, flaxseed, soy Whey-free margarine Fleischmann's low sodium, no salt margarine® Parkay diet spread® Meat drippings and poultry fat Homemade gravy made with allowed thickeners Lard
Herbs	All fresh or dried herbs, including: Basil Bay leaf Chervil Coriander leaf Dill weed Garlic powder Marjoram Mint Onion powder Oregano Parsley Poultry seasoning Rosemary Sage Savory Tarragon Thyme Cooked garlic and cooked ginger if tolerated

Sweeteners	Glucose
	Dextrose
	Fructose (fruit sugar)
	Levulose
	Honey
	Fruit conserves made with allowed fruits and sweetener
	In moderation, lactose free sugar substitutes, including Sugar
	  Twin®, Splenda®
	Note: Avoid aspartame® and sugar alcohols such as sorbitol,
	        xylitol, and mannitol

Beverages	Plain water and mineral water (carbonated mineral water may
	  cause gas and bloating)
	Herbal teas without spices, e.g., mint, peppermint,
	  chamomile, rosehip
	Cooked and cooled fruit juices diluted with water and
	  sweetened with allowed sweeteners, e.g., lemonade, limeade,
	  orangeade

Diet For Irritable Bowel Syndrome

Type of Food	Foods Allowed
Other	Baking soda Baking yeast Allergen free baking powder (see recipes) Cream of Tartar Salt Guar gum Plain gelatin

Nutritional Guidelines

To ensure an adequate intake of nutrients the following is advised:

Grains

Five servings daily of the allowed grains, especially the whole grains such as brown rice, wild rice, buckwheat, quinoa, amaranth, and millet should be eaten.

Milk and Milk Products

No milk products are allowed, but a good variety of meats and alternatives are included, which supply the same proteins as milk. Soy-based beverages and Rice Dream® can be used as substitutes for milk in recipes, beverages, and on cereals, but unless the nutrients are added artificially, these substitutes do not contain the calcium and Vitamin D that is in milk.

Since milk and milk products are the principal sources of calcium in the Western diet, when these foods are eliminated, it is difficult to obtain adequate amounts of daily calcium from dietary sources alone.

Vitamin D is required for uptake and utilization of dietary calcium. Adequate amounts of Vitamin D are usually obtained from the action of sunlight on the skin. One half hour per day of exposure to the sun will provide the daily Vitamin D requirements for an individual. In situations where the exposure to sunlight is limited, a supplementary source of Vitamin D is recommended.

Calcium Supplements

Supplementation of calcium is recommended when following a milk-free diet. Vitamin D is provided by skin exposure to sunlight, and a daily multivitamin/mineral usually provides 100% of the Recommended Daily Intake (RDI) or Recommended Daily Allowance (RDA) of the vitamin. Calcium carbonate provides 625-750 mg elemental Calcium per 2.5 mL (1/2 teaspoon). However, calcium gluconate, calcium citrate, and the Krebs cycle derivatives (fumarate, pyruvate, malate) appear to be more efficiently utilized supplements than calcium carbonate. In addition, some research studies indicate that they may interfere less with the absorption of iron and other trace elements than calcium carbonate alone. Supplements should contain allowed ingredients only (see Vitamins and Trace Minerals, below).

Vegetables

Vegetables must be cooked, but the variety is unlimited. Nutrients can be increased by using cooking water of vegetables in other dishes and with home made soups, meat and vegetable stews, and stir fries, or added to tomato juice as a beverage.

Fruits

Fruits must be cooked. They can be eaten alone (apple sauce, pear sauce, mixed fruit sauce), poached in a little water (poached pears, poached peaches), baked (baked apple, baked banana) or pureed and served as sauces on cooked grains. Raisins provide a quick and easy snack. Raisins, berries, and other fruits can be added to baked goods such as muffins, pancakes, and specialty breads.

Meat and Alternates

If three servings or more of meat and alternatives are included daily, most of the nutrient needs will be met.

Vitamins and Trace Minerals

Due to possible limitations of the diet, a daily multivitamin/mineral supplement is advised for insurance.

Supplements must be free from wheat, yeast, corn, lactose, sugar, and all artificial additives such as colors, flavors, and preservatives. The label will specify that the product is free from these ingredients. A few brands which make products that comply with these specifications include: Quest®, Jamieson®, Nulife®, Nutricology®, and Natural Factors®.

See Appendix II for Irritable Bowel Syndrome diet guidelines and sample recipes beginning page 377.

30

Urticaria and Angioedema

Urticaria

Urticaria is characterized by local pruritic (itchy) weals and erythema (reddening) in the skin.[1] Individual urticarial weals vary from one millimeter to several centimeters and may be found on any part of the body. The weals usually last less than four hours.

Some studies have indicated that disease conditions such as asthma, rhinitis, and eczema are more prevalent in subjects with urticaria than in other atopic subjects. Other studies have shown no correlation between urticaria and these conditions.[2,3]

Angioedema

Angioedema is similar to urticaria, but is characterized by larger edematous areas that involve swelling of the skin and mucous membranes. Areas most commonly affected are the eyelids, lips, and tongue. Other parts of the body possibly affected are the face, ears, under the chin, genitalia, hands, feet, trunk, and arms.[4] Angioedema is usually not itchy.[5]

Other symptoms that may occur at the same time as angioedema are headache, arthralgia, the sensation of a lump in the throat, hoarseness, shortness of breath, wheezing, nausea, vomiting, abdominal pain, and diarrhea.[2]

Causes of Urticaria and Angioedema

Histamine is thought to be the primary inflammatory chemical responsible for urticaria and/or angioedema.[6] Many factors, such as physical stimuli, drug intake, and diet, can increase circulating levels of this bioamine.[4] Dietary histamine is catabolized by diamine oxidases located in the mucosa of the small bowel, a step that controls total body histamine.

Some people with urticaria and/or angioedema have a defect that reduces diamine oxidase activity.[7] As a result, dietary sources of histamine may be a sizeable source of circulating histamine for these people.[8] If these foods can be avoided, the symptoms of chronic urticaria and/or angioedema may be alleviated.

In addition, foods and food additives may increase circulating histamine by stimulating the release of histamine in body tissues through immunological and/or non-immunological mechanisms.[9] Alleviation of symptoms may be achieved by identifying and avoiding these triggers.

IgE mediated urticaria occurs approximately 30 minutes after ingestion or inhalation of an allergen. As a result, the allergen is often obvious. Antigens that commonly provoke an IgE mediated urticaria are found in shellfish, nuts, chocolate, and drugs.[2] Inhaled allergens are rarely reported to be the cause of urticaria,[5] but a theory of "total allergy burden" suggests that they are implicated.[3] According to this theory, even though one allergen does not result in urticaria, the additive effect of several contact, inhaled, and ingested allergens produces urticaria. If this is the case, identification of each of the contributing allergens would be very difficult in practice.

Regulation of Histamine

Diamine oxidase and N-methyl transferase are responsible for the catabolism of histamine. Hepatic N-methyl transferases ensure a consistent post-hepatic level of blood histamine.[10] A deficiency of these enzymes leaves an excess of histamine in the circulation.

Food and Food Additives Inducing Urticaria and Angioedema

Food Allergens

The foods most commonly reported to induce urticaria are shellfish, fish, egg, nuts, chocolate, berries, tomatoes, cheese, milk, and wheat.[11] The mechanism of action may be immunological (allergy) or non-immunological (pharmacological).

Food Additives

Studies using food additive elimination diets have been reported to control urticaria in approximately 20 to 50% of subjects. The substances most commonly implicated in these studies have been tartrazine, sunset yellow, benzoates, and BHT and/or BHA. Naturally occurring salicylates and benzoates have also been implicated as contributors.

Histamine Releasing Food

Foods reported to release histamine directly from mast cells are uncooked egg white, shellfish, strawberries, tomatoes, chocolate, fish, pineapple, and alcohol.[12]

Food Containing Histamine

Histamine is formed in food from the decarboxylation of histidine by bacteria that possess the enzyme histidine decarboxylase. Aged protein containing foods and fermented foods commonly have increased histamine levels. Foods reported to be high in histamine are fermented cheeses (e.g., Camembert, Brie, Gruyere, Cheddar, Roquefort, Parmesan), brewer's yeast, shellfish, many fin fish, canned fish, tomato, spinach, red wine (especially Chianti), beer, unpasteurized milk (i.e., cow, goat, or human milk), chicken, dry pork sausage, beef sausage, ham, chocolate, fermented soy products, and all fermented vegetables, such as sauerkraut.[12,13] The amount of histamine in these foods varies with conditions under which they are processed and stored.

Histamine Restricted Diet

The diet designed to manage idiopathic urticaria and angioedema restricts the intake of foods and food additives that are known to increase histamine in the body, either by their intrinsic histamine content or by releasing endogenous histamine, (see *Histamine Restricted Diet*, page 160).

Controlled trials using this management strategy are presently underway and results are not yet available. However, this approach has proved effective in a number of affected people who failed to improve with other treatment modalities. Preliminary results indicate that people with urticaria in which the primary symptom is pruritus and who experience relief with the use of antihistamines, and people with facial angioedema, benefit most from this dietary management.

References

1. Atkins, F.M. Food induced urticaria. In: Metcalfe, D.D., Sampson, H.A., and Simon, R.A. (Eds), *Food Allergy: Adverse Reactions to Foods and Food Additives*. Blackwell Scientific Publications, Oxford, London, 1991. 129-138.

2. Soter, N.A. Acute and chronic urticaria and angioedema. J. Am. Acad. Dermatol. 1991 25:146-154.

3. Armenaka, M., Lehach, J., and Rosenstreich, D.L. Successful management of chronic urticaria. Clin. Rev. Allergy 1992 10:371-390.

4. Holgate, S.T., and Church, M.K. (Eds), *Allergy*. Gower Medical Publishing, New York, 1993. 21.1 22.12.

5. Burrall, B.A., Halpern, G.M., and Huntley, A.C. Chronic urticaria. Western J. Med. 1990 152(3):268-276.

6. White, M.V. The role of histamine in allergic disease. J. Allergy Clin. Immunol. 1990 86(4 part 2):599-605.

7. Lessof, M.H. Food, food additives and urticaria. Clin. Exper. Allergy 1991 21(Suppl.1):316-320.

8. Sattler, J., Hafner, D., Klotter, H., Lorenz, W., and Wagner, P.K. Food induces histaminosis as an epidemiological problem: plasma histamine elevation and haemodynamic alterations after oral histamine administration and blockade of diamine oxidase (DAO). Agents and Actions 1988 23(3/4):361-365.

9.   Murdoch, D.D., Lessof, M.H., Pollock, I., and Young, E. Effects of food additives on leukocyte histamine released in normal and urticaria subjects. J. Roy. Coll. Phys. London 1987 <u>21</u>(4):251-256.

10.   Moneret Vautrin, D.A. Food intolerance masquerading as food allergy: False food allergy. In: Brostoff, J., and Challacombe, S.J. (Eds), *Food Allergy and Intolerance*. Baillière Tindall, London, 1987. 836-849.

11.   Taylor, S.L. Histamine food poisoning: toxicology and clinical aspects. CRC Crit. Rev. Toxicol. 1986 <u>17</u>(2):90128.

12.   Finn, R. Pharmacological actions of foods. In: Brostoff, J., and Challacombe, S.J. (Eds), *Food Allergy and Intolerance*. Baillière Tindall, London, 1987. 425-430.

13.   Chandra, R.K. Food allergy. In: Shils, M.E., and Young, V.R. (Eds), *Modern Nutrition in Health and Disease*. Lea and Febiger, Philadelphia, 1988. 1298-1305.

Method: Histamine Restricted Diet for Control of Urticaria / Angioedema

Do not eat the following food during the 4 week trial elimination period.

Meat, Poultry, and Fish

- All seafood including shellfish or fin fish, fresh, frozen, smoked, or canned
- Egg (a small quantity in a baked product such as pancakes, muffins, cakes is usually tolerated)
- Processed, smoked and fermented meats such as luncheon meat, sausage, wiener, bologna, salami, pepperoni
- Leftover meat: Eat freshly cooked meat *only*.

Milk and Milk Products

- All fermented milk products, including cheese such as Cheddar, Colby, Blue cheese, Brie, Camembert, Feta, Romano, etc.
- Cheese products such as processed cheese, cheese slices, cheese spreads
- Yogurt, buttermilk, and kefir.

(Any milk product that is curdled rather than fermented is allowed, for example, cottage cheese, ricotta cheese, panir)

Fruits and Vegetables

Orange	Strawberries	Pineapple	Relishes	Tomatoes
Grapefruit	Raspberries	Dates	Pickles	Ketchup
Lemon	Cranberries	Raisins	Spinach	Tomato sauces
Lime	Loganberries	Prunes		
Cherries	Apricot	Currants		

Food Additives

- Tartrazine and other artificial food colors (see *Diet Restricted in Tartrazine*, page 181)
- Preservatives, especially benzoates, sulfites and BHA, BHT (see *Benzoate* and *Sulfite Restricted Diets,* pages 213 and 228 respectively).

Note: Many medications, and vitamin pills contain these additives, especially colors. Ask the pharmacist to recommend additive-free supplements and medications.

Seasonings

Cinnamon	Cloves	Nutmeg	Hot paprika (cayenne)
Chili powder	Anise	Curry powder	

Miscellaneous

- Fermented soy products (such as soy sauce, miso)
- Fermented food (such as sauerkraut)
- Tea (herbal or regular)
- Chocolate, cocoa, and cola drinks
- Alcohol (beer, ale, lager, cider, wine, hard liquor)
- Vinegar and foods containing vinegar such as pickles, relishes, ketchup, and prepared mustard

31

Diet and Migraine

Migraine headache is estimated to afflict 5 to 30% of the population. The incidence in women is three times as high as in men, and the condition is inherited in 60 to 80% of cases.[1]

Migraine may be defined as:

"Recurrent attacks of headache, widely varied in intensity, frequency, and duration. The attacks are commonly unilateral in onset; are usually associated with anorexia and, sometimes, with nausea and vomiting; in some cases are preceded by, or associated with, conspicuous sensory, motor, and mood disturbances; and are often familial." [1]

The causes of migraine are still unknown, even though many etiological theories have been proposed. Probably several different mechanisms are involved.[1]

Factors Precipitating Migraine Headaches

Migraine headaches may be triggered by a number of factors, including stress, bright lights, loud sounds, physical exertion, inhalation of chemicals such as petroleum derivatives, fasting, menstruation, and oral contraceptives. In addition, foods and food additives can cause migraine or play a part in causing the condition.

Less common allergens are:

Shellfish
Nuts
Fin fish
Tomato
Beef
Citrus fruits
Refer to *Table 5-2: Joneja Allergen Scale*, page 28.

Biogenic Amines[7]

The biogenic amines most likely to elicit symptoms are histamine, tyramine, phenylethylamine, and octopamine. Refer to Part III for a discussion of these substances and for the method for *Histamine and Tyramine Restricted Diets*, (see pages 160 and 153 respectively).

Histamine is found in:

Fish and shellfish
Fermented cheeses
Fermented soy products, soy sauce
Fermented beverages: wines (red and white) and beer
Dry pork and beef sausage (pepperoni, salami, bologna, etc.)
Tomato
Spinach
Egg white
Strawberries
Chocolate
Sauerkraut

Tyramine is found in:

Aged cheeses
Processed and fermented sausages
Sour cream
Wines (red and white)
Pickled herring
Smoked and pickled fish (e.g., smoked salmon)
Sauerkraut
Broad bean pods
Vinegar and foods containing vinegar such as pickles, relishes, and sauces
Avocado
Peanut
Chicken liver

Phenylethylamine is found in:

Chocolate
Aged cheeses
Red wines

Other Pharmacologically Active Chemicals

Other chemicals in foods known to trigger migraine headaches through pharmacological action are methylxanthines (e.g., caffeine), theobromine, and theophylline and aminophylline.

Methylxanthines are found in:

Coffee
Tea
Cola drinks

Nitrites

Nitrites[9] are other possible triggers, in particular potassium or sodium nitrite, which are used as food preservatives and coloring agents, (see *Nitrite and Nitrate Sensitivity*, page 241).
Nitrites are found in:

Cured meats such as:
- Wieners
- Salami
- Bologna
- Pepperoni
- Luncheon meats
- Ham
- Bacon

Smoked meats and fish such as:
- Smoked salmon
- Smoked bacon

Aged cheeses

Alcohol

There is evidence that the chemicals in alcoholic beverages are more frequent triggers for migraine headaches than the alcohol itself.[10]

10.   Raskin, N.H. Chemical headaches. Ann. Rev. Med. 1981 $\underline{32}$:63 71.

11.   Lipton, R.B., Newman, L.C., Cohen, J.S., and Solomon, S. Aspartame as a dietary trigger of headache. Headache 1989 $\underline{29}$:90 92.

Method: Test Diet for Migraine

General Description

The test diet should be followed for a minimum of four weeks or through a period in which at least three migraine headaches are usually experienced.

If there is significant improvement on the test diet, the diet should be followed by individual challenges of each food. This procedure is important to determine whether the food acts as a migraine trigger. If no headache is experienced on the challenge food, the food should be returned to the diet.

Test Diet for Migraine

Type of Food	Foods Allowed	Foods Restricted

Milk and Dairy	None except butter
	As a substitute:
	Rice Dream® (made with
	  brown rice and safflower oil)
	Coconut and other nut milks
	In recipes, allowed fruit juices
	  and vegetable water
		All fermented cheeses
		Cottage cheese
		Processed cheese
		Cream cheese
		All milk (homogenized, skim,
		  1%, 2%, buttermilk)
		Yogurt
		Cream
		Sour Cream
		Ice Cream

Breads and Cereals	Grains and Flours
	Rice, rye, buckwheat, oats,
	  bey, kasha, amaranth, quinoa,
	  tapioca, sago, arrowroot,
	  millet
		Wheat, wheat bran, wheat
		  germ, wheat berries,
		  Wheatena, spelt, triticale,
		  semolina, kamut, durum,
		  farina, couscous, matzoh,
		  "gluten enriched flour", bulgur,
		  corn, cornmeal, corn starch,
		  corn flour

	Breads and Baked Goods
	Made from allowed flours
	  and starches:
	  100% rye bread
	  Pumpernickel bread
	  Oat and oat bran bread
	  Rice bread
		All made with wheat or corn,
		  including white, whole wheat
		  or multigrain bread or baked
		  goods (muffins, pies, cookies,
		  etc.)
		Corn bread, muffins, etc.

	Crackers and Snacks
	Rice cakes and crackers
	  made with allowed ingredients
	Pure crisp rye crackers
		All made with wheat or corn,
		  including crackers, tortillas,
		  nachos, chips

Test Diet for Migraine

Type of Food	Foods Allowed	Foods Restricted
	Cereals Cream of Rice® Puffed rice Oatmeal Homemade granola and Muesli with allowed ingredients Any grain on the allowed list	All made with wheat or corn
	Pasta Buckwheat pasta Rice noodles and pasta Wild rice pasta Quinoa pasta	Wheat or corn pasta Legume pasta such as soy or mung bean pasta
Vegetables	Fresh, frozen or canned pure vegetables which are not overripe or spoiled Asparagus Bamboo shoots Beans, green/yellow Beets Broccoli Brussels sprouts Cabbage Cauliflower Celery Chard Cucumber Eggplant (aubergine) Lettuce Mushrooms Onions Parsnips Parsley Peas, green and snow Peppers (capsicum) Pumpkin Radish Rutabaga and turnip Squash, all types Zucchini (courgette)	Avocado Bean and wheat sprouts Broad beans Corn and corn on the cob Potato Spinach Sweet potato Tomato All overripe and spoiled vegetables Sauerkraut and other fermented vegetables Any pickled vegetables

Test Diet for Migraine

Type of Food	Foods Allowed	Foods Restricted
Fruit	Fresh, frozen, or canned pure fruits which are not overripe or spoiled All berries except strawberries and raspberries Apple Apricot Cherry Date Fig Kiwi Mango Melon, all types Nectarine Papaya (pawpaw) Peach Pear Pineapple Rhubarb	Overripe or spoiled fruit Strawberries Raspberries All citrus fruit, including: orange, lemon, lime, grapefruit, kumquat, tangerine, tangelo Banana Plum Prune Raisins
Meat, Poultry, and Fish	The following pure, fresh, frozen, or canned in water or oil: Lamb Game meats such as venison or moose All poultry, including: Chicken (except liver) Cornish game hen Duck Goose Turkey All very fresh or flash frozen fish if it is known not to be a migraine trigger	Pork, including ham and bacon Beef, including veal Processed and fermented meats, e.g.: Pepperoni Salami Bologna Hot dogs, wieners, smokies Frankfurters Luncheon meats Chicken liver All shellfish Smoked fish Pickled fish (e.g. herring)
Nuts and Seeds	All plain nuts and seeds	Nuts and seeds prepared with restricted foods, such as soy sauce, garlic, cheese or chocolate

Test Diet for Migraine

Type of Food	Foods Allowed	Foods Restricted
Eggs	Limited to small amounts in baking only Egg white is usually more reactive than the yolk	Omelette Poached Scrambled Fried Boiled Dishes in which egg is the principal ingredient, e.g.: Soufflé Quiche Eggnog Custard Meringue
Legumes	None	All, including: Peanut Licorice Soy: beans, flour, milk, tofu, soy sauce and any food in which soy is the main ingredient, especially fermented soy products Other dried peas and beans, especially pinto beans and black eyed peas
Fats and Oils	Butter Pure vegetable oils Pure vegetable shortening Allowed meat drippings Homemade gravy with allowed thickeners	Most margarine Lard Mayonnaise Prepared salad dressings Prepared gravies Prepared sauces
Spices, Herbs, and Seasonings	All as tolerated except those listed opposite	Packets and mixes with restricted ingredients Soy sauce and other fermented sauces Garlic Cinnamon Curry spices Cayenne Nutmeg Anise

Test Diet for Migraine

Type of Food	Foods Allowed	Foods Restricted
Sweets and Sweeteners	All except those listed opposite	Aspartame Chocolate and cocoa All candy bars containing chocolate Chocolate, cocoa, and cola drinks Chocolate laxatives Jams, jellies, etc., made with restricted fruits
Other	Baking powder Baking soda Cream of Tartar Baking yeast in moderation	Yeast and meat extracts: 　Marmite® 　Oxo® 　Bovril® 　Vegemite® Vinegar and all foods containing vinegar, e.g.: 　Pickles 　Relishes 　Sauces 　Salad dressings Wine (red is often more reactive than white) Brewer's and nutritional yeast
Beverages	Allowed fruit and vegetable juices Herbal tea without spices Plain and carbonated mineral water Carbonated beverages other than cola or root beer Distilled alcoholic beverages such as vodka, gin, rum with caution	Coffee Tea Cola drinks Root beer Restricted fruit and vegetable drinks Milk and milk beverages Drinks made with other restricted items, e.g., Bovril® Wine Beer Alcoholic beverages made with restricted foods, e.g., brandy, fruit liqueurs, coolers

32

Attention Deficit Disorder with Hyperactivity (ADDH)

The possibility that hyperactive behaviour in children is caused by food allergy or by a food component or additive is an idea that has been debated since the 1920's.[1]

The role of food allergy, especially reactions to wheat and corn, as a cause of fatigue, irritability, and behaviour problems was suggested in the 1940's. A well known proponent of a relationship between food and hyperactivity was Benjamin Feingold, who in 1975[2] claimed that behavioral and learning disorders in children were caused by food additives and salicylates in foods. Thereafter, the "Feingold diet" became very popular, until it fell into disrepute when other investigators were unable to reproduce Feingold's results.[3]

In recent years, a number of well conducted studies have addressed the role of food allergy and intolerance in learning and behavioral disorders in children.[4,5] A recent review of research in this field[6] discusses current thought on the link between diet and behaviour disorders. The reviewers state:

"It must be recognized that adverse effects of foods on behaviour may be either a manifestation of (probably pharmacologically based) food intolerance, or they may be psychologically based (e.g. via suggestion or adverse conditioning)."

Current opinions on the link between diet and behaviour include the following:

- Children suffering allergic reactions respond as any child responds to an acute or chronic illness.[1] They feel miserable, are irritable and restless, have difficulty sleeping, and may be unable to concentrate. The obverse of these symptoms is that children experience fatigue and listlessness.
- Food allergy is a direct physiological cause of behaviour changes. The hypersensitivity reaction releases inflammatory chemicals that can directly affect functions of the central nervous system.[4]
- Additives in foods such as azo dyes (e.g., tartrazine), preservatives (especially benzoates and BHA and BHT), flavor enhancers (especially glutamates), and artificial flavors have a direct physiological effect on central nervous system functions.[7]

Several explanations have been proposed for the significant improvement observed in a surprisingly large number of behaviorally disturbed children using a "hypoallergenic diet." These reasons include:

- When food allergens are excluded from the diet, an allergic child feels better and behaviour naturally improves.
- When food additives are excluded from a child's diet, the "junk food" is removed. The resulting diet is often more balanced and of higher nutritional value. The child's behaviour is a response to the more nutritious diet.
- When a specifically formulated diet is prescribed, parents take extra care in food preparation. The child feels special and commands more attention within the family. This change in status and family dynamics has a positive psychological effect on the child and behaviour improves.

Undoubtedly, all these factors have an influence on a child, especially an atopic child. Whether or not it has a scientific basis, this form of dietary management is justified if it improves the quality of life of the child and family and imposes no psychological, nutritional, or economic stress on a family already in a stressful situation.

The diet outlined in this chapter is designed to remove food allergens or specific food additives suspected on the basis of history or of dietary elimination. The prescribed diet must be nutritionally adequate, supplying equivalent nutrients from alternative sources.

The diet is followed for a period of four weeks. If significant improvement is achieved, an incremental dose challenge is implemented to identify specific food allergens and behaviour triggers, (see *Challenge Phase*, page 41).

References

1.   David, T.J. Behaviour problems. In: *Food and Food Additive Intolerance in Childhood.* Blackwell Scientific Publications, Oxford, London, 1993. 420-437.

2.   Feingold, B.F. Hyperkinesis and learning disabilities linked to artificial food flavours and colours. Am. J. Nurs. 1975 75:797-803.

3.   Harley, J.P., Ray, R.S., Tomasi, L., Eichman, P.L., Matthews, C.G., Chun, R., Cleeland, C.S., and Traisman, E. Hyperkinesis and food additives: testing the Feingold hypothesis. Pediatrics 1978 61:818-828.

4.   Egger, J., Carter, C.M., Graham, P.J., Gumley, D., and Soothill, J.F. Controlled trial of oligoantigenic treatment in the hyperkinetic syndrome. Lancet 1985 1:540-545.

5.   Kaplan, B.J., McNicol, J., Conte, R.A., and Moghadam, H.K. Dietary replacement in pre-school-aged hyperactive boys. Pediatrics 83:7-17.

6.   Robinson, J., and Ferguson, A. Food sensitivity and the nervous system: Hyperactivity , addiction and criminal behaviour. Nutr. Res. Reviews 1992 5:203-223.

7.   Egger, J. The hyperkinetic syndrome. In: Brostoff, J., and Challacombe, S.J. (Eds), *Food Allergy and Intolerance*. Baillière Tindall, London and Philadelphia, 1987.

Method: Hyperactivity Test Diet

General Description

This four week test diet is designed to restrict the foods and food additives most frequently linked to Attention Deficit Disorder with Hyperactivity (ADDH) in children. Although hyperactivity is only one of the symptoms associated with this disorder, it is the term most frequently applied to diets associated with ADDH.

If there is a significant improvement during the four week diet trial, foods will be systematically reintroduced to determine foods and additives that can precipitate a reaction, and to increase the variety of foods and nutrient value of the diet.

Mechanism of Sensitivity

The diet has been planned to remove the foods and food additives which may not be tolerated or be contributing to the problem. This diet is initially followed for four weeks.

If symptoms have not improved in this time, diet is unlikely to be a contributing factor, and there will be no benefit in following the dietary restrictions any longer.

If significant improvement is experienced, foods can be reintroduced individually to isolate the dietary offenders.

Symptoms of ADDH

The following symptoms may indicate the need for the Hyperactivity Test Diet:

- Trouble falling asleep at night
- Frequent awakenings during the night
- Bad breath despite good oral hygiene and absence of infection
- Frequent runny or stuffy nose despite lack of infection
- Headaches
- Several of the following symptoms: (typical of ADDH)

Restlessness or overactivity	Easily frustrated
Excitability	Demands must be met immediately
Impulsiveness	Inattentive and easily distracted
Disturbs other children	Cries often and easily
Failure to finish activities	Mood changes quickly and drastically
Short attention span	Temper outbursts and explosive and
Constant fidgeting	unpredictable behaviour

Foods and Food Additives Eliminated in the Test Diet

Foods

- Milk and milk products
- Wheat and corn
- Peanut
- Apple
- Orange
- Tomato

Benzoates

These chemicals are used as preservatives in many foods including ice cream, candies, baked goods, chewing gum, margarine, and pickles. They occur naturally in some foods including: prunes, tea, raspberries, cinnamon, anise, and nutmeg.

Artificial Colors

These will appear on labels as "artificial color" or simply "color" and are likely to be present in most packaged and commercially prepared foods.

Artificial Flavors

Monosodium glutamate (MSG) and anything with "glutamate" on the label indicates artificial flavors. They may be added to any commercially prepared foods, flavor packages, canned soup and soup mixes, and restaurant meals.

Butylated hydroxyanisole (BHA) and Butylated hydroxytoluene (BHT)

These are antioxidants that are added to many commercially prepared foods and packaged cereals, especially foods containing oils. "BHA" and "BHT" will appear on food labels.

Nitrites and Nitrates

These chemicals are used in cured meats as preservatives and to maintain color and flavor. They are likely to be present in cured ham, bacon, bologna, frankfurters, salami, pepperoni, and smoked fish. Avoid deli meats.

Propyl gallate

Propyl gallate is an antioxidant used in commercially prepared foods, especially those containing fats and oils such as ice cream, baked goods, and desserts. "Propyl gallate" will appear on food labels.

Sulfites

Preservatives used in a variety of foods such as dried fruits, grapes, frozen sliced mushrooms, sliced potatoes, baked goods, canned fish, pickles and relishes. "Sulfite" or "sulphite" will appear on food labels.

Caffeine

Caffeine is found in foods and beverages (coffee, tea, cola drinks, chocolate, cocoa).

Artificial Sweeteners

Aspartame in particular, is eliminated.

Other Restrictions

Sweeteners, such as sugar, syrups, jam, candy, are allowed in moderation. Fruit juices should be diluted by one half with water, and low sugar products are recommended. Products and foods with moderate amounts of sugar should be given at the end of the meal and should not be used alone for snacks.

Meals should be divided into at least six feedings to ensure that some food is taken about every 2 - 2½ hours.

Highly scented products such as perfumes, scented cleaners, and laundry products should be avoided. Children have been reported to react to scented markers and to products like Wite-Out® or Liquid Paper®, especially when they are toluene-based.

All food should be free from artificial colors, artificial flavors, and preservatives.

Test Diet For Hyperactivity

Type of Food	Foods Allowed
Milk and Dairy	Rice Dream® (made from brown rice and safflower oil) Coconut milk In recipes: substitute allowed fruit or vegetable juices, or homemade soup stock On toast, instead of butter use pure jelly, jam, honey, herb flavored olive oil On vegetables, use herbs and dressings made with allowed foods (see below) Light whipped butter made from clarified butter (see recipe below)

Breads and Cereals	Grains and Flours
	  Amaranth and amaranth flour
	  Arrowroot starch and flour
	  Barley and barley flour
	  Buckwheat and buckwheat flour
	  Chickpea or garbanzo flour (Besan)
	  Millet and millet flour (Bajri)
	  Oats and oat flour
	  Potato starch and flour
	  Quinoa and quinoa flour
	  Rice and rice flour
	  Rye and rye flour
	  Tapioca, tapioca starch, and flour
	  Wild rice and wild rice flour

	Breads and Baked Goods
	  100% rye bread and Pumpernickel bread
	  Rice bread
	  Bread made with allowed grains
	  Baked goods and specialty baking mixes containing allowed foods
	  Specialty breads:
	    Ener-G® rice, brown rice, or tapioca bread
	  Homemade baked goods made with allowed foods

	Crackers and Snacks
	  Pure rice crackers or rice cakes without restricted grains
	  RyVita Rye Krisp® (white package)
	  Wasa® Lite and Golden Crackers
	  Potato chips made with allowed oil, such as Nalley 100% Golden Light Chips®

Test Diet For Hyperactivity

Type of Food	Foods Allowed
	Cereals Cream of Rice® and rice bran Oatmeal Homemade granola or muesli with allowed ingredients Any of the allowed grains, cooked Puffed rice Puffed millet Puffed amaranth
	Pasta Rice noodles and pasta Brown rice pasta Wild rice pasta Mung bean pasta Quinoa pasta
Vegetables	Plain, fresh, frozen, and canned vegetables and their juices All vegetables are allowed, *except* tomato
Fruit	Plain fresh, frozen, and canned in fruit juice Plain fruit juices (no added sugar, preservatives, or color) All fruits are allowed *except*: Apple Dried fruits Grapes Orange Prunes Raisins Raspberries Fruit and dried fruit with sulfites
Meat, Poultry, and Fish	All plain, cooked, fresh, or frozen, meat, poultry, or fish Can be marinated in oil, herbs, lemon Plain fish such as tuna canned in water (check label for sulfites) *Avoid* all deli style meats, smoked or pickled meats and fish, and any breaded, creamed, or prepared with restricted ingredients
Eggs	All plain eggs *without* milk, cheese, wheat or other restricted ingredients
Nuts and Seeds	All plain nuts and seeds are allowed, *except* peanuts Any product labeled "nuts" should be *avoided*, as it may contain peanuts Nut and seed butters, e.g.: Almond butter Cashew butter Sesame tahini

Test Diet For Hyperactivity

Type of Food	Foods Allowed
Legumes	All *except* peanut, soy, and red beans, and products made from them Allowed legumes include: <table><tr><td>Black eyed peas</td><td>Lima beans</td></tr><tr><td>Broad beans (fava beans)</td><td>Navy beans</td></tr><tr><td>Chickpeas or garbanzos</td><td>Pinto beans</td></tr><tr><td>Cranberry beans</td><td>Romano beans</td></tr><tr><td>Great northern beans</td><td>White beans</td></tr><tr><td>Yellow and green split peas</td><td>Lentils</td></tr></table>
Fats and Oils	Pure vegetable oils, including canola, olive, sunflower, safflower, flaxseed Meat drippings and poultry fat Homemade gravy made with allowed foods Lard Light whipped clarified butter (see recipe)
Spices and Herbs	All fresh and dried pure herbs, including: <table><tr><td>Basil</td><td>Bay leaf</td></tr><tr><td>Chervil</td><td>Coriander leaf</td></tr><tr><td>Dill weed</td><td>Garlic powder</td></tr><tr><td>Marjoram</td><td>Mint</td></tr><tr><td>Onion powder</td><td>Oregano</td></tr><tr><td>Parsley</td><td>Poultry seasoning</td></tr><tr><td>Rosemary</td><td>Sage</td></tr><tr><td>Savory</td><td>Tarragon</td></tr><tr><td>Thyme</td><td></td></tr></table>All pure spices except cinnamon, cloves, nutmeg, and anise Allowed spices include: <table><tr><td>Allspice</td><td>Caraway</td></tr><tr><td>Cardamom</td><td>Cayenne</td></tr><tr><td>Celery seed</td><td>Coriander</td></tr><tr><td>Cumin</td><td>Fennel</td></tr><tr><td>Ginger</td><td>Mustard seed</td></tr><tr><td>Paprika</td><td>Pepper</td></tr><tr><td>Poppy seed</td><td>Red Pepper</td></tr><tr><td>Saffron</td><td>Turmeric</td></tr></table>
Sweets and Sweeteners	All sugar *except* icing sugar, used in moderation Unsulfured molasses Honey Pure maple syrup Pure fruit sauces made with allowed fruit and sugar Pure fruit conserves made with allowed fruit

Test Diet For Hyperactivity

Type of Food	Foods Allowed
Beverages	Rice Dream® Plain water Mineral water, carbonated and plain Herbal teas without spices, e.g., mint, peppermint, chamomile, rosehip Fruit drinks made with allowed fruits and sweeteners Drinks made with allowed fruit juice concentrates and carbonated mineral water
Other	Baking soda Allergen-free baking powder Cream of Tartar Salt Baking yeast Guar gum Plain gelatin

Nutritional Guidelines

This diet excludes all artificial colors, flavors and preservatives. Most packaged and commercially prepared foods are not allowed. Cook and use fresh or frozen ingredients without additives. Eliminate junk food and convenience food. By focusing on food without added sugar and other unnecessary flavorings a more nutritiously balanced diet will result.

Nutrients

This diet offers a good variety of foods in all food groups, except milk and milk products.

To ensure an adequate intake of nutrients, the child should eat five servings daily of a variety of the allowed grains, especially the whole grains such as brown rice, wild rice, oats, rye, amaranth, and quinoa as cereals, pastas, baked goods, and breads. Three or more servings of meat and alternatives per day will meet many nutrient needs.

Because children are often resistant to new foods, a multivitamin/mineral supplement is advised until a wider range of alternate foods is acceptable in the diet. A few brands which are made with allowed ingredients are: Quest®, Jamieson®, Nutricology®, and Nulife®. Make sure that the supplement is free from the following: wheat, corn, lactose, yeast, sugar, and additives such as artificial colors, flavors, and preservatives.

Rice Dream® can be used as a substitute in beverages and on cereal instead of milk. Rice Dream® does not contain the calcium and Vitamin D that are in milk. Supplementation of calcium is recommended. Calcium carbonate provides 625-750 mg elemental calcium per 2.5 mL (½ teaspoon). Calcium citrate malate or calcium gluconate appear to be more effective supplements than calcium carbonate.

33

Diet and Asthma

A large number of factors can trigger an asthma attack in a person prone to asthma.[1] These factors include: infection, exercise, exposure to cold air, weather changes, air pollution, inhalation of allergens (mold spores, pollens, house dust mites, animal dander), psychological factors (anxiety and stress, laughing and crying), and gastroesophageal reflux.

Most clinicians believe that, although an adverse reaction to a food or food additive may provoke or worsen an asthma attack, food is only one of many asthma triggers and is an uncommon cause of asthma in children.[2] It is uncommon for asthma to be the only symptom when food allergy or intolerance is involved in triggering an asthma attack. Sufferers usually experience other symptoms such as gastrointestinal disturbances (vomiting, loose stools and/or abdominal pain), rhinitis and skin reactions (urticaria and/or eczema).[3]

The prevailing directive is to avoid foods that have triggered asthma attacks. The faster the onset of the attack after eating the triggering food, the easier it is to identify the offending food.[1] However, the effect of avoiding that food or food additive on the underlying asthma is considered minimal.[1]

Foods Implicated in Provoking Asthma

The foods and food additives most commonly implicated in provoking asthma are:

Allergens[4]

- Cow's milk protein
- Egg

- Peanuts
- Wheat
- Corn
- Fish

In addition, any food that triggers an allergic response in an atopic individual could provoke an asthma attack.[1]

Food Additives[5]

- Sulfites
- Tartrazine
- Other food dyes
- Benzoates
- Monosodium glutamate (MSG)

Tyramine has also been implicated as an asthma trigger in adults. Persons who exhibit sensitivity to tyramine are reported to experience improvement in their asthma on a tyramine-restricted diet.[6]

Although it is important for persons with asthma who are sensitive to acetylsalicylic acid to avoid Aspirin®, there is no evidence that salicylates in foods provoke an asthma attack.[1]

References

1.   David, T.J. Asthma. In: *Food and Food Additive Intolerance in Childhood.* Blackwell Scientific Publications, Oxford, London, 1993. 291-316.

2.   Bock, S.A. Food-related asthma and basic nutrition. J. Asthma 1983 20:377-381.

3.   Novembre, E., Martino, M., and Vierucci, A. Foods and respiratory allergy. J. Allergy Clin. Immunol. 1988 81:1059-1065.

4.   Onorato, J., Merland, N., Terral, C., Michel, F.B., and Bousquet, J. Placebo-controlled double-blind food challenge in asthma. J. Allergy Clin. Immunol. 1986 78:1139-1146.

5.   Genton, C., Frei, P.C., and Pecoud, A. Value of oral provocation tests to aspirin, and food additives in the routine investigation of asthma and chronic urticaria. J. Allergy Clin. Immunol. 1985 76:40-45.

6.   Huwler, T., and Wuthrich, B. Tyramine-induced asthma. Allergy Clin. Immunol. News 1991 3:14-15.

34

Diet and Eczema

Adverse reaction to food or food additives is not considered to be a primary cause of eczema. However, in a number of cases, food components or additives can exacerbate pre-existing eczema.[1] An estimated 10% of children with eczema are considered likely to benefit from exclusion diets to treat their eczema.[2]

The key indicators in determining which atopic persons with eczema are likely to be helped by dietary manipulation are:[1]

- Established food allergy or intolerance

- Area of affected skin: persons with over 20% of the skin area affected are more likely than those with less affected skin

- Age: children under 2 years of age and exclusively breast-fed babies respond best to the elimination of dietary factors; children under 5 years of age respond better than older children

- Motivation on the part of the person or parent to try using diet to determine whether food is contributing to the eczema.

The time needed for an elimination diet to indicate whether food factors may be contributing to eczema is usually 6 weeks;[1] a shorter period is unlikely to produce any definitive changes in the appearance of the skin lesions.

Foods Implicated in Eczema

Foods and food additives most commonly implicated in causing or exacerbating eczema are listed below.

Allergens[1,3]

- Cow's milk proteins
- Egg
- Wheat
- Fish
- Legumes (particularly peanut, soy, and green pea)
- Nuts
- Tomato
- Berries
- Citrus fruits
- Currants
- And occasionally:[4]
  - Chicken
  - Beef
  - Pork
  - Potato

Food Additives[5]

- Artificial food colors
- Benzoates
- Sulfites

References

1. David, T.J. Atopic eczema. In: *Food and Food Additive Intolerance in Childhood*. Blackwell Scientific Publications, Oxford, London, 1993. 317-336.

2. Atherton, D.J. Diet and atopic eczema. Clin. Allergy 1988 18:215-228.

3. Sampson, H.A. Eczema and food hypersensitivity. In: Metcalfe, D.D., Sampson, H.A., and Simon, R.A. (Eds), *Food Allergy: Adverse Reactions to Foods and Food Additives*. Blackwell Scientific Publications, Oxford, London, 1991. 113-128.

4. Burks, A.W., Mallory, S.B., Williams, L.W., and Shirrell, M.A. Atopic dermatitis: Clinical relevance of food hypersensitivity reactions. J. Pediatrics 1988 113(3):447-451.

5. Freier, S. Paediatric gastrointestinal allergy. J. Hum. Nutr. 1976 30:187-192.

35

Diet and Nocturnal Enuresis (Bed Wetting)

There are a number of reports in the medical and scientific literature which link adverse reactions to foods and nocturnal enuresis. Food allergy as a cause of enuresis has not been objectively proven.[1] However, Gerrard reports that in his clinic, exclusion of milk and dairy products with a salicylate restricted diet led to an increase in bladder capacity, and that one third of the children in his study became dry.[2] Gerrard suggests that the bladder of the atopic individual may be in spasm in response to the release of inflammatory mediators that cause smooth muscle contraction, analogous to the bronchospasm of asthma. As a result, the bladder of the enuretic individual is unable to relax and accommodate the urine that accumulates at night.

Urgency and increased frequency of micturition in the adult has been suggested to be due to a reaction to coffee and tea in some individuals.[1,2]

Although a variety of foods have been implicated, including peas, chocolate, corn, citrus fruits, and food coloring,[3] cow's milk protein allergy has been the most frequently reported dietary cause of bed wetting in children.[4]

A limited time trial of total exclusion of milk and dairy products from the diet of a child who wets the bed might be worthwhile in cases where other methods of control have proved ineffective.

Avoidance of tea, coffee, and cola drinks for a trial period[1,4] may be worthwhile for adults who are bothered by urinary frequency and urgency, if all other causes for their problem have been ruled out.

References

1.   Sandberg, D. Food sensitivity: The kidney and bladder. In: Brostoff, J., and Challacombe, S.J. (Eds), *Food Allergy and Intolerance*. Baillière Tindall, London, 1987. 755-767.

2.   Gerrard, J.W. Cow's milk and breast milk. In: Brostoff, J., and Challacombe, S.J. (Eds), *Food Allergy and Intolerance*. Baillière Tindall, London, 1987. 344-355.

3.   Goldberg, B.J., and Kaplan, M.S. Controversial concepts and techniques in the diagnosis and management of food allergies. Immunology and Allergy Clinics of North America: Food Allergy. November 1991 11(4):863-884.

4.   Bahna, S.L., and Heiner, D.C. *Allergies to Milk*. Grune and Stratton, New York, 1980.

Part VI

Appendices

Appendix I

Few Foods Elimination Test Diet

Foods Allowed

All of the sources listed below should be free from all additives:

Protein

- Lamb
- Turkey

Grains

- Rice
- Tapioca
- Whole grains and flours made from these grains

Fruits

- Pears
- Pear juice
- Cranberries
- Cranberry juice (preferably extracted from cranberries with a juicer)

Vegetables

- Squash, all kinds
- Parsnips
- Sweet potatoes
- Yams
- Lettuce

Condiments

- Sea salt

Desserts

- Pudding made from tapioca beads or rice, fruit and fruit juice of allowed fruits, and agar-agar flakes.

Oils

- Canola oil
- Safflower oil

Beverages

- Distilled water in *glass* bottles (available from drug stores: use your own containers)
- Juice from the allowed fruits

Basic Elimination Diet Instructions

- Begin investigating by eating only the foods listed for 7 days, or the length of time as instructed. Keep a diary of your entire experience, listing the date, time, food eaten and how you feel. You will need to plan to shop ahead, having plenty of appropriate foods on hand. You may get bored, but you won't go hungry. There is no restriction on calorie intake unless you intentionally wish to lose weight. However, weight loss should not be a priority during this test period. It is important to remain healthy and as well-nourished as possible while investigating your specific responses to foods. The issue of weight loss can be addressed later if necessary.

- The menu is simple, without spices, butter or condiments, so don't start at Christmas, during a holiday season, around birthday parties or other important celebrations.

- Use as many fresh food sources as possible. Frozen is the next best alternative.

- Wash and cook food with distilled water only, not tap water as this may contain contaminants to which you are reacting.

- Use pots, pans, and containers that do not contain aluminum, Teflon® or Silverstone® interiors. These may add small amounts of chemical toxins that can confuse a possible food reaction with a chemical reaction.

- Avoid sources of chemicals in the following:
  Chewing gum
  Over-the-counter medications (unless you *really* need them)
  Breath mints
  Coffee
  Tea
  Diet drinks
  Mouth wash
  Cigarettes

Some food allergies and sensitivities are masked or hidden and only become obvious when you take out the commonly eaten food allergens for a period, and reintroduce them later. If this is the case for you, you may notice a period of withdrawal on the first three days of beginning your elimination test. Lots of rest, Vitamin C, alkali salts (page 373) and water, will help to minimize this experience. You will notice that some of your symptoms start to clear and you should be free of food reactions by the fifth or sixth day. Keep track of these experiences in your exposure diary.

- If you know that you have had an adverse reaction to any food on the list, or have had a positive skin test reaction to any of the foods, another low allergenicity food will be substituted.

- This test diet is nutritionally inadequate and must not be continued for more than fourteen days. You will be given explicit instructions about how long to follow this eating plan before moving on to the challenge phase of the test.

Elimination Diet Menus

Note: Turkey may used in place of lamb as desired in any of the menus and recipes.

Breakfast Food Ideas:

Rice cakes, rice crackers, Cream of Rice® cereal, puffed rice cereal with fruit sauce, rice, fried sweet potatoes, yams, parsnips, squash or a combination, plain wild rice waffles, rice-anola (granola), cranberry and pear juice or sauce, tapioca pudding, fruit agar mold.

Suggested Menus

Day	Breakfast	Lunch / Dinner
1	Fluffy Rice Poached Pears	Lamb Souvlaki Steamed Rice Lettuce, Zucchini, and Pear Salad Oil-based Salad Dressing Cranberry Sauce Fruit Agar Mold
2	Cream of Rice Cereal Berry Mold	Lamb Lettuce Wraps Rice Noodles Boiled Yams and Parsnips Fresh Pear
3	Plain Wild Rice Waffles with Fruit Butter Mixed Pear and Cranberry Cup	Lamb Meatballs Spaghetti Squash Rice Cakes Boston Leaf Lettuce and Zucchini Slices Fruit Slush
4	Hash Brown Sweet Potatoes Fresh Pear	Stir Fried Vegetables with Lamb on Rice Red Leaf Lettuce with Pear Slices Tapioca Pudding Fruit Sauce
5	Cream of Rice Cereal Cranberries in Pear Juice	Grilled Lamb Tenderloin Baked Squash with Pears Baked Parsnips Zucchini Sticks Fruit Juice Popsicles
6	Tapioca Pudding Rice Cakes Cranberry/Pear Juice	Stuffed Chayote Squash Hash Brown Sweet Potatoes Romaine Lettuce, Zucchini, and Pear Salad Fruit Agar Mold
7	Plain Wild Rice Waffles with Fruit Sauce	Lamb Stew Rice Noodles Fresh Pear
8	Hash Brown Sweet Potatoes Poached Pears	Stuffed Zucchini Parsnip and Yam Casserole Mixed Pear and Cranberry Cup
9	Rice Anola with Fruit Sauce Rice Cakes Berry Mold	Lamb Rice Paper Wraps Cranberry Sauce Lettuce Salad Oil Based Salad Dressing Poached Pear

Suggested Menus

Day	Breakfast	Lunch / Dinner
10	Sweet Potato Pancakes Tapioca Pudding Cranberry / Pear Juice	Lamb Patties Fruit Sauce Rice Stir Fried Zucchini Agar-agar Jelly
11	Puffed Rice Cereal Pear and Cranberry Sauce Rice Crackers	Broiled Lamb Chops with Pears Puréed Parsnips, Squash, and Sweet Potatoes Rice Fruit Juice Tapioca Pudding
12	Cream of Rice Cereal Poached Pears with Cranberry Sauce	Marinated Grilled Lamb Baked Sweet Potatoes or Yams with Pear Juice Rice Brown Rice Pudding
13	Hash Brown Sweet Potato Berry Mold	Spaghetti Squash with Spaghetti Squash Meat Sauce Rice Crackers Glazed Parsnips Tapioca Pudding with Fruit Sauce
14	Rice Anola with Fruit Sauce Tapioca Pudding	Roast Lamb Stuffed with Rice Baked Parsnips and Acorn Squash Fresh Pear

Recipe List

Note: In all recipes using lamb, turkey may be substituted. Safflower oil may be substituted for canola oil if desired.

Meat

Lamb

Broiled Lamb Chops with Pears
Grilled Lamb
Lamb Lettuce Wraps
Lamb Meatballs
Lamb Patties
Lamb Rice Paper Wraps
Lamb Souvlaki
Lamb Stew
Marinade for Lamb
Roast Lamb Stuffed with Rice
Roast Leg of Lamb
Spaghetti Squash Meat Sauce
Stir Fry Vegetables with Lamb
Stuffed Chayote Squash
Stuffed Zucchini

Grains

Rice

Acorn Squash Stuffed with Rice
Brown Rice Pudding
Brown Rice Noodles
Caramelized Rice
Fluffy Rice
Long Grain Wild Rice
Plain Wild Rice Waffles
Rice Anola (Granola)
Rice Noodles
Rice Wrappers
Roast Lamb Stuffed with Rice
Steamed Rice
Stuffed Chayote Squash
Stuffed Zucchini
Wild Rice Noodles

Tapioca

Fruit Juice Tapioca Pudding
Non-dairy Tapioca Pudding
Tapioca Pudding

Fruits

Agar-agar Jelly
Berry Agar Mold
Brown Rice Pudding
Fruit Agar Mold
Fruit Drink
Fruit Juice Popsicles
Fruit Juice Tapioca Pudding
Fruit Slushes
Lettuce, Zucchini and Pear Salad
Mixed Pear and Cranberry Cup
Non-dairy Tapioca Pudding
Poached Pear
Tapioca Pudding

Vegetables

Lettuce Salad

Lettuce, Zucchini, and Pear Salad

Parsnips

Baked Parsnips
Glazed Parsnips
Puréed Parsnips, Squash, and Sweet Potatoes
Stir Fried Zucchini and Parsnips
Parsnip and Yam Casserole

Squash

Acorn Squash Stuffed with Rice
Baked Squash
Baked Squash with Pears
Lettuce, Zucchini, and Pear Salad
Puréed Parsnips, Squash, and Sweet
  Potatoes
Spaghetti Squash Pasta
Stir Fried Zucchini
Stir Fried Zucchini and Parsnips
Stuffed Chayote Squash
Stuffed Zucchini
Zucchini and Yam Casserole
Zucchini Rice

Yam/Sweet Potatoes

Baked Yams or Sweet Potatoes with
  Pear Juice
Fried Yams with Pears
Hash Brown Sweet Potatoes
Mashed Sweet Potatoes
Puréed Parsnips, Squash, and Sweet
  Potatoes
Sweet Potato Milk
Sweet Potato Pancakes
Parsnip and Yam Casserole
Zucchini and Yam Casserole

Non-dairy Milk for Baking

Sweet Potato Milk
Flavored Squash Milk
Squash Milk

Condiments

Sauces and Glazes

Spaghetti Squash Meat Sauce
Cranberry Pear Sauce
Cranberry Sauce
Fruit Butter or Topping
Fruit Sauce
Basic Glaze

Oils and Dressings

Oil Based Salad Dressing

Desserts

Agar-agar Jelly
Berry Agar Mold
Brown Rice Pudding
Fruit Agar Mold
Fruit Juice Popsicles
Fruit Juice Tapioca Pudding
Fruit Slushes
Mixed Pear and Cranberry Cup
Non-dairy Tapioca Pudding
Pear Crisp
Poached Pear
Tapioca Pudding

Beverages

Fruit Drink

Elimination Test Diet Recipes

Meat Recipes

Roast Leg of Lamb

1 leg of lamb
Sea salt

Season lamb with sea salt. Place fat side up on rack in roasting pan. Insert meat thermometer. Roast at 325°F (160°C) 30-35 minutes per lb (500 g). Meat thermometer should read 125°F (52°C) for medium or 182°F (83°C) for well done.

Nutrition Information for 1 Serving : Kcal 219, Protein 22g, Carbohydrate 0g, Fat 14g

Roast Lamb Stuffed with Rice - *Makes 6 servings*

Follow recipe for roast leg of lamb, but use a crown roast instead, and fill the center with cooked rice and cranberries just before serving.

Nutrition Information for 1 Serving : Kcal 973, Protein 71g, Carbohydrate 29g, Fat 61g

Lamb Souvlaki - *Makes 4 servings*

1½ lb (750 g) cubed lamb
Sea salt to taste - ½ tsp (2 mL)
Canola oil
Assorted cubed zucchini and yellow squash (optional)

Soak wooden skewers in water for 30 minutes prior to use. Salt cubed lamb if desired. Thread cubes onto skewers and brush with oil. Broil or grill over hot coals for 10 minutes, turning occasionally or until desired degree of doneness.

If desired, alternate cubed lamb with cubes of assorted squash. Brush with oil before grilling or broiling.

Nutrition Information for 1 Serving : Kcal 650, Protein 45g, Carbohydrate 7g, Fat 49g

Lamb Stew - *Makes 5 servings*

2 lbs (1 kg) lamb shoulder or leg cut into cubes
1 cup (250 mL) zucchini, cubed
1 cup (250 mL) yams, peeled and cubed
1 cup (250 mL) summer squash, peeled and cubed
Rice noodles
¼ cup (60 mL) canola oil
2 cups (500 mL) water
Sea salt to taste

Heat canola oil in frying pan. Add lamb cubes and brown on all sides. Drain excess oil, but retain lamb gravy. Transfer to stew pot. Add vegetables, water, and salt. Bring to the boil. Cover, reduce heat and simmer 1 hour. Add rice noodles broken into short pieces. Simmer a further 10-15 minutes until noodles are tender.

Nutrition Information for 1 Serving : Kcal 738, Protein 43g, Carbohydrate 31g, Fat 48g

Spaghetti Squash Meat Sauce - *Makes 4 servings*

½ lb (250 g) ground lamb
1 medium pear, peeled and sliced
1 cup (250 mL) cooked cranberries
1 cup (250 mL) pear juice
Sea salt to taste

Brown lamb in skillet. Add sliced pear, cooked cranberries, and pear juice. Season with salt. Bring to boil, reduce heat and simmer until sauce thickens (about 10-15 minutes). Pour over cooked spaghetti squash pasta.

Nutrition Information for 1 Serving : Kcal 271, Protein 18g, Carbohydrate 24g, Fat 11g

Marinade for Lamb - *Makes 4 servings*

4 tbsp (60 mL) cranberry juice
2 tbsp (30 mL) canola oil
2 tbsp (30 mL) water
1 tsp (5 mL) sea salt

Combine ingredients in a bowl. Pour over meat or combine with meat in a plastic bag; cover and refrigerate 1 hour or overnight.

Nutrition Information for 1 Serving : Kcal 35, Protein 0g, Carbohydrate 1g, Fat 4g

Grilled Lamb

Use lamb tenderloins or loins. Broil or grill over hot coals 3-4 minutes for tenderloins, 6 minutes for loins or until meat is still pink inside, turning once or twice.

Nutrition Information for 1 Serving : Kcal 263, Protein 19g, Carbohydrate 0g, Fat 20g

Lamb Lettuce Wraps - *Makes 4 servings*

1 head Boston or Leaf lettuce
½ lb (250 g) ground lamb
½ cup (125 mL) zucchini, grated
1 cup (250 mL) cooked rice (brown or white)
½ cup (125 mL) yellow squash (i.e., acorn or butternut), grated
2 tbsp (30 mL) canola oil
1 tsp (5 mL) sea salt

Heat canola oil. Brown ground lamb. Add grated zucchini, squash, and salt and cook for 4-5 minutes. Add rice and continue to cook mixture until rice is hot. Cut large lettuce leaves down center vein.   On narrow end of each lettuce leaf place a tbsp (15 mL) of rice/lamb mixture and roll into a cylinder shape. May be served hot or cold.

Nutrition Information for 1 Serving : Kcal 313, Protein 17g, Carbohydrate 19g, Fat 18g

Lamb Rice Paper Wraps

Use rice paper as wrapper in Lamb Lettuce Wraps. These thin flexible wrappers are available from Chinese or Vietnamese grocers. In a large pot of hot water soak 1 round of rice paper until softened. Remove from water and place of work surface. Place 3-4 tbsp (45-60 mL) of lamb/rice mixture on one edge of paper. Roll gently, tucking in edges of paper as it is rolled. Serve warm or cold.

Broiled Lamb Chops with Pears - *Makes 4 servings*

4 lean lamb chops
4 pears halved and cored

Score fat edges of chops; place on rack in broiling pan. Broil 3" (2.5 cm) from heat 8-10 minutes; turn. Broil 5-8 minutes. Place pear halves beside chops for last minutes of cooking.

Nutrition Information for 1 Serving : Kcal 183, Protein 16g, Carbohydrate 12g, Fat 8g

Lamb Patties - *Makes 4 servings*

1 lb (500 g) ground lamb
1 tsp (5 mL) sea salt

Add salt and press ground lamb into patties. Grill over hot coals or broil on rack 3" (7.5 cm) from heat 4-6 minutes on each side. Turn when juices begin to form on top of meat.

Nutrition Information for 1 Serving : Kcal 320, Protein 28 g, Carbohydrate 0g, Fat 22g

Stuffed Zucchini - *Makes 4 servings*

1 cup (250 mL) cooked rice
2 medium zucchini
1½ lb (750 g) ground lamb
4 tbsp (60 mL) canola oil
2 tsp (10 mL) sea salt

Slice zucchini in half lengthwise. Scoop out insides, leaving ¼" (0.5 cm) rim. Chop zucchini innards. Heat oil and brown lamb. Add chopped zucchini and salt and sauté until tender. Remove from heat. Add rice and mix. Scoop filling into zucchini halves. Bake 40 minutes at 350°F (180°C).

Nutrition Information for 1 Serving : Kcal 696, Protein 45g, Carbohydrate 21g, Fat 47g

Stir Fry Vegetables with Lamb - *Makes 4 servings*

½ lb (250 g) lamb cubes
2 cups (500 mL) thinly sliced mixed winter squash (i.e. acorn, butternut, Hubbard)
1 cup (250 mL) sliced summer squash (zucchini, Italian marrow)
½ tsp (2 mL) sea salt
1 cup (250 mL) cooked diced sweet potatoes and yams
3 tbsp (45 mL) canola oil

Heat 1 tbsp (15 mL) of canola oil and brown lamb in hot oil on all sides. Remove lamb from pan. Add remaining oil and salt and heat. Add winter squash and sauté for 5 minutes. Add summer squash and sauté for 2 minutes. Return lamb to pan and add yams/sweet potatoes. Sauté together until vegetables are tender and lamb is cooked. Serve over rice, rice noodles, or spaghetti squash.

Nutrition Information for 1 Serving : Kcal 362, Protein 15g, Carbohydrate 23g, Fat 24g

Lamb Meatballs - *Makes 4 servings*

½ lb (250 g) ground lamb
½ cup (125 mL) grated zucchini
½ tsp (2 mL) sea salt

Combine all ingredients. Shape into bite size meatballs. Arrange on ungreased baking sheet and bake uncovered in 400°F (200°C) oven for 20 minutes <u>or</u> heat 1 tbsp (15 mL) of canola oil in fry pan and fry meatballs, turning frequently.

Nutrition Information for 1 Serving : Kcal 164, Protein 14g, Carbohydrate 1g, Fat 11g

Grains

Rice Information

White rice flour has been made from polished rice where the outer brown skin, containing nutrients, has been removed. The outer layer removed in this process is sold as rice polish (which is the equivalent of wheat germ). Like wheat germ, rice polish is removed to give the rice flour a longer shelf life, but at the expense of nutritional value. It is preferable to use freshly ground brown rice flour or appropriately stored (refrigerated or frozen) brown rice flour, although the recipes work with white rice flour.

Rice Recipes

Short and Long Grain Brown Rice

Place rice in a pot and fill it with water. Hand-rub the rice together and swirl it around to remove excess starches, dirt, and stray rice husks. Pour off all the water. Repeat the process once or twice until the water remains relatively clear. Add 2 to 2¼ cups (500-560 mL) water per 1 cup (250 mL) of rice. Bring to a boil over medium heat. Simmer on low heat for 45 to 60 minutes until done.

Wild Rice

This is one of the few main dish grains that sometimes requires soaking before cooking. Wash and then soak 1 cup (250 mL) rice in 2 cups (500 mL) water and let sit 2 to 4 hours. Only by experimentation can one determine if rice needs pre-soaking.   Many varieties can be cooked without pre-soaking. If the rice remains hard after 1 to 1½ hours, turn the heat off, let it sit until cool and then cook again until tender. Next time - pre-soak if using the same wild rice. Cook the same as brown rice for about 60 minutes or more. Wild rice is very expensive and rich tasting, so it is usually mixed with brown rice. Cook the two rices separately and mix before serving, or cook wild rice for 15 to 20 minutes and then add brown rice to it and cook together for another 45 to 60 minutes.   Add extra water if needed.

Steamed Rice - *Makes 4 servings*

1 cup (250 mL) rice
2 cups (500 mL) boiling water
1 tsp (5 mL) sea salt
1 tsp (5 mL) canola oil

Wash rice in colander and drain. Heat oil and add rice and salt. When well-covered with oil, add boiling water. Mix well and cover.   Let simmer on lowest heat for 15-20 minutes for white rice, 40-45 minutes for brown rice.

Nutrition Information for 1 Serving : Kcal 142, Protein 3g, Carbohydrate 29g, Fat 1g

Fluffy Caramelized Rice - *Makes 4 servings*

1 cup (250 mL) rice
2 cups (500 mL) boiling water
½ tsp (2 mL) sea salt

Caramelize rice by heating in a dry pan on a burner, or in the oven until a golden brown. Pour into salted boiling water. Cook in a large saucepan with a tight fitting lid. Do not uncover while it is cooking. Simmer for 50 minutes. Hold the lid and shake the saucepan up and down to fluff it. Let simmer 10 more minutes and turn out carefully onto a platter or shallow dish. Use less water for a dry, fluffy rice. Brown short grain rice done this way and topped with fresh sliced pear and fruit sauce is suitable for breakfast. Brown long grain or brown Basmati rice prepared in this manner and served with cranberries and/or pears is suitable for dinner.

Nutrition Information for 1 Serving : Kcal 109, Protein 2g, Carbohydrate 23g, Fat 1g

Rice Anola - *Makes 4 servings*

1½ cups (375 mL) rolled rice
¼ cup (60 mL) brown rice flour
¼ cup (60 mL) rice polishings (optional)
½ cup (125 mL) hot water
¼ tsp (1 mL) salt

Combine ingredients in a bowl. Spread on a cookie sheet. Bake at 250°F (120°C) for one hour or until lightly browned and dry. When cool, add ½ tbsp (7 mL) oil. Use as granola, serving with fruit sauces.

Nutrition Information for 1 Serving : Kcal 132, Protein 3g, Carbohydrate 29g, Fat 1g

Rice Wrappers

These thin flexible wrappers are available from Asian specialty food stores and in most major grocery chains. Wrap them around vegetables or with filling such as ground lamb, rice and cranberries. Use instead of wheat or corn tortillas. To prepare, briefly dip the dry wrapper in cold water and handle carefully.

Bread Replacement Recipes

Plain Wild Rice Waffles - *Makes 4 servings of 2 waffles each*

1⅓ cups (335 mL) wild rice
2 cups (500 mL) water-hot if necessary

For each blender batch, soak wild rice in water overnight. When ready to make waffles, blend the wild rice until fine, 3 minutes or more.

Now add:
½ cup (125 mL) warm cooked wild rice (not packed)
½ tsp (2 mL) sea salt or more

Blend 2 minutes and add 1 scant cup (250 mL) water. Blend briefly. Plug in waffle iron. Let batter sit 10 minutes or so to thicken. When iron is hot (medium setting), re-blend batter and pour into the lightly greased iron. If the batter is too thick to flow evenly, add slightly more water and blend briefly.

Do not overfill the waffle iron, as this batter boils over easily. Leave the iron open 15 seconds or so, then lower lid slowly to avoid splattering.

Re-blend batter before each filling and check its thickness.

Cook 10-12 minutes or until slightly browned. You may need to adjust the temperature control. Freeze and toast to serve. Serve with fruit sauces or fruit butter.

Makes about 8 waffle pieces in a 2 piece waffle iron.

Nutrition Information for 1 Serving : Kcal 206, Protein 9g, Carbohydrate 43g, Fat 1g

Preparing Rice Noodles

Bring a large pot of water to a boil. When it is bubbling hard, add the noodles. Most noodles expand to 2-3 times their size.

After adding the noodles, wait for the water to boil again, then turn down the heat and ensure the water continues to simmer. Cook until tender and serve with sauce. Do not to overcook the noodles.

Rice Noodles (Canasoy, Eden, and Chinese Stores) cook in about 8-10 minutes.

Brown Rice Noodles (Pastariso) cook in about 8-11 minutes.

Wild Rice Noodles (Northern Lights): the package says to cook 2-4 minutes, but cooking 8-14 minutes produces better results.

Tapioca Information

When tapioca is used in a recipe, it is small grain (minute) tapioca. Recipes using tapioca flour, specify tapioca flour as an ingredient as opposed to tapioca. Tapioca is a useful, usually non-allergenic, thickener.

Tapioca Recipes

Tapioca Pudding - *Makes 4 servings*

2 cups (500 mL) cranberry or pear juice, or a combination (cranberry juice must be extracted from cranberries in a juicer)
4 tbsp (60 mL) tapioca

Soak tapioca in juice for 15 minutes. Heat to boiling point. Stir occasionally until mixture begins to thicken. Cool and top with sliced fruit or fruit sauce.

Nutrition Information for 1 Serving : Kcal 104, Protein 0g, Carbohydrate 26g, Fat 0g

Non-dairy Tapioca Pudding - *4 servings*

2 cups (500 mL) squash milk
4 tbsp (60 mL) tapioca
Sliced pears

Soak tapioca in squash milk for 15 minutes. Heat to boiling point. Stir occasionally until mixture begins to thicken. Do not allow to burn. Cool. Add sliced fruit and serve warm.

Nutrition Information for 1 Serving : Kcal 63, Protein 1g, Carbohydrate 15g, Fat 0g

Fruit Juice Tapioca Pudding

The same as Non-dairy Tapioca Pudding above, using fruit juice such as pear juice instead of squash milk.

Nutrition Information for 1 Serving : Kcal 119, Protein 0g, Carbohydrate 30g, Fat 0g

Fruits

Fruit Recipes

Fruit Slush - *Makes 1 serving*

1 cup (250 mL) pear or cranberry juice (extracted from cranberries in a juicer)
4-5 ice cubes (made with distilled water)

Put in blender and mix well.

Nutrition Information for 1 Serving : Kcal 150, Protein 0g, Carbohydrate 39g, Fat 0g

Poached Pear - *Makes 1 serving*

1 pear, cut in half. Place in a bowl and add a small amount of water. Microwave until soft.
or:
Put pear halves in a saucepan and add water to cover the bottom of the pan. Cover with lid and cook at low heat until soft.

Nutrition Information for 1 Serving : Kcal 98, Protein 1g, Carbohydrate 25g, Fat 1g

Mixed Pear and Cranberry Cup - *Makes 4 servings*

4 pears
2 cups (500 mL) cranberries
1 cup (250 mL) pear juice

Cube pear, add cranberries and juice. Mix in a microwave proof bowl and microwave for 4 minutes until soft.

Nutrition Information for 1 Serving : Kcal 128, Protein 4g, Carbohydrate 29g, Fat 1g

Vegetables

Vegetable Recipes

Lettuce / Salad

Lettuce, Zucchini, and Pear Salad - *Makes 4 servings*

2 cups (500 mL) lettuce
1 cup (250 mL) zucchini, thinly sliced
1 large or 2 small pears, peeled, cored and sliced
Oil-based salad dressing (see recipe)
Sea salt to taste

Combine first three ingredients in salad bowl. Pour canola oil over salad. Add salt. Toss. Serve chilled.

Nutrition Information for 1 Serving : Kcal 162, Protein 1g, Carbohydrate 10g, Fat 14g

Non-dairy Milk for Baking

Squash Milk - *For baking only*

6 medium zucchini
water

Blend above ingredients in food processor/blender. Add sufficient water to make a liquid similar to milk.

Nutrition Information for 1 Cup : Kcal 37, Protein 2g, Carbohydrate 8g, Fat 1g

Flavored Squash Milk - *For baking only*

6 medium zucchini
pear juice

Blend above ingredients in food processor/blender. Add sufficient pear juice to make a liquid similar to milk.

Nutrition Information for 1 Cup : Kcal 112, Protein 2g, Carbohydrate 28g, Fat 1g

Sweet Potato Milk - *For baking only*

1 sweet potato, peeled
water

In food processor/blender, add ½ cup (125 mL) water with the sweet potato. Blend to a smooth consistency. Add more water until a liquid, milk-like consistency is obtained.

Nutrition Information for 1 Serving : Kcal 39, Protein 1g, Carbohydrate 9g, Fat 0g

Parsnip Information

Unlike carrots, parsnips are eaten cooked because they are too fibrous to be pleasant when eaten raw. Their flavor is sweetest when just tender, so do not overcook.

Preparation: Cut off root and leaf ends. Trim major rootlets or knobs. Scrub or peel.

Cooking: Parsnips can be boiled, baked, steamed, or microwaved.

Times:
    Baked: 20 to 30 minutes in a 350°F(180°C) oven.
    Boiled: 5 to 15 minutes.
    Microwave: 4 to 6 minutes in covered dish
    Steamed: Whole parsnips: 20-30 minutes; Cut up parsnips: 5 to 15 minutes.

Cooking times are approximate and depend on the age and tenderness of the vegetables. Older vegetables take longer.

Parsnip Recipes

Baked Parsnips - *Makes 4 servings*

Peel, then cut in half, 4 medium-sized parsnips. Place in oiled, oven-proof dish. Oil parsnips with 2 tbsp (30 mL) canola oil. Sprinkle with ¼ tsp (1 mL) sea salt. Add ¾ cup (200 mL) water. Cover and bake at 350°F (180°C) for 45 minutes or until tender.

Nutrition Information for 1 Serving : Kcal 155, Protein 2g, Carbohydrate 23g, Fat 7g

Glazed Parsnips - *Makes 4 servings*

¾ lb (375 g) parsnips
¾ oz (25 g) canola oil
1 tbsp (15 mL) pear concentrate
sea salt to taste

Top, tail and peel the parsnips, then cut them into quarters lengthwise. Plunge them into fiercely-boiling water for 4 minutes (but no longer) then drain them and set aside. Put the oil in a small saucepan over a low heat, then stir in pear concentrate and season with sea salt. Remove from heat and set aside. Put the parsnips in an ovenproof dish, pour the sauce mixture over and toss until well covered. Bake in the middle of a moderate oven at 350°F(180°C) for ½ hour.

Nutrition Information for 1 Serving : Kcal 40, Protein 0g, Carbohydrate 6g, Fat 2g

Parsnip and Yam Casserole - *Makes 4 servings*

2 tbsp (30 mL) canola oil
1 cup (250 mL) yams, peeled and sliced
1 cup (250 mL) parsnips, peeled and sliced
½ cup (125 mL) cranberries
½ cup (125 mL) pear juice
sea salt to taste

Heat oil in ovenproof saucepan. Add yams and parsnips. Stir and fry for 5 minutes. In a separate saucepan, bring pear juice and cranberries to a boil and simmer 15 minutes. Add cooked cranberries to yams and parsnips. Add salt. Bake in 375°F (190°C) oven for 30 minutes

Nutrition Information for 1 Serving : Kcal 157, Protein 1g, Carbohydrate 24g, Fat 7g

Stir Fried Zucchini and Parsnips - *Makes 4 servings*

¼ cup (60 mL) canola oil
2 cups (500 mL) zucchini sliced thinly
1 cup (250 mL) parsnips peeled and sliced
¼ cup (60 mL) pear juice
sea salt to taste

Heat oil in frying pan or wok. Add zucchini and parsnips. Stir and fry for 7 minutes. Add pear juice and salt. Cover. Reduce heat and steam 5 minutes.

Nutrition Information for 1 Serving : Kcal 176, Protein 4g, Carbohydrate 14g, Fat 14g

Puréed Parsnips, Squash, and Sweet Potatoes - *Makes 4 servings*

In separate saucepans, boil until tender, drain, and peel after cooking (peeling the vegetables after cooking retains more nutrients than peeling before):

⅓ lb (170 g) parsnips
⅓ lb (170 g) sweet potatoes
⅓ lb (170 g) winter squash

Purée each cooked vegetable in a food processor. Add salt to taste. Combine vegetables by stirring lightly to retain the individual colors of the vegetables. Garnish with 1 lettuce leaf chopped finely.

Nutrition Information for 1 Serving : Kcal 85, Protein 2g, Carbohydrate 20g, Fat 0g

Squash Information

Summer Squash

Distinguished by their edible skins and seeds, summer squash vary widely in shape and skin color. All types have a mild, delicate flavor that makes them largely interchangeable in use. Despite the name, summer squash are generally available almost all year round.

Most popular among the group is the zucchini (also called Italian squash or courgette), typically straight, slim, and dark green.   Some newer zucchini varieties are solid yellow in color. English squash looks like a fatter, paler zucchini, while global squash is rounded. Other favorite kinds of summer squash include yellow straight-neck; yellow, curving crookneck; and pale green, dark green, white or yellow (Sunburst) pattypan, scallop, or scallopine squash, shaped something like a top with a scalloped edge.

Season: All year; peak July through September.

Selection: Select small to medium-size, firm squash with smooth, glossy, tender skin. Squash should feel heavy for their size.

Storage: Refrigerate, unwashed, in a plastic bag for up to 5 days.

Preparation: Trim off and discard ends. Rinse squash, but do not peel. Leave whole, dice, or cut into slices or julienne strips.

Cooking Methods

Boiling:

In a 3-quart (3.75 L) pan, boil 1 to 1 ½ lb (500-750 g) whole squash, covered, in 1" (2.5 cm) water until tender when pierced (8 to 12 minutes). Drain.

Boil 1 to 1½ lb (500-750 g) of 1/4" (0.5 cm) slices in ½" (1 cm) water for 3 to 6 minutes. Drain.

Microwaving:

Cut 1 to 1½ lb. (500-750 g) squash into ¼" (0.5 cm) slices. Arrange in a 1¼" (3 cm) nonmetallic baking dish. Add 1-2 tbsp (15-30 mL) canola oil, cover. Microwave on **high** (100%) for 6 to 7 minutes, stirring after 3 minutes. Let stand, covered, for 3 minutes. Squash should be tender when pierced.

Steaming:

Arrange whole squash or ¼" (0.5 cm) slices on a rack. Steam until tender when pierced (10 to 12 minutes for whole squash, 4 to 7 minutes for slices).

Stir-frying:

Cut squash into ¼" (0.5 cm) slices. Stir-fry up to 5 cups (1250 mL), using 1 tbsp (15 mL) canola oil, for 1 minute. Add 2 to 4 tbsp (30-60 mL) liquid, cover, and cook until tender crisp to bite (3 to 4 more minutes).

Winter Squash

Selection: Choose hard, thick-shelled squash that feel heavy for their size. Banana and Hubbard squash are usually sold cut; select pieces with thick, bright yellow-orange flesh. The smaller pumpkins are the best for eating; choose larger ones for decorative uses or serving containers.

Storage: Store whole squash, unwrapped, in a cool (50°F, 10°C), dry, dark place with good ventilation for up to 2 months. Wrap cut pieces in plastic wrap and refrigerate for up to 5 days.

Preparation: Rinse. Cut acorn, butternut, Chinese, Delicata, Golden Acorn, Japanese (Kobocha) squash, or pumpkin in half lengthwise; or cut a "lid" off Japanese squash or pumpkin. Cut Sweet Dumpling in half cross-wise; use top half as lid. Cut banana or Hubbard squash into serving-size pieces.

Remove and discard seeds and fibers. Bake unpeeled. For other cooking methods, peel with a sharp knife and cut into cubes, spears, or slices.

Cooking Methods

Boiling:

Prepare all squash as previously directed, then peel and cut into ½" (1 cm) thick slices. In a wide frying pan, boil 1½ to 2 lb (750g to 1 kg) squash, covered, in ½" (1 cm) of water until tender when pierced (7 to 9 minutes). Drain.

Baking:

Prepare all squash as previously directed. Place, cut side down, in a greased , rimmed baking pan. Bake all except pumpkin, covered, in a 400 to 450°F (200-230°C) oven until flesh is tender when pierced (1 to 1¼ hours).

Microwaving:

As previously directed, prepare 2 medium-size squash such as acorn or butternut (about 1½ lbs, 750g each) or a 1 lb (500 g) piece of squash such as banana. (Pumpkin is not recommended for microwaving.) Place squash, cut side up, in a 9" x 13" nonmetallic baking dish. Spread cut surfaces with 1 to 2 tbsp (15-30 mL) canola oil. Cover. Microwave on HIGH for 10-13 minutes, rotating dish ½ turn after 5 minutes. Squash should be tender when pierced.

Steaming:

Prepare all squash as previously directed, then peel and cut into ½" (0.5 cm) slices. Arrange on a rack. Steam until tender when pierced (9-12 minutes).

Serving Suggestions:

Serve with heated pear or cranberry juice poured on top or mixed with cooked pears or cranberries or as a salad with lettuce and cold rice.

Spaghetti Squash

Spaghetti squash separates into strands when cooked-hence the name. And like spaghetti, this squash is an ideal base for all types of sauces.

Selection: Spaghetti squash should have a hard, thick shell and feel heavy for its size.

Storage: Store whole squash, unwrapped, at room temperature for up to 2 months.

Preparation: Rinse; do not peel. Then proceed as directed for baking or microwaving.

Cooking Methods

Baking:

Pierce shell of medium-size squash in several places to allow steam to escape. Place whole squash in a rimmed baking pan. Bake, uncovered, in a 350ºF (180ºC) oven for 45 minutes; turn squash over and continue to bake 15 to 45 more minutes until shell gives to pressure.

Microwaving:

Cut 1 small spaghetti squash (1¼ lb, 625 g) in half lengthwise; remove seeds. Place squash, cut sides up, in a 9" x 13" nonmetallic baking dish. Spread cut surfaces with 1 to 2 tbsp (15-30 mL) canola oil; cover. Microwave on HIGH for 10-12 minutes, rotating each piece ½ turn after 5 minutes. Let stand, covered, for 5 minutes. Shell should give to pressure.

Scrape out pulp with a fork - it will separate into strands resembling spaghetti.

Serving Suggestion:

Spaghetti Squash Pasta served with Spaghetti Squash Meat Sauce (see Lamb Recipes).

Squash Recipes

Baked Squash - *Makes 4 servings*

3 cups (750 mL) cubed acorn squash
canola oil

Wash squash, remove seeds. Cut into halves or squares, brush with oil. Place cut side down in shallow pan. Bake at 350°F (180°C) for 30 minutes, turn. Brush again with oil, bake 30 minutes longer or until tender. Season lightly with salt.

Nutrition Information for 1 Serving : Kcal 106, Protein 2g, Carbohydrate 22g, Fat 3g

Baked Squash with Pears - *Makes 4 servings*

1 acorn squash (or any winter squash)
canola oil
1 tsp (5 mL) sea salt
2 pears

Bake whole squash at 375°F (190°C) for 30-40 minutes or until almost soft. Remove from oven, cut in half, scoop out seeds. Brush with oil. Sprinkle with salt. Peel and core pears. Grate enough to fill squash cavities. Mound grated pears into squash halves and continue to bake at 375°F (190°C) 25-30 minutes or until tender.

Nutrition Information for 1 Serving : Kcal 102, Protein 1g, Carbohydrate 24g, Fat 2g

Stuffed Chayote Squash - *Makes 4 servings*

2 chayote squash
½ cup (125 mL) cranberries
¾ lb (375 g) lean ground lamb

Wash squash well and cut in half lengthwise. Simmer in small amount of sea salted water until tender, 40 to 50 minutes. Drain and cool. Scoop out pulp and seeds, leaving a ¼" (0.5 cm) shell. Chop pulp and seeds and set aside. Heat 1 tbsp (15 mL) canola oil in a large frying pan. Add the lamb. Sauté lamb in the oil until just pink. Remove from heat and add the chopped chayote pulp and cranberries. Mix thoroughly and mound in the chayote shells. Put squash into shallow baking dish, add ¼" (0.5 cm) water, and bake, uncovered, at 350°F (180°C) about 30 minutes, or until mixture is cooked and lightly browned.

Nutrition Information for 1 Serving : Kcal 299, Protein 15g, Carbohydrate 7g, Fat 24g

Spaghetti Squash Pasta - *Makes 4 servings*

Boil the squash whole for 1 hour or more until tender, or cut it in half lengthwise and bake it for 45-60 minutes. Then scoop out the pulp, as above, and serve it with cranberry-pear sauce or lamb.

Nutrition Information for 1 Serving : Kcal 80, Protein 2g, Carbohydrate 18g, Fat 1g

Acorn Squash Stuffed with Rice - *Makes 4 servings*

3 large acorn squash cut in half, seeds and membranes removed
2 tbsp (30 mL) canola oil
3 cups (750 mL) rice (cooked)
1 pear, cored and sliced
For garnish; ¼ cup (60 mL) cranberries

Preheat oven to 375ºF (190ºC) and oil a 2-3 liter baking dish. Rub the cut surface of the squash with oil. Fill with the rice, until the mixture flows over the sides. Cover the remaining exposed edges of the squash with the pear slices. Place the squash in the baking dish, flat side up and fill the dish with ½" (1 cm) of water. Cover the dish and bake for 45 minutes until the squash is tender and succulent. Serve topped with cranberries.

Nutrition Information for 1 Serving : Kcal 415, Protein 7g, Carbohydrate 84g, Fat 8g

Zucchini Rice - *Makes 4 servings*

3 tbsp (45 mL) canola oil
1 cup (250 mL) chopped zucchini
1 cup (250 mL) long grain brown rice
sea salt to taste
2 cups (500 mL) water

Heat canola oil in saucepan. Add zucchini. Stir and fry for 3 minutes. Add rice; stir and fry 3 minutes. Add water and salt. Bring to the boil. Cover. Reduce heat and simmer 1 hour.

Nutrition Information for 1 Serving : Kcal 269, Protein 4g, Carbohydrate 38g, Fat 12g

Zucchini and Yam Casserole

Substitute 1 cup (250 mL) sliced zucchini for parsnips in Parsnip and Yam recipe.

Nutrition Information for 1 Serving : Kcal 156, Protein 3g, Carbohydrate 22g, Fat 7g

Stir-fried Zucchini

Prepare as for Stir-Fried Zucchini and Parsnips, replacing parsnips with zucchini.

Nutrition Information for 1 Serving : Kcal 151, Protein 1g, Carbohydrate 8g, Fat 14g

Yam and Sweet Potato Information

Nutrition: Sweet potatoes are an excellent source of Vitamin A, a good source of Vitamin C and potassium. One sweet potato, baked or boiled in its skin, has about 165 calories.

Selection: Choose firm, well-shaped sweet potatoes with bright, uniformly colored skin.

Storage: Store, unwrapped, in a cool (50°F, 10°C), dry, dark place with good ventilation for up to 2 months or at room temperature for up to 1 week.

Preparation: Scrub well. Leave whole; or peel, then slice, dice, or shred.

Cooking Methods

Baking:

Pierce skin in several places; rub with canola oil. Arrange in a single layer in a rimmed baking pan. Bake, uncovered, in a 400°F (200°C) oven until soft when squeezed (45 to 50 minutes).

Boiling:

In a 3-quart (3.75 L) pan, boil 4 whole medium-size (3", 7.5 cm diameter) sweet potatoes, covered, in 2" (5 cm) water until tender throughout when pierced (20 to 30 minutes). Drain.

Microwaving:

Pierce skin of medium-size sweet potatoes with a fork. Place on a double layer of paper towels on floor of microwave; if cooking more than two at a time, arrange like spokes. Microwave on HIGH, turning halfway through cooking. Allow 4 to 5 minutes for 1 potato; add 2 to 3 minutes to the total cooking time for each additional potato. Let stand for 5 to 10 minutes, wrapped in foil or a clean towel. Potatoes should feel soft when squeezed.

Steaming:

Arrange whole medium-sized (3", 7.5 cm diameter) sweet potatoes on a rack. Steam until tender throughout when pierced (30 to 40 minutes).

Yam and/or Sweet Potato Recipes

Hash Brown Sweet Potatoes - *Makes 4 servings*

4 sweet potatoes or yams
2 tsp (10 mL) canola oil
dash sea salt

Boil or steam potatoes until tender crisp when pierced (about 10-15 minutes) in their jackets. Chill. Peel. Shred or grate. Toss in oil and salt. Pat into thin patties. Brown in a Teflon skillet over medium heat 10-12 minutes. Turn. Brown 8-10 minutes longer or to desired brownness. For extra crispness, using 2 spatulas, cut horizontally through center of patty; flip one half over the other.

Nutrition Information for 1 Serving : Kcal 136, Protein 1g, Carbohydrate 28g, Fat 2g

Baked Yams or Sweet Potatoes with Pear Juice

Preheat oven to 425°F (220°C).   Scrub the potatoes and rub with oil. Puncture once with a fork. Bake for 40 minutes - 1 hour, until tender all the way through when pierced. When they are done, slit open and mash ⅓ cup (75 mL) of pear juice into each potato.

Nutrition Information for 1 Serving : Kcal 161, Protein 2g, Carbohydrate 39g, Fat 0g

Mashed Sweet Potatoes - *Makes 4 servings*

3 medium sweet potatoes
1 tbsp (15 mL) canola oil
¼ tsp (1 mL) sea salt
3 tbsp (45 mL) fruit juice (pear or cranberry)

Drop peeled sweet potatoes into boiling water to cover and simmer about 25 minutes or until cooked. Push potatoes through ricer or mash. Add oil, salt, and juice. Beat with a fork or whisk until very light.

Nutrition Information for 1 Serving : Kcal 125, Protein 1g, Carbohydrate 22g, Fat 4g

Sweet Potato Pancakes - *Makes 4 servings*

4 medium peeled, grated sweet potatoes and/or yams
2 tbsp (30 mL) rice flour
½ tsp (2 mL) sea salt
3 tbsp (45 mL) canola oil

Combine grated potato, rice flour and sea salt.* Heat oil in skillet.   Drop potato mixture by spoonful into oil. Flatten with back of spoon. Fry until brown and crisp on both sides.

*Add more flour 1 tsp (5 mL) at a time if more required to make mixture stick together.

Nutrition Information for 1 Serving : Kcal 225, Protein 2g, Carbohydrate 32g, Fat 10g

Fried Yams with Pears - *Makes 4 servings*

2 cooked yams or sweet potatoes, sliced ¼" (0.5 cm) thick
2 tbsp (30 mL) canola oil
2 pears, peeled, cored, sliced

Heat oil. Add yams and fry until golden on each side. Just before serving, add pears and cook just until warm.

Nutrition Information for 1 Serving : Kcal 167, Protein 1g, Carbohydrate 26g, Fat 7g

Condiment Recipes

Sauces and Glazes

Basic Glaze - *Makes 1 serving*

¼ cup (60 mL) allowed fruit juice
1 tbsp (15 mL) canola oil

Combine ingredients and bring to a boil. Simmer three minutes. Remove from heat. When cool, drizzle over chosen food.

Nutrition Information for 1 Serving : Kcal 156, Protein 0g, Carbohydrate 9g, Fat 14g

Cranberry Sauce - *Makes 4 servings*

1 cup (250 mL) pear juice
2 cups (500 mL) fresh or frozen cranberries

Add pear juice to cranberries in a small saucepan. Heat to boiling, reduce heat until cranberries are cooked and sauce thickens.

Nutrition Information for 1 Serving : Kcal 158, Protein 8g, Carbohydrate 32g, Fat 0g

Fruit Butter Or Topping - *Makes 4 servings*

½ cup (125 mL) dried pear (without additives) finely chopped
½ cup (125 mL) water

Combine the ingredients in a covered saucepan. Bring to a boil, then simmer for 15 minutes over low heat. Turn off heat and let stand, covered, 30 minutes or longer. The fruit absorbs more water as it cools. Add extra water or juice as necessary. Keep refrigerated between servings.

This chunky spread is a great sweetener on pancakes, cereals, and ice creams. Experiment by substituting it for other sweeteners in breads and cookies. The mixture can be stirred to soften it, or blended or mixed in a food processor to make a smoother topping. Prepared in a food processor, the spread can be used as a sandwich spread instead of honey or jelly.

Nutrition Information for 1 Serving : Kcal 40, Protein 0g, Carbohydrate 11g, Fat 0g

Fruit Sauce - *Makes 4 servings*

½ lb (250g) fresh/frozen cranberries
or ½ lb (250g) peeled, cored, dried pears (without additives)
1 cup (250 mL) cranberry or pear juice (Cranberry juice must be extracted from cranberries with a juicer)

Wash and prepare selected fruit. Put in pan with fruit juice, cover and simmer over low heat for 12-20 minutes, or until fruit breaks down. Chill before serving as an accompaniment to main dishes, topping or pudding or spread for bread etc.

Nutrition Information for 1 Serving : Kcal 71, Protein 0g, Carbohydrate 18g, Fat 0g

Cranberry Pear Sauce - *Makes 4 servings*

1 cup (250 mL) pear juice
1 small unpeeled, sliced pear
½ to 1 cup (125-250 mL) cooked cranberries

Blend together the juice and pear. Add the cranberries until the mixture thickens.

Nutrition Information for 1 Serving : Kcal 72, Protein 0g, Carbohydrate 19g, Fat 0g

Desserts

Agar-agar Jelly

¼ oz or 30g (about 6-7 tbsp, 90-105 mL) agar-agar flakes
or 2 - 2½ tbsp (30-40 mL) agar-agar powder
1 cup (250 mL) cool water
1 - 1½ quarts (1250-1875 mL) pear juice

Optional: cut pears, or cranberries

Mix the agar flakes in the water and heat up to a boil, stirring as it heats. Once it boils, turn down the heat and simmer until most of the agar is dissolved and it thickens. Stir regularly. Make sure the fruit juice is at room temperature. Pour the juice in a glass or metal bowl and **strain** the agar mixture into it. Stir it and mix everything well. Chill thoroughly until it hardens and gels. When the jelly is partially set, about 30-40 minutes or more, add cut fruit to it if desired. Jelly is usually ready to eat in 1½ to 3 hours. Some juice may settle to the bottom of the bowl when the jelly is spooned out-this is natural for agar jelly.

*Note: Most citrus juices do not "set well" with agar. Avoid them. Agar is a great gelatin substitute.

Nutrition Information for 1 Serving : Kcal 55, Protein 0g, Carbohydrate 15g, Fat 0g

Berry Agar Mold - *Makes 4 servings*

2 tbsp (30 mL) agar-agar flakes
1 cup (250 mL) cranberry juice (extracted from cranberries with a juicer)
1 cup (250 mL) cold water
1 cup (250 mL) hot water

Mix agar-agar flakes with cold water and let sit for 1 minute. Add hot water. Boil 2 minutes, let cool and add juice and sweetener. Cover bottom of glass mold with berries. Pour part of jelly over fruit and allow to set. Repeat process to form layers of fruit and jelly.

Nutrition Information for 1 Serving : Kcal 38, Protein 0g, Carbohydrate 10g, Fat 0g

Fruit Agar Mold - *Makes 4 servings*

2 tbsp (30 mL) agar-agar flakes
1 cup (250 mL) cold water
1 cup (250 mL) hot water
1 cup (250 mL) cranberry or pear juice or a combination of whole cranberries or sliced pears or a combination. (Cranberry juice must be extracted from cranberries in a juicer.)

Mix agar-agar flakes with cold water and let sit for 1 minute. Add hot water. Boil for 2 minutes, let cool and add juice. Cover bottom of glass mold (or bowl) with fruit. Pour part of jelly over fruit and allow to set. Repeat process to form layers of fruit and jelly.

Nutrition Information for 1 Serving : Kcal 39, Protein 0g, Carbohydrate 10g, Fat 0g

Brown Rice Pudding - *Makes 4 servings*

1 cup (250 mL) cooked brown rice
¾ cup (175 mL) squash
⅛ cup (30 mL) chopped pears

Mix all ingredients. Pour into deep casserole dish. Bake 20 minutes at 325°F (160°C) Serve hot with additional squash milk.

Nutrition Information for 1 Serving : Kcal 63, Protein 1g, Carbohydrate 14g, Fat 0g

Fruit Slush

1 cup (250 mL) pear or cranberry juice (extracted from cranberries in a juicer)
4-5 ice cubes (made with distilled water)

Put in blender and mix well.

Nutrition Information for 1 Serving : Kcal 150, Protein 0g, Carbohydrate 39g, Fat 0g

Fruit Juice Ice Pops

Make ice pops using pear or cranberry juice (extracted from cranberries in a juicer).

Nutrition Information for 1 Serving : Kcal 72, Protein 0g, Carbohydrate 18g, Fat 0g

Pear Crisp

Use unbaked rice anola over sliced pear to make a Pear Crisp.

Nutrition Information for 1 Serving : Kcal 208, Protein 4g, Carbohydrate 48g, Fat 1g

Oils

Oil-based Salad Dressing - *Makes 4 servings*

¼ cup (60 mL) canola oil
½ tsp (2 mL) sea salt
¼ cup (60 mL) cranberry juice (extracted from cranberries in a juicer) or pear juice

Mix all ingredients well. Serve on lettuce.

Nutrition Information for 1 Serving : Kcal 129, Protein 0g, Carbohydrate 2g, Fat 14g

Beverages

Fruit Drink

1 cup (250 mL) water
¼ cup (60 mL) pear or cranberry juice or combination. Cranberry juice must be extracted from cranberries in a juicer.

Mix and chill.

Nutrition Information for 1 Serving : Kcal 120, Protein 8g, Carbohydrate 22g, Fat 0g

Other

Alkali Salts

Mix together 2 tablespoons of sodium bicarbonate (baking soda) and 1 tablespoon of potassium bicarbonate. Store the mixture in a screw-capped jar.

Take ½ teaspoonful of the mixture in ½ cup warm water when an adverse reaction starts. This can be repeated after 20 to 30 minutes if the reaction has not subsided.

Potassium bicarbonate is available at most larger drug stores. Some specialty pharmacies sell pre-mixed alkali salts with Vitamin C.

Nutritional Content of Recipes

Recipe Name	Page #	kcal Per Serving	Grams Protein Per Serving	Grams Carbo. Per Serving	Grams Fat Per Serving
Acorn Squash Stuffed with Rice	365	415 kcal	7g	84g	8g
Agar-agar Jelly	370	55 kcal	0g	15g	0g
Baked Yams or Sweet Potatoes with Pear Juice	367	161 kcal	2g	39g	0g
Baked Parsnips	359	155 kcal	2g	23g	7g
Baked Squash with Pears	364	102 kcal	1g	24g	2g
Baked Squash	364	106 kcal	2g	22g	3g
Basic Glaze	368	156 kcal	0g	9g	14g
Berry Agar Mold	371	38 kcal	0g	10g	0g
Broiled Lamb Chops with Pears	350	183 kcal	16g	12g	8g
Brown Rice Pudding	371	63 kcal	1g	14g	0g
Fluffy Caramelized Rice	353	109 kcal	2g	23g	1g
Cranberry Sauce	369	158 kcal	8g	32g	0g
Cranberry-Pear Sauce	370	72 kcal	0g	19g	0g
Flavored Squash Milk	358	1 cup= 112 kcal	1 cup= 2g	1 cup= 28g	1 cup= 1g
Fried Yams with Pears	368	167 kcal	1g	26g	7g
Fruit Butter or Topping	369	40 kcal	0g	11g	0g
Fruit Sauce	369	71 kcal	0g	18g	0g
Fruit Juice Ice pops	372	72 kcal	0g	18g	0g
Fruit Drink	373	120 kcal	8g	22g	0g
Fruit Juice Tapioca Pudding	356	119 kcal	0g	30g	0g
Fruit Slush	356	150 kcal	0g	39g	0g
Fruit Agar Mold	371	39 kcal	0g	10g	0g
Glazed Parsnips	359	40 kcal	0g	6g	2g

Nutritional Content of Recipes

Recipe Name	Page #	kcal Per Serving	Grams Protein Per Serving	Grams Carbo. Per Serving	Grams Fat Per Serving
Grilled Lamb	350	263 kcal	19g	0g	20g
Hash Brown Sweet Potatoes	367	136 kcal	1g	28g	2g
Lamb Meatballs	352	164 kcal	14g	1g	11g
Lamb Souvlaki	348	650 kcal	45g	7g	49g
Lamb Stew	349	738 kcal	43g	31g	48g
Lamb Lettuce Wraps	350	313 kcal	17g	19g	18g
Lamb Patties	351	320 kcal	28g	0g	22g
Lettuce, Zucchini, and Pear Salad	357	162 kcal	1g	10g	14g
Marinade for Lamb	349	35 kcal	0g	1g	4g
Mashed Sweet Potatoes	367	125 kcal	1g	22g	4g
Mixed Pear and Cranberry Cup	357	128 kcal	4g	29g	1g
Non-dairy Tapioca Pudding	356	63 kcal	1g	15g	0g
Oil-based Salad Dressing	372	129 kcal	0g	2g	14g
Parsnip and Yam Casserole	359	157 kcal	1g	24g	7g
Pear Crisp	372	208 kcal	4g	48g	1g
Plain Wild Rice Waffles	354	206 kcal	9g	43g	1g
Poached Pear	356	98 kcal	1g	25g	1g
Puréed Parsnips, Squash and Sweet Potatoes	360	85 kcal	2g	20g	0g
Rice Anola	354	132 kcal	3g	29g	1g
Roast Lamb Stuffed with Rice	348	973 kcal	71g	29g	61g
Roast Leg of Lamb	348	219 kcal	22g	7g	14g
Spaghetti Squash Pasta	365	80 kcal	2g	18g	1g
Spaghetti Squash Meat Sauce	349	271 kcal	18g	24g	11g

Nutritional Content of Recipes

Recipe Name	Page #	kcal Per Serving	Grams Protein Per Serving	Grams Carbo. Per Serving	Grams Fat Per Serving
Squash Milk	357	1 cup= 37 kcal	1 cup= 2g	1 cup= 8g	1 cup= 1g
Steamed Rice	353	142 kcal	3g	29g	1g
Stir Fried Zucchini	366	151 kcal	1g	8g	14g
Stir Fry Vegetables with Lamb	351	362 kcal	15g	23g	24g
Stir Fried Zucchini and Parsnips	360	176 kcal	4g	14g	14g
Stuffed Chayote Squash	364	299 kcal	15g	7g	24g
Stuffed Zucchini	351	696 kcal	45g	21g	47g
Sweet Potato Milk	358	39 kcal	1g	9g	0g
Sweet Potato Pancakes	368	225 kcal	2g	32g	10g
Tapioca Pudding	355	104 kcal	0g	26g	0g
Zucchini Rice	365	269 kcal	4g	38g	12g
Zucchini and Yam Casserole	365	156 kcal	3g	22g	7g

Appendix II

Irritable Bowel Syndrome (IBS) Diet
General Guidelines

Every meal and snack must contain at least one food from each of the following categories:

Note: Because a number of basic foods are excluded, in order to supply an adequate balance of nutrients, the following categories contain foods which traditionally would not be included in that particular group.

Protein (PRO):

Meat of any type
Poultry
Fish
Shellfish
Egg
Nut spreads
Seed spreads
Tofu

Grain (GRA):

Any allowed whole grain
Whole grain flour as allowed
Lentils, split peas and any skinless
   legumes
Lentil, pea or bean flour
Potato

Fruits and Vegetables (FR/VEG):

All cooked as allowed

Irritable Bowel Syndrome (IBS) Examples of Balanced Meals

Breakfast

Vegetable Omelette

PRO: Egg
GRA: Potato
FR/VEG: Assorted vegetables, fruit juice

Saute in an omelette pan in clarified butter, or a combination of clarified butter and olive oil:

Zucchini grated
Mushrooms, thinly sliced
Red and green peppers, chopped finely
Parsley, chopped
Carrots, grated
Garlic, pressed, to taste

Whip together two or three eggs until foamy. Add to the above cooked ingredients. Add salt and herbs to taste. Cook until set on the bottom. Slide onto a plate, cooked side down. Invert into the omelette pan, uncooked side down. Cook a further minute or two until set on the bottom. Fold over into a half circle. Slide onto a heated plate. Garnish with parsley and serve with hashbrown potatoes and heated and cooled fruit juice. Do not eat garnish unless it is cooked.

Enriched Scrambled Eggs

PRO: Egg
GRA: Potato, rice bread, rice/soy bread
FR/VEG: Green onions, black olives, fruit juice

Saute in clarified butter:

Green onions or chives, chopped small
Black olives
Garlic, pressed, to taste

Beat two or three eggs together with a fork. Add to the cooked vegetables. Stir until cooked and firm. Add salt to taste. Garnish with parsley and serve with hash brown potatoes or toasted rice or rice/soy bread and fruit juice, heated and cooled.

Pancakes

½ cup rice flour   ½ cup soy flour
1 tbsp allowed baking powder   1 tbsp honey or fructose
½ tsp salt   ¼ cup allowed oil
1 cup Rice Dream or soy milk   2 eggs

Sift dry ingredients three times and set aside. Beat the eggs, oil, and milk together until well blended. Add to the flour and beat until batter is smooth. Heat a non stick pan. Pour 1-2 tablespoon of batter for each pancake. When air bubbles appear on the surface and the bottom is golden, flip to cook on the other side. These freeze well and can be reheated in a toaster.

Pancakes with Variations

PRO: Nut or seed butter
GRA: Flours used in pancake batter
FR/VEG: Fruit included in pancake batter
          Puréed cooked fruit as topping
          Fruit juice

Make batter according to recipe. Add frozen or fresh berries such as blueberries, strawberries, raspberries, or any fruit allowed, chopped into small pieces. Cook individual pancakes on skillet (fruit will cook at the same time). Spread two tsp of any nut or seed butter on each hot pancake. Top with any cooked fruit, sweetened with honey to taste. Serve with heated and cooled fresh or frozen fruit juice.

Breakfast Cereals

PRO: Nut or seed butters
          Soya beverage (if tolerated)
GRA: Cooked cereal grain
FR/VEG: Fruit cooked or canned in fruit juice
          OR 100% fruit jam sweetened with honey
          Fruit juice, cooked and cooled

Alternative whole grain (amaranth, quinoa, buckwheat, millet, brown rice) OR puffed whole grain (rice, millet, amaranth) cooked in water or fruit juice (see below)*.

1 cup of cooked grain, add 2-3 tsp of a nut or seed butter. Add cooked fruit, honey, Rice Dream, Soya beverage, or Mocha Mix.

*Cooking Alternate Grains

Cook amaranth, millet, quinoa and buckwheat grain like brown rice.

Combine a cup of grain with 2¼ or 2½ cups of water. Bring to the boil, lower heat and simmer for 45-60 minutes depending on the texture desired. The grains can be cooked in large batches (for example, four cups of grain), and frozen in one cup quantities. The cooked grain can be reheated in the microwave and provides the basis for an instant breakfast cereal.

Quick Blender Drink

PRO: Tofu: nut or seed butter
GRA: Rice bran
FR/VEG: Cooked fruit

In a blender combine:

Medium or soft tofu (from produce section of grocery store)
Any cooked fruit
2- 4 tbsp sesame tahini, seed or nut spread
1 tbsp boiled lime juice
1 tbsp of honey or to taste
2 tbsp rice bran
Soy milk as desired if mixture is too thick

Blend until well combined.

Snacks or Lunch Box

Brown rice cakes spread with nut or seed spread, 100% fruit jam, honey to taste (PRO: nut or seed spread, GRA: brown rice, FR/VEG: 100% fruit jam)

Rice crackers spread with nut or seed spread and vegetable spread (recipes below) (PRO: nut or seed spread; GRA: rice cracker; FR/VEG: vegetable spread)

Rice cakes spread with meat spreads (recipes below) (PRO: meat, poultry or fish; GRA: Rice cake; FR/VEG: vegetables or fruits)

Rice cakes or crackers spread with nut or seed and fruit spreads (recipes below) (PRO: Nut or seed spreads; GRA: Rice cake or crackers; FR/VEG: fruits)

Vegetable or Fruit Pancake Sandwiches

PRO: Nut or seed butter
GRA: Flours used in pancake batter
FR/VEG: Grated vegetables (carrot, zucchini, red and green peppers, etc)
          OR Chopped fruit (apple, pear, peach, apricot, nectarine, pineapple)
          OR Berries (blueberry, strawberry, raspberry)

Make batter according to recipe. Add grated vegetables or chopped fruit or berries.
Cook individual pancakes on griddle. Make square pancakes for variety. Cool on a cake rack.

For lunch box sandwiches, spread with nut or seed butters and honey or 100% fruit jam without sugar, but add honey to taste if desired. Include heated and cooled fruit juice and cooked fruit in a small container for a complete lunchbox meal.

Dinner

(FR/VEG) Stir fried vegetables, including bean sprouts, with (PRO) chicken, tofu, fish or shellfish, (GRA) served with rice
(GRA) Rice pasta or any pasta made from suggested grains, (PRO) homemade meat and (FR/VEG) tomato sauce with additional vegetables

(GRA) Rice or alternative grain pasta with (PRO) tuna and (FR/VEG) black olive sauce
(PRO) Bouillabaisse (fish and shellfish stew) with a variety of (FR/VEG) vegetables served with (GRA) toasted rice or alternate grain breads

(PRO) Roast meat or poultry with a variety of (FR/VEG) vegetables, served with (GRA) French fries or baked potato

(PRO) Steamed, poached, or broiled fish with a (FR/VEG) variety of vegetables and (GRA) rice

(PRO) Broiled steak, (GRA) French fries and a (FR/VEG) variety of vegetables

(PRO) Meat and (FR/VEG) vegetable kebabs served with (GRA) rice

Recipes

Butter

Clarified Butter

Heat regular butter gently until it melts. Milk solids will sink to the bottom (they may also rise to the top as "foam"). Skim off the top foam and discard. Allow the milk solids to settle to the bottom and pour off the clear oil. Discard the bottom solids.

The clear yellow oil is clarified butter.

Clarified butter is very hard and difficult to spread once it has solidified. Making a light whipped butter with the addition of a polyunsaturated vegetable oil, such as canola oil, makes the product softer and reduces the saturated to unsaturated fat ratio which is beneficial in cholesterol lowering diets.

Light Whipped Butter

Add canola oil to the liquid clarified butter after it has cooled and just started to solidify in the following proportion:

½ cup canola oil to 1 cup of clarified butter

Whip together in a blender, food processor, or by hand. Pour into a plastic container and refrigerate.

Nut and Seed Butters and Milks

Peanut, Nut, and Seed Butters

225g shelled raw peanuts
Canola oil (sufficient to make spreading consistency)

Spread nuts on a baking sheet. Roast gently at bottom of oven until the nuts under the skins are golden brown. Rub skins off using a soft cloth. Grind nuts as fine as possible in a blender or food processor.

Add sufficient oil to make a spreading consistency while processing. Store in fridge. Stir before use as oil separates out.

Note: Use fresh peanuts. Check for mold. Store in a tin or in a dry place. Use quickly.

This recipe may be used to make butters from any other nuts or seeds.

Nut and Seed Milks

2½ cups nuts
4 cups water

Place in a blender or food processor. Process until the mixture becomes a smooth liquid.

Noodles

Chickpea Noodles

4 oz chickpea flour
1 tsp herbs as preferred (optional)
2 tbsp clarified butter, melted
Water
Salt to taste

Mix flour and seasonings. Add sufficient water to make a stiff dough. Roll out on a floured surface as thinly as possible. Cut into long, narrow strips. Cook in rapidly boiling salted water for 10 to 15 minutes. Coat with melted clarified butter and sprinkle with herbs.

Serve with any pasta sauce made with allowed ingredients, including a protein and vegetable.

Appetizers, Spreads and Condiments

Hummus as a Dip or Spread

PRO: Sesame tahini
GRA: Chick peas, rice cakes
FR/VEG: Various vegetables

1 can chick peas (garbanzo beans) in water. Drain and reserve *half* of the liquid
4 tbsp sesame tahini
1-3 cloves pressed garlic (to taste) cooked in 1 tbsp lemon juice

Put all ingredients with half of the liquid from the chick peas into a blender. Blend on high until completely smooth. Spread on rice cakes or serve with a variety of cooked vegetables (carrot, celery, strips of red and green peppers, whole string beans, mushrooms, cauliflower and broccoli florets).

Quick Cooked Vegetable Dressing or Meat Marinade

2 tbsp olive or pure vegetable oil
2 tbsp heated lemon juice
2 tbsp water
¼ tsp garlic powder
Honey (optional)
Salt to taste

In a small jar with a screw top, combine all ingredients and mix well. Good on cooked vegetables or as a marinade for meat.

Variation : Add ¼ - ½ tsp dried herbs for variety.

Vegetable Spreads

Combine clarified light whipped butter with one of the following vegetables:

(1) Puréed cooked carrot with honey
(2) Cooked mashed yams with honey
(3) Grated zucchini and chopped parsley or cilantro, cooked
(4) Green peas and chopped mint, cooked
(5) Mashed cooked mixed vegetables with herbs
(6) Cooked mushrooms chopped finely with cooked green onion or chives
(7) Cooked, mashed lentils with cilantro

Whip with a fork, or in a food processor or blender until well mixed. Add salt, cooked pressed garlic, or herbs to taste.

Fish or Meat Spreads with Fruit or Vegetables

Combine clarified light whipped butter with one of the following mixtures:

(1) Canned fish (tuna, sardine, salmon) with cooked lemon juice to taste
(2) Chopped ham with canned pineapple
(3) Finely chopped cooked chicken or turkey with cooked cranberries
(4) Chicken or turkey livers cooked and with chopped cooked onions or chives
   Whip with a fork, or in a food processor or blender until well mixed. Add salt, cooked pressed garlic and herbs to taste.

Fruit Spreads

Combine the following in a food processor, blender, or mix by hand:

(1) Any cooked fruit with honey.
(2) Mashed cooked banana with nut or seed butter
(3) Nut butters with raisins soaked in boiling water
(4) Nut butters and puréed canned peaches or apricots
(5) Apple sauce (apples cooked in a little water and mashed) with nut or seed butters
(6) Pear sauce (pears cooked in a little water and mashed) with nut or seed butters
(7) Cooked, mashed berries with nut or seed butters

Note: If tomato is not tolerated, many of the recipes containing tomato (salsa, pasta sauce, ketchup can be made quite successfully by substituting ripe mangoes in place of the tomatoes.

Salsa

2 ripe Roma tomatoes	1 garlic clove, chopped
1 tbsp cilantro	¼ cup chopped cucumber
Juice from ½ lime	Salt to taste

For salsa, process ingredients in food processor, using pulse button, until chopped and combined. Do not purée. Cook in microwave or heat to boiling in a saucepan. Cool. Serve with patties.

If tomato is not tolerated, a very successful salsa can be made by substituting ripe mango for the tomato in the above recipe.

Tomato Ketchup

2 large or 3 medium, ripe tomatoes		1 clove garlic, sliced
¼ cup canola oil		1 tbsp honey
1 tbsp lemon juice	OR	Distilled vinegar
¼ tsp onion powder	OR	½ tsp grated onion
¼ tsp oregano		Salt to taste

Place whole tomatoes in boiling water. Remove from water and peel off skins. Remove seeds and discard. Place in blender. Add all other ingredients. Process on high speed until blended (2-3 minutes). Pour into saucepan. Bring to the boil. Reduce heat and simmer until thickened (about 10-15 minutes). Cool and pour into plastic or glass tomato ketchup dispenser.

Note: If tomatoes are not tolerated, substitute ripe mangoes for the tomatoes in the above recipe.
Cook mango before adding additional ingredients.

Mock Caviar

1 lb eggplant	1 garlic clove, crushed
3 tbsp olive oil	1 tbsp lemon juice
Salt to taste	

Char eggplant. Place under a hot grill, and turn from time to time until skin is black and inside is soft. Scrape off skin and discard. Purée eggplant. Put in bowl and stir in other ingredients. Mix well.

Chill until required.

Substitutes for Restricted Flours in Recipes

In place of restricted grain flour in recipes, combinations of alternative flours make better cakes, cookies, breads, pancakes, and waffles than a single flour alone.

For example, tapioca plus soy flours are available as pastry and bread mixes (Good 'N' Easy mixes). A combination of rice, soy, potato, and arrowroot (or tapioca,) starch make an acceptable bread mix. Use one cup of the mix in place of 1 cup wheat flour in recipes.

Combining "light", "intermediate" and "heavy" flours in the ratio below will give a better baked product than using any single flour.

Heavy flours	Intermediate flours	Light flours
Soy	Potato	White rice
Buckwheat	T'ef	Tapioca
Millet (bajri)	Brown rice	Arrowroot
Amaranth		Sago
Chickpea		
Channa (besan)		
Moong bean		
Any nut		
Quinoa		

Combine in a ratio:

⅔ cup heavy flour   ¼ cup light flour   ¼ intermediate flour

Breads and Baked Goods

Bread for Bread Machine

Ingredients:

2½ cups flour mixture*
2 tsp baking powder
2 tsp guar gum
½ tsp salt
1 pkg fast rising yeast
2 tsp sugar
1 egg
1 cup + 2 tbsp warm water
½ tsp lemon juice
2 tbsp canola oil

Place 1 cup of warm water, sugar and 1 package of yeast in the bread machine and leave for 30 minutes to allow the yeast to begin fermenting. The mixture will be foamy after 30 minutes.

In a mixing bowl combine flour mixture, baking powder, salt, and guar gum. Mix well and add to the ingredients in the bread machine.

In a small bowl beat the egg until well mixed and add 2 tablespoons of warm water and lemon juice. Mix well and add on top of the flour mixture in the bread machine.

Process on 4 hour French Bread cycle. Makes one loaf.

*Flour Mixture:

1¼ cup soya bean flour
1¼ cup brown rice flour
1 cup millet flour (bajri)
¾ cup tapioca starch
¾ cup potato flour

Mix together and place in an airtight container. This mixture will make 2 loaves of bread.

Bread with Variations

Bran and Raisin Bread

Substitute: Rice bran instead for ¼ cup of rice flour in the flour mixture
                 Grape juice instead of lemon juice.

Add: ½ cup raisins to the dry ingredients

Cranberry Bread

Substitute: Orange juice instead of lemon juice

Add: ½ cup cranberries (fresh or frozen) to the dry ingredients

Blueberry Bread

Substitute: Lime juice instead of lemon juice

Add: ½ cup blueberries (fresh or frozen) to the dry ingredients

Herb Bread

Add: 2 tbsp mixed herbs to the dry ingredients
                 OR Mixture of sweet basil, rosemary and parsley to make 2 tbsp
                 OR Any preferred mixture of herbs (leaves and flowers of edible plants)

Pizza Dough

2 cups rice flour	¾ cup water
2½ tsp allergen free baking powder	3 tbsp pure olive oil
½ tsp salt	

Sift together flour, allergen free baking powder and salt in a large bowl. Add water and olive oil and mix well with a fork until combined. Shape into a ball with wet hands, and add a little more water if necessary. Turn dough onto rice floured work surface and knead 2-3 minutes. Roll out to desired thickness and place on oiled pizza pan.

Either top with sauteed, drained meat and/or vegetables or cook without topping at 450°F for 10 minutes or until crust is golden brown.

If cooked without toppings, this crust can be served with herbed olive oil, jam, jelly or honey or cooked fruit or berries.

Makes one 12" pizza.

Restricted Grains Baking Powder

Baking powder contains starch which may be from a restricted grain. To make your own combine:

(1)	Baking soda	1 part (⅔ cup)
	Cream of Tartar	2 parts (⅔ cup)
	Ground rice or brown rice flour	1 part (⅓ cup)

Mix and sift ingredients together. Use in same quantities as baking powder in recipes.

(2)	Baking soda	1 part (⅓ cup)
	Cream of Tartar	2 parts (⅔ cup)
	Arrowroot starch	2 parts (⅔ cup)

Mix well and store in an airtight container.
1 tsp regular baking powder = 1½ tsp arrowroot baking powder

Quinoa Blueberry Nut Loaf

PRO: Egg, tofu, nut butter
GRA: Quinoa, rice flour
FR/VEG: Dates, orange juice and rind, blueberries

½ cup clarified butter
2 large eggs
1 cup quinoa flour
1 tsp baking powder
½ cup cooked quinoa, cooled
½ cup chopped pitted dates
¾ cup medium tofu
¼ cup orange juice

¾ cup honey
1½ cups rice flour
1 tsp baking soda
¼ tsp salt
1 cup blueberries
2 tbsp peanut or nut butter
1 tsp grated orange rind
honey

In bowl, cream butter and sugar. Beat in eggs, one at a time. In another bowl, combine flours, baking soda, baking powder, salt, and quinoa. Add blueberries, dates, and nut butter, toss to coat with flour.

Combine tofu, orange rind, and juice. Add flour mixture and tofu mixture alternately to butter mixture, stirring just until dry ingredients are moistened. Spoon into greased and floured 9 x 5 x 3 inch loaf pan.

Bake at 350° F for 50 to 60 minutes or until done. Turn loaf out on to wire rack and brush top lightly with honey.

Banana Muffins

PRO: Eggs
GRA: Flour mix
FR/VEG: Banana

½ cup clarified butter
2 eggs
1½ cup sifted *flour mix**
2 tbsp hot water
2-3 tsp corn and wheat free baking powder

½ to ¾ cup honey
1 cup ripe bananas (3 med size)
1 tsp baking soda
1 tbsp vanilla

Cream margarine and sugar. Add eggs and bananas. Mix well. Stir in flour. Dissolve soda in hot water, add to banana mixture. Stir in vanilla. Fill greased muffin tins 2/3 full. Bake at 350°F for approximately 20 minutes or until golden brown.

Makes 24 medium muffins (16-18 large).

* Flour Mix

1 cup rice flour
¼ cup soya flour
2 tbsp amaranth flour

2 tbsp tapioca or arrowroot flour
1 tbsp carob powder (optional)

Orange and Date Muffins

Wet ingredients:

1 orange, including rind
½ cup orange juice
½ cup chopped dates
1 egg
½ cup clarified butter
½ cup honey

Flour mix:

1 cup brown rice flour
2 tbsp arrowroot flour
5 tbsp tapioca flour/starch
1 tbsp guar gum
1 tbsp baking powder
1 tbsp baking soda
¼ tsp salt

Cut orange into pieces, grind in blender. Add orange juice, dates, egg, butter and honey. Blend until well mixed. Put into mixing bowl. Sift flour ingredients together. Add wet ingredients to flour mixture and mix well. Pour into muffin cups in a muffin tin. Bake at 400°F for 15 minutes.

Makes about 15 medium size muffins.

Fudgey Carob Brownies

Dry ingredients:

Sift together
1 cup amaranth flour
½ cup carob powder
⅓cup arrowroot powder
2 tsp Cream of Tartar
1 tsp baking soda
½ tsp salt

Wet ingredients:

¾ cup honey
¼ cup water
⅓ cup canola oil
2 tsp real vanilla extract

Sift the dry ingredients together and beat the wet together separately. Slowly beat the dry into the wet ingredients and scoop the batter into a lightly oiled and floured 8" x 8" or 9" x 9" square baking pan (the pan can be floured with tapioca flour or arrowroot powder). Bake for 25 or 30 minutes at 350°F.

The brownies should be moist and tender, do not overbake. When done, set to cool before cutting and removing from the pan. Store in the fridge.

Carob Fudge Topping

⅔ cup almond milk
⅓ cup honey
¼ cup carob powder
2 tsp arrowroot powder
Dash of salt
½ tsp real vanilla flavoring   (If flavoring is not available, vanilla extract may be used, however it must be heated with the rest of the ingredients.)

Blend all the ingredients except the vanilla. Bring to a boil and simmer 5 minutes, stirring constantly until the mixture thickens. Add vanilla. Remove from heat and serve hot or chilled.

Shortbread

6 oz rice flour or tapioca flour
4 oz clarified butter
2 oz fructose (fruit sugar)
2 oz (2 tbsp) almond butter

Beat all ingredients in a bowl or food processor to form a stiff dough. Roll out to ¼ inch thickness on a floured surface. Cut into 2 inch (5 cm) rounds. Place on an oiled baking sheet. Bake at 325°F (170°C) for about 25 minutes. Sprinkle with fructose. Cool and serve.

Soups, Stocks, and Stews

Ground Meat Soup

PRO: Meat (chicken turkey, beef, pork, lamb)
 GRA: Rice or rice noodles
 FR/VEG: Various frozen or fresh vegetables

In a saucepan or wok, brown 500 grams ground meat (beef, pork, lamb, chicken or turkey). Add two large chopped tomatoes, and any fresh or frozen vegetables, chopped or grated (for example: onion, garlic, carrot, zucchini, green or red peppers, mushrooms, celery, peas, green or yellow beans).

Add 3-4 cups water and bring to a boil. Add 1 cup white or brown rice or rice noodles. Reduce heat and simmer for 30 minutes or until rice is cooked. Add herbs and salt to taste. Serve with toasted rice bread or rice cakes.

Meat and Lentil Soup

PRO: Pork shoulder (or any poultry or meat desired)
GRA: Lentils or split peas
FR/VEG: Various

Place pork shoulder in a large pot and cover with water. Bring to the boil, add herbs to taste. Reduce heat and simmer 1½ hours. Remove pork shoulder. Remove bone, cut meat into cubes and return meat to the soup. Add 1 cup washed lentils or yellow or green split peas. Add various chopped or grated fresh or frozen vegetables (see above). Bring to the boil, reduce heat to simmer and cover. Simmer 30 minutes or until legumes are completely cooked.

Lentil Stew

PRO: Lentils
GRA: Lentils
FR/VEG: Basic vegetable mix (see recipe page ???)

Basic vegetable mix
2 cups red lentils
4 medium tomatoes, chopped
4 cups water
2 tbsp cilantro, fresh, chopped
Salt to taste

Wash lentils and drain. Bring lentils, tomatoes, and water to a boil. Cover, reduce heat and simmer for 20 minutes. Add more water if lentils become too dry. The consistency should be a thick soup.

Add vegetable mix and cilantro to the cooked lentils, stir, and simmer for a further 10 minutes.

Add salt and pepper to taste. Serve with fresh bread or rolls made with alternate flour.

Root Vegetable and Lentil Stew

PRO: Lentils
GRA: Root vegetables
FR/VEG: Assorted vegetables

3 tbsp olive oil	2 garlic cloves, crushed
4 ½ cup (1 ½ lb parsnip, carrot, turnip, swede peeled and diced)	1 cup tomatoes, canned
	3 cups stock (see recipe below)
3 onions, large	2 tbsp lemon juice
2 celery sticks, sliced	½ cup parsley
2 cups split red lentils, dried	Salt to taste

Wash lentils and drain. Heat 2 tablespoons oil in a large saucepan. Add 3 onions, celery, and root vegetables. Fry without browning for about 5 minutes. Add lentils and garlic. Cook gently for 4-5 minutes, stirring often. Mix in tomatoes and stock, cover, and simmer gently for 30 minutes.

Add lemon juice, parsley, and salt. Simmer until vegetables and lentils are soft.

Easy Vegetable Stock

Use any combination of washed, trimmed: onion skins, potato and carrot peelings, celery strings and leaves, parsley stems, green bean and tomato ends, outer lettuce leaves.

Save trimmings in a plastic bag in the freezer until ready to use.

In a saucepan, add enough water to just cover trimmings. Add a bay leaf and pepper, and bring to a boil. Simmer for 30 minutes. Strain, and add salt to taste. Use instead of consommé or soup base.

Freeze leftovers immediately in ice cube trays.

Green Vegetable Stock

Use a mixture of greens for this stock. Choose two of the following:

Spinach	Kale
Swiss chard	Mustard greens

8 cups lightly packed, coarsely shredded greens	1 large onion, chopped
1 small head green cabbage, coarsely shredded	1 tsp thyme, fresh
	1 bay leaf
2 medium leeks, including green tops, sliced	12 cups water
	Salt to taste
2 large stalks celery, fresh, chopped, including greens	
3 large garlic cloves, minced or pressed	

Combine all ingredients in large iron pot. Bring to a boil. Cover, reduce heat, and simmer for 1 ½ hours. Strain and discard vegetables.

Makes 8 cups. Stock freezes well.

Root Vegetable Stock

2 tbsp canola or olive oil	3 large carrots, sliced
2 large stalks celery, including leaves, sliced	1 large turnip, diced
	½ cup parsley, chopped
2 large onions, chopped	1 bay leaf
1 tsp thyme, fresh chopped	12 cups water
2 garlic cloves, minced or crushed	
Salt to taste	

In large iron pot, fry onions, celery, carrots, and turnip over medium heat for about 15 minutes until vegetables are golden, but not brown. Add water, parsley, bay leaf, thyme, garlic, peppercorns, and salt. Bring to a boil, cover, reduce heat and simmer for 1½ hours.

Strain and discard vegetables.

Makes about 10 cups. Can be frozen for future use.

Hearty Vegetarian Borscht

GRA: Potato
FR/VEG: Assorted vegetables

2 tbsp canola oil
2 large garlic cloves, minced
8 large fresh tomatoes peeled, chopped
2 medium carrots, sliced thinly
6 medium beets, cut in thin strips
1 celery heart, sliced including leaves
1 red or yellow pepper thinly sliced

2 medium onions, sliced thinly
12 cups vegetable stock (see recipe above)
4 medium potatoes, peeled and diced
2 cups green pepper, shredded
1 cup red cabbage, ,shredded
¼ cup dill weed, fresh
Salt to taste

In Dutch oven, saute onions and garlic until soft but not brown, about 5 minutes. Add fresh tomatoes, bring to boil, cover and simmer for 10 minutes. Add vegetable stock, and all vegetables except cabbage. Bring to the boil, reduce heat, cover, and simmer until vegetables are tender (about 20 minutes). Add cabbage, dill weed, salt, and pepper.

Simmer covered until cabbage is tender (about 10 minutes).

Minestrone Soup

PRO: Lentils
GRA: Lentils, potato, rice macaroni
FR/VEG: Assorted vegetables

3 tbsp canola or olive oil
1½ cups celery, chopped
1½ cups potatoes, diced
1½ cups turnip (1 medium)
2 cups tomatoes, chopped
8 cups vegetable stock
2 cloves garlic minced or pressed
1½ cups rice pasta (macaroni)
2 tbsp parsley, fresh, chopped

1 cup onion, chopped
1½ cups zucchini, chopped
1½ cups carrots, thinly sliced
2 cups green cabbage, shredded
2 cups red lentils, cooked
1 tsp rosemary, dried and crushed
1 tsp oregano, dried and crushed
1 tsp thyme ,dried and crushed
Salt to taste

Heat oil in large iron pot. Add onion, garlic, and celery and cook until onion is soft, about 5 minutes. Add potatoes, carrots, tomatoes, stock, and herbs. Bring to a boil. Cover, reduce heat, and simmer for 20 minutes. Add turnip and zucchini. Continue to simmer for 20 minutes more. Add lentils and their cooking liquid, and rice pasta. Bring to a boil. Cover, reduce heat and simmer until macaroni is cooked (about 15 minutes). Season to taste with salt and pepper.

Serve with freshly baked bread or rolls made with alternate flours.

Substitutes for Restricted Grains as a Thickener

To replace 2 tbsp of wheat flour as a thickener in soups, sauces, gravies, and puddings, use **one** of the following:

1 tbsp potato starch or flour

OR rice flour
OR arrowroot starch or flour
OR gelatin
OR 2 tbsp quick-cooking tapioca or tapioca flour
OR ¼ cup uncooked rice
OR 1 egg

Entrees

Whenever possible, use iron cookware as this will increase the iron content of any food cooked in it, especially if the food is acidic.

Most of the dishes freeze well. They can be made in large quantities and stored in the fridge or freezer for future use.

Quick Fix Meals

Starting with a simple vegetable stir fry mixture, a number of different main dishes can be made quickly by adding a variety of protein sources and varying the seasonings.

The following recipes will provide 4-6 servings, if used alone, or 6-8 servings if additional dishes are served alongside.

Basic Vegetable Mix

3 tbsp canola oil
2 garlic cloves, minced or pressed
1 cup zucchini, chopped
½ cup green pepper, chopped
½ cup red pepper, chopped

1 cup onion, chopped
1 cup celery, chopped
1 cup carrots, sliced thinly
1 cup mushrooms, thinly sliced

Heat oil in large iron pot. Add onions and garlic. Fry for 3 minutes. Add all other vegetables, except mushrooms. Fry for 5 minutes. Add mushrooms. Fry for 5 minutes.

Vegetable Mix Variations

Herbed Vegetable Rice

PRO: Tofu, fish
GRA: Rice
FR/VEG: Assorted vegetables

Basic vegetable mix (above)
2 cups long grain white rice
 (preferably Basmati)
1 lb (450-500 g) tofu

4 cups water
Salt to taste
2 tbsp herbs (thyme, rosemary, oregano, dill)

Soak rice in hot water for 10 minutes to remove excess starch or use brown rice. Drain. Add rice to cooked vegetable mix. Stir well to coat rice and fry for 3-5 minutes. Add water. It should be about one inch above the level of the rice and vegetables. Add salt if used and bring to a boil. Cover pot and turn heat down to simmer. Add herbs as desired. Simmer for 30 minutes until rice is soft for white rice or simmer for 45-60 minutes if using brown rice.

Cut tofu into ½ inch cubes. Fry in canola oil until outside is brown and slightly crispy. Serve together.

When used as an accompaniment to strong flavored dishes, use fewer varieties of vegetables in the basic vegetable mix (for example, use only onions, green peppers and celery).

Variation:Vegetable rice is a good accompaniment to any broiled or baked fish instead of tofu.

Vegetarian Spaghetti

PRO: Tofu
GRA: Noodles
FR/VEG: Assorted vegetables

Basic vegetable mix
3 cups tomatoes, chopped, or homemade
tomato sauce (below)
Herbs: chopped fresh, or dried
1 tsp basil
1 tsp rosemary

1 tsp parsley
1 tsp oregano
500g restricted grain spaghetti
  (rice, mung bean, pea, or lentil
  noodles)
Salt to taste

Prepare basic vegetable mixture and use as base for spaghetti sauce. Cut tofu into ½ inch cubes and fry in canola oil until outside is slightly brown, set aside. To spaghetti sauce add tomatoes or tomato sauce, herbs. Bring to boil and reduce heat. Add tofu and simmer for 20 minutes. Cook spaghetti according to package directions.

Pour sauce over spaghetti and mix.

Variation: Instead of tofu, substitute shellfish in sauce.

Fresh Tomato Sauce

3 tbsp olive oil
1 large onion, chopped
2 cloves garlic, minced or pressed
1 red pepper, seeded and chopped
8 tomatoes, peeled and chopped

1 tbsp basil, fresh or dried
2 tbsp parsley, fresh or dried
1 tsp thyme
Salt to taste

Fry onions and garlic in oil until soft, but not browned, about 5 minutes. Add red pepper and fry for 1-2 minutes. Add tomatoes, herbs, salt, and pepper. Bring to boil and stir and continue cooking until tomatoes are soft. Reduce heat and simmer uncovered until sauce thickens, about 30 minutes.

Ratatouille (vegetable stew)

PRO: Tofu
GRA: Rice or other grain noodles
FR/VEG: Assorted vegetables

2 tbsp canola oil
2 large garlic cloves, minced
1 large green pepper, sliced
8 large tomatoes, chopped
¼ cup parsley, fresh, chopped
4 cups eggplant chopped into
  1 inch cubes
Salt to taste

1 large onion, sliced thin
3 cups zucchini, sliced thinly
1 cup mushrooms, sliced
½ inch cubes tofu, chopped
2 tbsp cilantro, fresh, chopped
1 tsp basil, dried

Cut eggplant into 1 inch cubes. Cover with salt. Place in strainer. Cover with lid and let drain for 30 minutes to remove bitter juices. Cut tofu into ½ inch cubes and set aside. In large pot or Dutch oven, saute onion and garlic in oil until soft but not brown. Add eggplant, zucchini, green pepper, and mushrooms. Stir and saute 5 minutes. Add tomatoes, stir, bring to the boil. Reduce heat.

Add tofu, cover, and simmer for 15 minutes until tomatoes are softened and liquid has increased. Add parsley, cilantro, basil, salt, and pepper.

Cover and simmer for 15 minutes longer until vegetables are soft. For faster cooking, use canned tomatoes instead of fresh and reduce cooking time 10 minutes.

Accompany with rice or rice noodles for a well balanced meal.

Quinoa Stuffed Potatoes

PRO: Tuna or chicken
GRA: Potato, quinoa
FR/VEG: Onion, olives, zucchini, tomato

2 large russet potatoes
1 cup cooked quinoa
4 sun dried tomato halves (in oil), chopped
¼ cup finely chopped green onion
½ cup sliced black olives
½ tsp fresh rosemary
3 tbsp tuna or chopped roast chicken

1 cup shredded zucchini
2 garlic cloves, chopped

Bake potatoes at 400° F for 60 minutes or until tender. Slash top of each potato and carefully scoop out pulp without breaking skin, reserve potato shells. Mash hot potato and mix with quinoa.

Drain one tablespoon oil from sun dried tomatoes and heat in fry pan. Add zucchini and sun-dried tomatoes. Saute for about one minute. Add garlic, green onion, and black olives and cook for 1-2 minutes. Add tuna or chopped chicken. Add zucchini mixture to potato mixture. Season with rosemary and salt.

Spoon potato mixture into reserved shells. Heat in oven until piping hot. Makes two servings.

Tofu Quinoa Fritters

PRO: Tofu, sesame tahini
GRA: Quinoa
FR/VEG: Tomato, cucumber, olive, onion, shallots, lime juice

2 cups cooked quinoa, cooled
2 tbsp finely chopped shallots
1 tbsp sesame tahini
¾ cup vegetable oil

½ cup crumbled extra firm tofu
¼ cup finely chopped parsley
2 tbsp finely chopped cilantro
Salt to taste

In bowl, combine quinoa, shallots, sesame tahini, tofu, and salt. In another bowl mix together chopped parsley and cilantro. Shape quinoa mixture into small patties, pressing firmly so mixture holds together. Roll each patty in chopped parsley/cilantro mixture to coat both sides lightly. Heat oil in 10 inch frying pan over medium high heat until hot but not smoking. Fry patties in oil, turning as they color. Remove from frying pan and drain on paper towels.

Serve hot with tomato salsa. Makes 24 patties.

Chickpea Batter

2 oz chickpea flour
1 tsp canola oil
1 tsp allergen free baking powder
4 tbsp (more if necessary) water

Mix all ingredients together to make a thick smooth coating batter. Makes about 150 mL.

Vegetable Fritters

Any tolerated vegetables such as: zucchini, carrot, onion, green or red peppers, sliced potatoes, mushrooms, cauliflower or broccoli florets
.

Peel or wash vegetables. Slice into ¼ inch thick rings or strips. Dip into chickpea batter until well coated.

Deep fry in canola oil at 375° F until crisp and brown (about 3-4 minutes). Drain on paper towel.

Serve with a protein source (fish, poultry, tofu) to make a complete meal.

Battered Fried Fish and Chips

PRO: Fish
GRA: Chick pea flour
FR/VEG: Tomato (if ketchup is used), any cooked vegetables as tolerated

White fish fillet (cod, sole, halibut, snapper) 2-4 3 oz portions
Chickpea batter
Potatoes cut into sections for French fries
Canola oil for frying

Coat each fish fillet with batter. Deep fry in canola oil at 375°F until crisp and golden. Drain on paper towels. Fry French fries in oil and drain.

Serve hot with salt and homemade tomato ketchup (see recipe page 386).

Stuffed Eggplant

GRA: Rice
FR/VEG: Assorted fruit, vegetables

2 (1 lb each) eggplants
2 garlic cloves, crushed
1 medium onion, chopped fine
1 tsp grated orange rind
½ cup water
2 cups rice, cooked

2 tbsp margarine or oil
1 medium red bell pepper, chopped
1½ cup dried fruit, chopped (prunes, pitted
  dates, apples, apricots)
Salt to taste

Place margarine, garlic, red pepper and onion in two quart (2L) microwaveable casserole.

Cover and microwave at HIGH (Full power) for 3-5 minutes or until pepper and onion are tender.

Add dried fruit, dates, water, salt, orange rind and rice. Mix well. Microwave at HIGH, uncovered, for 2-3 minutes or until hot.

Cut eggplants in half lengthwise. Scoop out pulp (use in soup or other vegetable dishes), leaving 3/4 inch (2 cm) thick shells. Fill eggplant shells with rice mixture. Place in 13 x 9 inch microwaveable baking dish. Cover loosely with wax paper and microwave at HIGH for 12-15 minutes or until eggplants are soft but not mushy. Let stand for 3 minutes before serving.

Makes four servings.

Eggplants Stuffed with Lentils and Mushrooms

PRO: Lentils
GRA: Lentils
FR/VEG: Assorted vegetables

2 (1 lb each) eggplants	1 onion, large, chopped
Olive oil	2 tsp lemon juice
2 garlic cloves, crushed	½ cup mushrooms, wiped and sliced
1¼ cup (14 oz) lentils, cooked, drained	Salt to taste
2 tbsp parsley chopped	Few dried "bread" crumbs (from restricted grain list)

Cut eggplants in half. Scoop out insides. Sprinkle the insides of the eggplant skins and pulp with salt.

Let drain for 30 minutes for bitter juices to be removed. Wash eggplants, pat dry. Preheat oven to 350°F. Fry eggplant skins in a little oil to soften. Arrange in oiled shallow casserole dish. Fry onion, garlic, eggplant pulp in 3 tbsp of oil in a large saucepan for 10 minutes. Add mushrooms and cook for 4-5 minutes. Mix in lentils, lemon juice, parsley, salt to taste.

Fill eggplants skins with mixture. Sprinkle crumbs on top. Bake in oven for 30-40 minutes.

Artichokes and Peas

GRA: Peas
FR/VEG: Assorted vegetables

4 medium globe artichokes	Cut lemon half
4 tbsp canola oil or olive oil	1 medium onion, chopped
1 tbsp fennel leaves, fresh, chopped	3 cups green peas, fresh, shelled
Salt to taste	

Wash artichokes in salted water. Cut off stalks at the base of the leaves, and trim the tops so that the artichokes are about 2 inches (5 cms) high. Slice the artichokes into ½ inch wedges. Remove the choke, and rub cut surfaces with the lemon half to prevent discoloration. Heat oil in saucepan. Add onions and fry gently until soft and translucent. Add fennel leaves, artichoke wedges, and 4 tbsp of water. Add salt. Cover, reduce heat, and cook over low heat for 15 minutes. Add peas.

If mixture appears dry add 2 tbsp more water. Cover pan and simmer gently for 15 minutes more or until vegetables are tender, but not too soft.

Apple Stuffed Acorn Squash

1 acorn squash
¼ cup raisins
1½ tsp grated fresh lemon rind
⅓ cup honey

2 cooking apples
1 tbsp fresh lemon juice
4 tbsp clarified light butter
Salt to taste

Cut squash in half lengthwise and scoop out seeds. Place in baking dish, cut side down, and add ¼ inch (1 cm) of boiling water. Bake at 400°F (200 C) for 20 minutes.

Pare, core, and dice apples. Mix apples, raisins, lemon juice, lemon rind, two tbsp clarified butter and honey. Brush squash halves with remaining two tbsp butter.

Sprinkle squash with salt. Fill squash halves with apple mixture. Place squash in baking dish and add ½ inch (1 cm) of boiling water. Cover and bake 30 minutes longer. If desired, garnish with apple and lemon slices. Makes four servings.

Buckwheat and Mushrooms

1 cup roasted buckwheat
2 tbsp yeast extract
2 onions, large, chopped
1 tbsp olive oil
1½ cup mushrooms,
 (washed and sliced)
Sea salt to taste

1¼ cup water
1 tbsp tomato purée
2 celery sticks, sliced
4 garlic cloves, crushed
Tamari (wheat free soya sauce)

Bring buckwheat, water, yeast extract and tomato purée to boil. Cover, turn heat to low. Leave for 15 minutes until buckwheat is fluffy and water is completely absorbed. While waiting, fry onions and celery in oil until soft. Add garlic and mushrooms, fry for 3-4 minutes more. Gently add cooked buckwheat to mixture.

Season with tamari and salt as necessary.

Variation: Use 1 cup mushrooms and 1 cup skinned, sliced tomatoes. Make as above.
      Add tomatoes with mushrooms when frying.

Desserts

Cooked Fruits

Fruit Kebabs

PRO: Tofu
GRA: Rice
FR/VEG: A variety of tolerated fruits

Alternate a variety of fruits on a metal skewer, such as the following:

Whole strawberries	Melon (cantaloupe, watermelon, honeydew)
Pineapple chunks	Apple pieces
Pear cubes	Kiwi fruit (use a quarter or half fruit)
Orange sections	Grapes (seedless varieties)

Cook on a barbecue until fruits are well cooked on the inside and crisp on the outside. Brush with liquid honey and reheat.

This can be made into a complete meal, such as breakfast by serving with tofu whipped with honey and lime juice heated and cooled, and rice pudding made with fruit juice instead of milk.

Poached Pears

Peel and core pears. Cut into halves lengthways. Place in a saucepan with sufficient water to cover fruit. Bring to a boil. Cover with a lid. Reduce heat. Simmer for about 10 minutes.

Drizzle melted honey over pears and serve with cooking water, which will be nicely pear flavored. Eat hot or cold.

Alternatively, the cooking water can be added to other dessert recipes requiring liquid as additional flavor and sweetener.

Baked Apples

Core apples, but leave skin intact. Reserve stem with a small amount of skin and apple attached.

Place cored apples in baking pan. Place honey inside hole left by removal of the core. Place reserved stem on top of hole to cover it.

Bake in 350°F oven for 25 minutes, or until flesh feels soft and well cooked when tested with a skewer.

Serve hot, with melted honey from the pan drippings spooned over the top. (The skin is usually not eaten).

For variety, the hole can be filled with other fruit such as blueberries, raisins mixed with peanut or nut butter, or any chopped or puréed fruit, added before cooking.

Baked Bananas

Peel bananas and cut in half lengthwise. Place cut side down in a baking or casserole dish. Drizzle honey over slices. Bake in 350°F oven for 20 minutes.

Serve hot with honey, peanut or other nut butters on top.

Appendix III

Cookbooks with Recipes Suitable for Allergen-restricted Diets

The All Natural Allergy Cookbook. Dairy-Free Gluten-Free. J.M. Martin.   Harbour Publishing, Madeira Park, BC, 1991.
- Gluten and dairy free recipes, (some recipes do contain gluten).
- Moderate ingredient list, simple instructions.
- Symbols indicating the allergen status of each recipe, (egg, gluten, soy, yeast grain, baking powder, and soda free).
- Variations for some recipes.
- Substitution recipes for flour, baking powder, egg, thickeners, milk, and clarified butter.
- Product source information provided.

All Natural Allergy Recipes: Breads, Desserts and Main Dishes - Gluten and Dairy-free.
J.M. Martin.   J.M.M. Publications, PO Box 4391, Vancouver BC, V6B 3Z8. 1986.
- Gluten and dairy-free recipes.
- Moderate ingredient list, long detailed instructions.
- Symbols indicating egg, gluten, wheat, soy, yeast, baking powder, and soda free status of each recipe.
- Substitution recipes for baking powder and nut and soy milks.
- Product source information provided.

Allergic People Eat Desserts Too! E.B. Milinusic. Mycel Project Management Services Inc., Calgary, AB, 1991.
- All recipes free of wheat, corn, gluten, eggs, dairy, and additives.
- Few ingredients, simple instructions.
- Must read recipes to identify other allergens.
- Substitution recipes for baking powder, butter, cream, egg, gluten flour, non-dairy milk products, vanilla, sweeteners, and yogurt.

The Allergy Cookbook: Diets Unlimited for Limited Diets. Allergy Information Association. Methuen Publications, Agincourt, Ontario, 1986.
- Recipes may be milk, egg, wheat, gluten, corn, sugar, and salicylate free.
- Many ingredients, simple instructions.
- Symbols with each recipe indicate which allergens the recipe contains, which allergens it is free from, and which allergens it can be free from if recipe is made using an alternative ingredient.
- Substitution recipes for egg, milk, wheat, and gluten.

The Allergy Cookbook: Foods for Festive Occasions. Allergy Information Association. Methuen Publications, Agincourt, Ontario, 1985.
- Recipes may be milk, egg, wheat, gluten, and corn free.
- Recipes may be sugar or additive reduced, (free of artificial color, artificial flavor, BHA/BHT, sulfites, sodium benzoates, caramel, or MSG).
- Symbols with each recipe indicate which allergens the recipe contains, which allergens it is free from, and which allergens it can be free from if recipe is made using an alternative ingredient.
- Substitution recipes for egg, milk, wheat and gluten.

The Allergy Cookbook. Tasty, Nutritious Cooking Without Wheat, Corn, Milk Or Eggs. R.R. Shattuck. The New American Library of Canada Limited, Scarborough, ON, 1986.
- Recipes are corn, egg, milk, wheat, and gluten free.
- Moderate ingredient list, simple instructions.
- Chart prior to each section and each recipe has symbols indicating allergen free status.
- Some recipes have variations.
- Substitution hints.

Allergy Cooking With Ease. N.M. Dumke. Starburst Publishers, Lancaster, PA, 1992.
- Recipes are designed to be wheat, milk, egg, corn, soy, yeast, sugar, grain, and gluten free.
- Easy to use recipes.
- Written description of allergen free status after each recipe.
- Variations (especially with different flours) for some recipes.
- Table of recipes and their appropriateness for each diet detailed at the end of the book.

The Allergy Diet. How to Overcome Your Food Intolerance. E. Workman, J. Hunter and V. Alun Jones. Macdonald and Co. Ltd., London, 1988.
– Offers recipes free of wheat, milk, and egg.
– Few ingredients, simple instructions.
– Symbols to identify allergen free status of each recipe.
– Labeling guidelines.
– No substitution recipes.
– Exclusion diet basics.

The Allergy Discovery Diet: A Rotation Diet for Discovering Your Allergies to Food.
J.E. Postley, M.D., with J. Barton. Doubleday , New York, 1990.
– No specific allergens identified.
– Consists of an elimination diet and reintroduction phase. The reintroduction phase does not include challenges of individual food components but combination foods. This practice is not recommended for the identification of food allergies.

The Allergy Kitchen 1: Savoury Soups. E. Ratner. Allergy Publications Inc., Menlo Park, CA, 1988.
– All recipes milk, egg, corn, and soy free. Suggestions on how to make recipes gluten free.
– Includes suggestions on how to modify recipes if you can use milk or eggs.
– From the American Allergy Association.

The Allergy Self Help Cookbook. M.H. Jones. Rodale Press, Emmaus, PA, 1984.
– Wheat, egg, corn, yeast, and sugar free recipes.
– Many ingredients, long complicated recipes.
– No indication of allergen free status with the recipe.
– Alternative flours suggested.
– Guidelines for eating out.
– Following rotary diet plan not necessary.

Baking with Amaranth. Marge Jones, PO Box 257 Deerfield, IL 60015. 1985
– Corn, wheat, milk, yeast, and egg free recipes.
– Moderate ingredient list, simple instructions.
– Indication of free status of each recipe.
– Many variations for some recipes.
– Baking powder substitution recipe included.
– Product source information provided.

Beyond the Staff of Life, K. Adler. Naturegraph Publishers, Happy Camp CA, 1990.
– Wheat and milk free recipes
– Few ingredients, simple instructions.
– No indication of other possible allergens in the recipes.

Cookies Naturally. With allergy related substitutes, nutrient analysis and diabetic choices.
S. Hartung. Cookies Naturally, 32 Layton St., Kitchener, ON. 1989.
  – Milk, egg, flour, and honey free recipes.
  – Few ingredients, simple instructions.
  – Must read recipes to identify other allergens.
  – Substitution recipes for flour, citrus, sugar, milk, egg, and baking powder.
  – Nutrient analysis (energy, protein, fat, carbohydrate, cholesterol, and fibre) and diabetic choices indicated for each recipe.

Dairy Free Cookbook. J. Zukin. Prima Publishing, Rocklin, CA, 1991.
  – Dairy free recipes.
  – No other allergens noted.
  – Nutritional analysis of each recipe with calories, protein, fat, carbohydrate, sodium, and cholesterol per serving.
  – Includes suggestions for eating out and shopping dairy free.
  – Easy to read recipes.

Diets To Help Gluten and Wheat Allergy. R. Greer. Thorsons Publishers Limited, San Francisco, 1993.
  – Gluten and wheat free recipes.
  – Few ingredients, simple instructions.
  – No indication of other allergens that may be present.
  – Substitutions for cereals, binders, and bran.
  – Lists of foods allowed and those to avoid.

Dr. Berger's Immune Power Cookbook. S.T. Berger. Nal Books, New York, 1986.
  – Developed to eliminate cow's milk and milk products, wheat, brewer's and baker's yeast, egg, corn, soy products and sugar cane.
  – Few ingredients, simple instructions.
  – Allergen-free status of each recipe is not indicated.

Food Allergies. M.L. Dobler. American Dietetic Association, USA, 1991.
  – Corn, egg, milk, soy, and wheat free recipes.
  – Moderate ingredient list, step by step instructions.
  – "No" list indicating allergen-free status of each recipe.
  – Nutrition evaluation including calories, protein, fat, carbohydrate, sodium, and cholesterol provided.
  – Meal planning suggestions.
  – Label reading guidelines.

Food Intolerance. J. Hunter, V. Alun Jones, and E. Workman. The Body Press, Tucson, AZ, 1986.
- Offers recipes free of wheat, milk, and egg.
- Few ingredients, simple instructions.
- Symbols with each recipe indicate allergen free status.
- No substitution recipes.
- Exclusion diet basics.

Freedom From Allergy Cookbook. R. Greenberg and A. Nori. Blue Poppy Press, Vancouver, BC, 1990.
- Wheat, yeast, milk, egg, corn, soy, and additive free recipes.
- Few ingredients, simple instructions.
- No indication of allergen free status of each recipe.
- Alternative list for included allergens.
- Snack ideas.
- Alternative food source list.
- Menu suggestions.

The Gluten-free Diet Book: A Guide to Celiac Sprue, Dermatitis Herpetiformis and Gluten-free Cookery. P. Rawcliffe and R. Rolph. NC Press Ltd., Toronto, ON, 1985.
- Recipes are wheat and gluten free.
- **Note:** The authors are British and recipes may use buckwheat flour or oats.

The Gluten-free Gourmet. Living Well Without Wheat. B. Hagman. Henry Holt and Company, New York, 1990.
- Gluten free recipes.
- Few ingredients, easy to follow instructions.
- No other allergens noted.
- Hidden sources of gluten indicated.
- Flour substitutions.
- Guidelines for traveling and eating out.
- Listings of product sources.

Gluten Intolerance. A Resource Including Recipes. American Dietetic Association. USA, 1985.
- All recipes are wheat-free but not all are gluten-free. Recipes can be made gluten-free by making the appropriate flour substitutions.
- Many ingredients, simple instructions.
- "No" list with each recipe, indicating allergen-free status.
- Flour substitutions.
- Some variations.
- Lists of allowed packaged and prepared foods.
- Product information sources.
- Lists other cookbooks suitable for allergen-restricted diets.

Going Against the Grain. Wheat-free Cookery. P. Potts. Central Point Publishing, Oregon City, OR, 1992.
- Wheat free recipes.
- Few ingredients, very simple instructions.
- No indication of other allergens that may be in recipes.
- Flour substitutions.

Hyperactive Child. Beat Hyperactivity and Other Food Sensitivities with Quick and Easy Meals. J. Ash and D. Roberts. Thorsons Publishers Limited, , Northamptonshire, 1990.
- Grain, gluten, milk and egg free recipes.
- Many ingredients, simple instructions.
- Allergen free status of each recipe indicated.
- Substitution recipes for baking powder and soda, gluten and grain free flours, cow's milk, egg, and soy.
- Lists recipes by specific diet restrictions.

Lactose Intolerance. A Resource Including Recipes. American Dietetic Association. USA, 1985.
- Lactose-free recipes.
- Many ingredients, simple instructions.
- "No" list with each recipe indicating allergen-free status.
- Some variations.
- Product information sources provided.
- Lists other cookbooks suitable for allergen-restricted diets.

The Milk-free Kitchen: Living Well Without Dairy Products. B. Kidder. Henry Holt, New York, USA, 1990.
- Cow's milk-free recipes. Some recipes use goat's milk or sheep milk cheese.
- Sour cream substitution recipe included.
- List in appendix indicates which baked goods and dessert recipes are also egg-free.
- No indication of other allergens that may be present.

Now You Eat It...Now You Don't. Kitchen Magic Food Substituting for the Allergic. L. Weiss. Keats Publishing Inc., New Canaan, CT, 1994.
- Recipes can be free of wheat, egg, gluten, sugar, and dairy products.
- Few ingredients, simple instructions.
- Symbols with each recipe to indicate allergen free status.
- Substitution recipes for flour, egg, baking powder, and dairy products.

The Rice Flour Cookbook. J. Kisslinger. Kisslinger Publications, Sidney, BC, 1986.
- Recipes are designed to be gluten and wheat free.
- Reviewed by the Canadian Celiac Association and Mavis Malloy, RDN.

Special Food for Special People. Recipes for Allergy Diets Food Rotation*. L. Smedley and A. Thrash. Lydia Smedley, Site 9 Comp 8 RR 3, Kamloops BC, V2C 5K1, 1985.
- No indication of allergens present in each recipe except for warnings for gluten.
- Few ingredients, step by step instructions.
- Nutrient information for each recipe includes calories and protein.
- Speciality food sources.
- It is not necessary to follow the rotary diet meal plan.

The Wheat and Gluten Free Cookbook. J. Noble. Vermilion, London, England, 1993.
- Recipes are wheat and gluten free.
- Nutrient analysis of each recipe for calories, protein, fat, and carbohydrate.
- Most recipes incorporate Nutricia products that may not be readily available in stores.

Wheat, Milk and Egg-Free Cooking. R. Greer. Thorsons Publishers Limited, London, 1989.
- All recipes are wheat, milk, and egg free.
- Many ingredients, detailed instructions.
- No indication of other possible allergens in the recipes.
- Baking powder substitution recipe.
- Provides lists of terms indicating foods that contain wheat, eggs, and milk.

Wheatless Cooking (including gluten-free recipes). L. Coffey. Ten Speed Press, Berkeley, California, 1985.
- Recipes are all wheat free, with notations if they are also gluten free.
- Substitution recipes for egg and alternative flours.
- Few ingredients, easy step by step instructions.
- No indication of other allergens that may be present.

The Yeast Connection Cookbook. A Guide to Good Nutrition and Better Health. W.G. Crook and M.H. Jones. Professional Books, Jackson, TN, 1989.
- Yeast, wheat, rye, and corn free recipes.
- Few ingredients, easy instructions.
- Symbols indicate allergen free status of each recipe, (corn, milk, egg, wheat, legumes, and yeast).
- Variations for some recipes.
- Substitution recipes.
- Product sources detailed.

Sources of Allergy Recipes for Children

Your Food-allergic Child: A Parents' Guide. J.E. Meizel. Mills and Sanderson, Bedford, MA, 1988.
- No consistent indication of allergen free status of each recipe.
- Includes wheat free playdough recipe and other children's favorites e.g. dairy or egg or nut free ice creams and cookies.
- Includes information of FDA labeling and additive codes, descriptions of additives, and product information.

The following cookbooks have not been reviewed and their availability is not known:

The Allergy Baker. C. Rudoff. Prologue Publications, Menlo Park, CA, 1981.

Caring and Cooking for the Allergic Child. L. Thomas. Sterling Publishing, New York, 1987.

Cooking for the Allergic Child. J. Moyer. Grove Printing, Belle Fonte, PA, 1987.

Cooking Without - Recipes for the Allergic Child (and Family). M. Williams. The Gimbal Corp., Ambler, PA, 1989.

Delicious and Easy Rice Flour Recipes. M. Wood. Charles C. Thomas, Springfield IL. 1979.

About the Author

Janice M. Vickerstaff Joneja, Ph.D., R.D.N., is the co-ordinator of the Allergy Nutrition Program located at Vancouver Hospital and Health Sciences Center, Vancouver, British Columbia, Canada. The program includes an outpatient clinic where people can obtain help in the identification and management of their adverse reactions to foods. The outpatient clinic records an average of 500 patient visits per year. In addition, the outreach program provides information on current research in food allergy for health care professionals such as physicians, public health nurses, and dietitians, in the form of seminars, lectures, workshops, and publications.

Dr. Joneja also conducts research in adverse reactions to foods and supervises graduate student research in this field.

Dr. Joneja holds a doctoral degree (Ph.D.) in medical microbiology from the University of Birmingham, England. Most of her research has been in the area of immunology and oral microbiology. She is also a registered dietitian/nutritionist (R.D.N.).

She has held university appointments as Assistant Professor at the University of British Columbia in the Department of Microbiology and the Department of Oral Biology (Faculty of Dentistry), Adjunct Assistant Professor, Department of Biochemistry and Microbiology, University of Victoria (B.C.), and is currently an Adjunct Professor in the School of Family and Nutritional Sciences, University of British Columbia. She has also conducted research in immunology and taught oral microbiology at the University of Colorado Medical Sciences Center and Medical School, in Denver.

Since 1986, Dr. Joneja has been extensively involved in research, education, and writing in the area of food allergy and food intolerance, particularly the immunological and biochemical reactions involved in these conditions. The fact that her two children have had severe allergies from birth has been a strong impetus in her work.

Dr. Joneja is the author and co-author of a number of publications on microbiology, immunology, and allergy, including the book *Understanding Allergy, Sensitivity, and Immunity: A Comprehensive Guide*, published by Rutgers University Press, New Brunswick, New Jersey, USA, in June 1990 (reprinted 1994). Dr. Joneja is the author of *Managing Food Allergy and Intolerance: A Practical Guide*, published by McQuaid Consulting Group, Vancouver, B.C., Canada, 1995, and by J.A. Hall Publications, Vancouver, B.C., Canada, 1997.

Index

Acetylsalicylic acid
    see Salicylate sensitivity, 187
Additive effect
    and migraine, 317
Adrenalin
    Anakit®, 17
    and anaphylactic reaction, 17
    Epipen®, 17
Alcohol
    and food additive intolerance, 12
    and MSG sensitivity, 235
    effect on migraine, 315
    effect on uptake of food allergens, 6
Allergenic Cross-reactivity, 19
Allergenic potential
    of foods, 23
Allergenicity of foods
    scale, 28
Allergens
    hidden sources, 24
Allergy
    and breast-feeding, 248
    and colic, 249
    and family history, 246
    avoidance of multiple food
     allergens, 139

    in children, 245
    in infancy, 245
    predictors, 246
    symptoms of, 4
    to barley, 111
    to corn, 111
    to egg, 105
    to food; definition, 1
    to fungi, 143
    to grain, 111
    to milk, 79
    to mould, 143
    to nickel, 165
    to oats, 111
    to peanut, 127
    to rice, 111
    to rye, 111
    to soy protein, 133
    to tree nuts, 127
    to wheat, 111
    to yeast, 143
Anaphylactic reaction, 5, 15
    avoidance of, 17
    definition, 15
    foods implicated in , 16
    Medic-Alert®, 18

occurrence of , 16
symptoms of, 5, 15
treatment of, 17
Anaphylactoid reaction
see Anaphylactic reaction, 3
Anaphylaxis
see Anaphylactic reaction, 5
Angioedema , 305
and histamine, 306
causes of, 306
food triggers, 306
Antibodies
IgA, 80
IgE, 1, 30, 80
IgG , 80
IgM , 80
sIgA, 248
Antihistamine
and anaphylactic reaction, 17
Antioxidants
BHA, 219
BHT, 219
Aspartame
role in triggering migraine, 316
Asthma
and diet, 335
and tyramine, 336
food additives implicated in, 336
foods implicated in , 335
Atopy, 1
Attention deficit disorder with hyperactivity
(ADDH)
see Hyperactivity, 325
Azo dyes
tartrazine, etc., 178
Bed-wetting
see Nocturnal enuresis, 339
Benzoate Sensitivity, 205
management of, 207
symptoms of, 207
Benzoates
and skin rashes, 207
benzoic acid, 205

benzoyl peroxide, 206
benzyl and benzoyl compounds, 208
occurrence in foods, 205
parabens, 208
sensitivity to, 205
sodium benzoate, 205
sources of, 213
use in foods, 205, 206, 208
BHA and BHT
sources of , 221
BHA and BHT sensitivity, 219
diet for, 221
Biogenic amines
dopamine, 150
epinephrine, 150
histamine, 149
norepinephrine, 150
octopamine, 149
phenylethylamine, 149
tyramine, 149
vasoactive amines, 149
Blood tests
ELISA (enzyme linked
immunosorbent assay), 30
FAST (fluorescent allergosorbent
test), 30
RAST (radioallergosorbent test), 30
Breast-feeding
and food allergy, 248
introducing solid foods, 251
mother's diet during, 248
sensitization by, 248
Calcium
absorption of, 98
daily requirements, 100, 101
dietary sources, 81
in milk, 81
Calcium citrate malate, 81
Calcium gluconate, 81
Candida albicans
sensitivity to, 145
Carbohydrate malabsorption
see disaccharide intolerance, 269

Celiac disease
 and grain, 112
 diagnosis of, 112
Challenge phase, 41
 Challenge Test Checklist, 56
 sequence of testing foods, 43
Challenge with suspected trigger food, 37
Childhood
 risk of allergy, 245
Chinese restaurant syndrome
 see MSG sensitivity, 233
Colic , 249
Coloring agents
 artificial color, 178
 azo dyes, 178
 see also tartrazine sensitivity, 11
 sensitivity to, 177
 use in foods, 177
Combined Allergic Reactions, 6
Contact allergy
 see: Type IV hypersensitivity, 3
Controversial tests
 biokinesiology, 30
 electroacupuncture, 30
 Vega Test, 30
Cookbooks
 for the allergic, 409
Corn-free Diet, 114
Crohn's Disease, 281
 and diet, 281
 and elemental diets, 282
 and immunology , 283
 diet for, 283, 286
 prevalence of, 281
 treatment of, 281
Cross-reactivity, allergenic, 19
 between plant species, 20
Dairy products
 adverse reaction to, 79
DBPCFC, 31
Diagnosis of food allergy and intolerance, 32
Diary of food intake and symptoms
 see Exposure diary, 35

Diet
 and asthma, 335
 and eczema, 337
 and nocturnal enuresis, 339
 BHA and BHT-restricted, 221
 corn-free, 114
 disaccharide-restricted, 273
 egg-free, 107
 Few foods elimination diet, 341
 Food colouring-restricted, 181
 for angioedema, 309
 for Crohn's disease, 286
 for hyperactivity, 328
 for IBS, 297
 for migraine, 319
 for urticaria, 309
 free from multiple allergens, 139
 grain-restricted, 113
 nickel-restricted, 174
 peanut-free, 129
 soy-free, 135
 sulfite-restricted, 228
 tartrazine-restricted, 181
 to eliminate suspected allergens, 36
 tyramine-restricted, 153
 wheat-free, 113
Digestive tract
 immaturity, 6
 inflammation , 6
 permeability, 5
Disaccharide intolerance, 269
 congenital, 271
 diet for, 273
 primary , 271
 secondary, 272
Dose-related response
 and migraine, 317
Double-blind Placebo-controlled Food
    Challenge, 31
Eczema
 and diet, 337
 food additives implicated in, 338
 foods implicated in, 338

Egg allergy, 105
    diet for, 107
Egg proteins
    egg white, 105
    egg yolk, 105
    heat stability of, 105
Egg replacers, 107
Elemental diets
    in Crohn's disease, 282
Elimination test diet, 36
Exercise
    effect on allergy, 6
Exposure diary, 39
    instructions, 39
    of food intake and symptoms, 35
    of infant food intake, 249
    of maternal food intake, 249
Feingold diet
    see hyperactivity, 325
Few Foods Elimination Diet, 32, 36, 341
    nutritional content of recipes, 374
    recipes, 348
Food additive intolerance
    sensitivity to alcohol, 12
    sensitivity to odors, 13
Food additives
    and asthma, 336
    antioxidants , 11
    coloring agents, 11
    definition, 11
    effect on hyperactivity, 325
    emulsifiers, 11
    flavor enhancers, 11
    GRAS list , 11
    humectants, 11
    intolerance of, 12
    preservatives, 11
    ripening agents , 11
    sources, 11
    stabilizers, 11
    texturizers, 11
    uses, 11

Food allergy
    definition, 1
    diagnosis of, 32
    management of, 32
    prevention of, 32
Food allergy tests, 29
    biokinesiology, 30
    blood tests, 30
    controversial tests, 30
    electroacupuncture, 30
    laboratory tests, 29
    skin tests, 29
    Vega Test, 30
Food colors
    erythrosine, 11
    see also tartrazine sensitivity, 177
    tartrazine, 11
Food Dye and Coloring Act, 177
Food dyes
    see tartrazine sensitivity, 177
Food hypersensitivity
    see Food allergy, 1
Food intolerance
    definition, 7
    diagnosis of, 32
    management of, 32
    prevention of, 32
    see also Food allergy, 1
Formula, infant
    see infant formulae, 250
    Composition of Infant Formulae, 264
Frequency of Exposure
    effect on allergy, 7
Galactosaemia
    see lactose intolerance, 85
Galactose
    see lactose intolerance, 85
Glucose
    see lactose intolerance, 85
Glutamate
    see MSG sensitivity, 234
Gluten complex, 111

Hidden sources of allergens, 24
Histamine, 3
    occurrence in food, 159, 307
    physiological role, 158
    role in triggering migraine, 314
Histamine sensitivity, 158
Hormone Levels
    effect on allergy, 7
Hydrolysed plant protein (HPP), 113,114,
    134
Hydrolysed vegetable protein (HVP), 113,
    114
Hyperactivity
    and food additives, 325
    and salicylates, 325
    Feingold diet, 325
    mechanism of, 328
    symptoms of, 328
    test diet for, 328
Hypersensitivity , 1
    Type I hypersensitivity , 1
    Type IV hypersensitivity, 3
IBS, 291
    diagnosis of , 291
    diet for, 297
    management of, 292
    mechanism of, 297
    symptoms of, 291, 297
Incidence of Allergy, 5
Infancy
    risk of allergy, 245
Infant formulae
    Alactamil®, 251, 265
    Alimentum®, 250, 266
    Aptamil, 264
    composition of, 264
    disaccharide-free, 251
    Enfalac, 264
    Follow Up, 265
    Good Start®, 250, 265
    hydrolysed milk casein , 250
    hydrolysed whey protein, 250
    I-Soyalac, 265
    Isomil, 265

    lactose-free, 251
    Milumil, 264
    Next Step, 264
    Nursoy, 265
    Nutramigen®, 250, 266
    Pregestimil®, 250, 266
    Prejomin, 266
    Prosobee®, 251, 266
    Similac, 264
    SMA, 264
    soy-based, 250
    Soyalac, 265
Inflammatory mediators, 2
    histamine, 3
    leukotrienes , 3
    prostaglandins , 3
Intestinal tract
    see digestive tract, 5
Intolerance
    of disaccharides, 269
    of food additives, 12
    of lactose, 79, 83
Irritable bowel syndrome
    see IBS, 291
Irritable colon
    see IBS, 291
Kwok's syndrome
    see MSG sensitivity, 233
Lactase deficiency
    congenital, 271
    incidence of, 84
    primary, 84
    secondary, 84
Lactation
    mother's diet during, 248
Lactose intolerance, 79, 83, 271
    and Lactaid®, 85
    diagnosis of, 84
    tests for, 85
    treatment of, 85
Lecithin, 134, 206
Leguminosae, 127, 133
Leukotrienes, 3
Management of food allergy and intolerance,

Lactation
    mother's diet during, 248
Lactose intolerance, 79, 83, 271
    and Lactaid®, 85
    diagnosis of, 84
    tests for, 85
    treatment of, 85
Lecithin, 134, 206
Leguminosae, 127, 133
Leukotrienes, 3
Management of food allergy and intolerance,
        32
Mandalona
    and peanut allergy, 128
MAOI
    drugs, 150
    effect on tyramine metabolism, 150
Menstruation
    effect on migraine, 316, 317
Migraine
    and alcohol, 315
    and aspartame, 316
    and diet, 311
    and dose-related response, 317
    and histamine, 314
    and menstruation, 316, 317
    and nitrites, 315
    and stress, 317
    and the additive effect, 317
    definition, 311
    diet for, 319
    food triggers, 312
    incidence, 311
    triggers, 311
Milk allergy, 79
    management of, 81
Milk proteins
    heat stability of, 80
Milk substitutes, 82
Milk-free diet, 89
Monoamine oxidase inhibitors
    see MAOI, 150

Monosodium glutamate
    see MSG, 233
Mold allergy, 143
MSG
    occurrence in food, 235
MSG sensitivity, 233
    and acetylcholine, 234
    and alcohol, 235
    management of, 235
    mechanism of, 234
    symptoms of, 234
Multiple food allergens
    diet free from, 139
Nickel
    and contact dermatitis, 165, 167
    and iron, 166
Nickel allergy, 165
    management of, 165
Nitrate and nitrite sensitivity, 241
    symptoms of, 241
Nitrates and nitrites
    occurrence in food, 241
    role in triggering migraine, 315
    Diet for, 243
Nocturnal enuresis
    and coffee, tea, 339
    and diet, 339
    and food allergy, 339
    foods implicated in, 339
Nutrients in common allergens, 73
Pediatric allergy, 245
    breast-feeding, 248
    Composition of Infant Formulae, 264
    infant formulae, 250
    introducing solid foods, 251
    preventive measures, 254
    sensitization to allergens, 245
    symptoms indicating , 249
Parabens
    sensitivity to, 208
    use in foods, 208
Peanut allergy, 127
    and anaphylactic reaction, 129

and Mandalona, 128
and tree nuts, 127
diet for, 129
symptoms of , 128, 129
Predictors of allergy, 246
cord blood, IGE levels, 246
family history, 246
IgE in cord blood, 246
prenatal sensitization, 247
sensitization of the fetus, 247
Preservatives, 11
benzoates, 11, 205
sorbates, 11
sulfites, 11, 225
Prevention of food allergy and intolerance, 32
Prostaglandins , 3
Proteins in wheat, 111
albumins, 111
gliadins, 111
globulins, 111
glutenins, 111
Relatedness of food allergens, 20
Ripening agents
ethylene, 11
Rotation diets, 67
sample, 71
Salicylate sensitivity, 187
mechanism of, 188
symptoms of, 188
Salicylates
effect on hyperactivity, 325
in medications, supplements and
toiletries, 188
occurrence in food, 187
Secretory IgA
see Antibodies: sIgA, 248
Sensitivity
to ASA, 187
to benzoates, 205
to BHA and BHT , 219
to biogenic amines, 149
to food coloring, 177
to histamine, 158

to MSG, 233
to nitrates, 241
to nitrites, 241
to salicylates, 187
to sulfites, 225
to tartrazine, 177
to tyramine, 150
Sequence of testing foods, 43
Solid foods
introduction of, 251
Soy milk, 82
Soy protein
sources of, 134
Soy protein allergy, 133
symptoms of, 133
Spastic colon
see IBS, 291
Sprue
see Celiac disease, 112
Stress
effect on allergy, 7
effect on migraine, 317
Sulfite sensitivity, 225
and asthma, 225
and steroid dependency, 225
diet for, 228
symptoms of, 225
Sulfites
detection of , 227
use in foods, 226, 228
use in medications, 226, 229
Symptoms of allergy, 4
digestive tract, 4
nervous system, 4
respiratory tract, 4
skin, 4
Tartrazine, 177
Tartrazine sensitivity
and ASA sensitivity, 179
and dietary salicylates, 179
mechanism of , 179
symptoms of, 179
Tests for food allergy, 29

biokinesiology, 30
blood tests, 30
controversial tests, 30
electroacupuncture, 30
ELISA, 30
FAST, 30
laboratory tests, 29
RAST, 30
skin tests, 29
Vega Test, 30
Tests for lactose intolerance, 85
Blood Glucose Level Test, 85
Fecal Reducing Substances Test, 85
Hydrogen Breath Test, 85
Textured vegetable protein (TVP), 114, 134
Total allergen load, 306
Tyramine
and asthma, 336
food sources, 151
Tyramine sensitivity, 150
and chronic urticaria, 150
and MAOI drugs, 150
and migraine headache, 150

causes of , 150
diet for, 153
symptoms of, 151
Uptake of Food Allergens, 6
alcohol, effect on, 6
exercise, effect on, 6
Urticaria , 305
and histamine, 306
causes of, 306
food triggers, 306
IgE-mediated, 306
Wheat allergy
symptoms of, 112
Wheat proteins, 111
albumins, 111
gliadins, 111
globulins, 111
glutenins, 111
Yeast
Candida albicans, 144
Saccharomyces, 143
Yeast allergy, 143

J.A. Hall Publications

J.A. Hall Publications was founded in 1997 in Vancouver, BC, Canada. Our mission is to provide high quality health science publications, based on scientific research and applied clinical practice. In addition to our publications, we organize workshops and provide distance education programs for health care professionals.

Detecting and managing food allergies and intolerances is a new area of dietary practice. Janice Joneja, Ph.D., R.D.N. is internationally recognized for her expertise on the topic. Dr. Joneja's scientifically based research and clinically trialed methods are well respected and used by renowned allergists in the US, the UK, and Canada.

Dr. Janice Joneja's continuing education programs are available on audio and video tapes. Dr. Joneja is available on a limited basis to deliver workshops. To arrange a workshop or a speaking engagement in your area, please contact us.

You are invited to visit J.A. Hall Publications' web site at **www.HallPublications.com**. We are committed to offering timely and up-to-date information about food allergies and food intolerances. Complimentary copies of the *Joneja Food Allergen Scale* and a FREE copy of *Sequence of Adding Solid Foods for the Allergic Infant* are available from the web site.

We like to hear from our customers. Please send us your comments by e-mail to info@hallpublications.com.

For complete information about our products and workshops, please contact us in Canada at:

Telephone:	(North America) toll-free 1-888-993-6133
	(International) 1-604-738-9424
Fax:	(North America) 1-888-881-1128
	(International) 1-604-738-9425
Internet:	www.HallPublications.com
e-mail:	info@hallpublications.com.

Publications and Distance Education Programs
by Janice Joneja, Ph.D., R.D.N.

Managing Food Allergy & Intolerance: A Practical Guide ISBN 0-9682098-0-7
- Practice-ready manual-with 280 pages of client information sheets to copy for your patients
- Designed for busy health care professionals who counsel people with food allergies or intolerances.
- Full of scientific explanations and practical applications.
- Recognized as the most complete & comprehensive manual available on the topic today.
- Nutritionally balanced diet plans for every known food sensitivity.
- Professionally formatted with tables & charts.
- Used by recognized food allergy experts around the world

581 pages, 8.5 x 11; 3 ring binder with tabs; referenced and indexed; tables and charts, publication date December, 1995, reprinted May ,1998, January, 1999. Weight: 6.5 lbs.

#1001	North America:	$149 USD
	UK and Europe:	contact Gazelle Book Services (UK) Tel +44 (0)1524 68765
#1012	CD-ROM: HTML format	$149 USD

DISTANCE EDUCATION (Examination optional - additional payment required with submission of completed examination- certificate issued on successful completion of examination)

FOOD ALLERGY & INTOLERANCE: MECHANISMS AND MANAGEMENT

This essential course for clinicians covers all aspects of this new area of dietetic practice. Topics include immunological mechanisms; anatomy, physiology & immunology of the digestive tract; physiological mechanisms of food intolerance; food additives, symptoms & diagnosis; allergenic potential of foods; cross reactivity of allergens; food biotechnology; desensitization techniques; oral tolerance; diets for specific conditions, including grain, wheat, corn, milk, lactose intolerance, egg, peanut, soy, nickel, sulfite, artificial colors; pediatric food allergy- prevention and management from birth to five years and specific food allergy; therapeutic diets for ADHD, eczema, nocturnal enuresis, asthma, urticaria & angioedema, migraine, Crohn's disease; diet for digestive tract disorder- irritable bowel syndrome. Scope and depth of course equivalent to a 3.0 credit university course. (1999)

#1008	16 hours/ Audio cassette set (13 tapes) in an album, workbook with lecture overheads, workshop copy of Dietary Management of Food Allergies & Intolerances:	$245 USD
#1012	Audio cassette set in an album and workbook only :	$199 USD (for those who have the reference book)

BABIES, CHILDREN & FOOD ALLERGIES

Explains how the immune response works and why and how babies develop food allergies. Discusses the practical aspects of prediction, prevention, identification and management of food allergies in children from birth to five years. (1999)

#1003	4.5 hours/ Video set (2 videos), workbook with lecture overheads, workshop edition of Dietary Management of Food Allergies & Intolerances:	$135 USD
#1007	Video tapes in an album and workbook only:	$ 98 USD (for those who have the reference book)

J.A. HALL PUBLICATIONS
9500 Erickson Drive Suite502
Burnaby, BC, Canada V3J 7B5
website: www.HallPublications.com

Quantity	Cat #	Unit Price	Total

Order by Phone, Fax, Internet, or Mail

Call toll free 1-888-993-6133 Or 604-738-9425

FAX 1-888-881-1128 Or 604-738-9425

North America add $16 USD shipping; overseas charged at cost

Subtotal	
Shipping	
GST (Canada)	
Total	

Ship To: (please print)

Name

Company

Address

City   Prov/State   Postal Code/Zip

Country   E-mail

☐ VISA   Account No.
☐ MasterCard

Exp. Date